# Health Promotion
## *and* Health Education
## *in* Nursing

# Health Promotion *and* Health Education *in* Nursing

Ruth Cross

**S** Sage

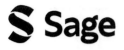

1 Oliver's Yard
55 City Road
London EC1Y 1SP

2455 Teller Road
Thousand Oaks, California 91320

Unit No 323-333, Third Floor, F-Block
International Trade Tower Nehru Place
New Delhi – 110 019

8 Marina View Suite 43-053
Asia Square Tower 1
Singapore 018960

Editor: Laura Walmsley
Editorial Assistant: Sahar Jamfar
Production Editor: Gourav Kumar
Copyeditor: Mary Dalton
Proofreader: Derek Markham
Indexer: KnowledgeWorks Global Ltd
Marketing Manager: Ruslana Khatagova
Cover Design: Sheila Tong
Typeset by KnowledgeWorks Global Ltd
Printed and bound by CPI Group (UK) Ltd,
Croydon, CR0 4YY

At Sage we take sustainability seriously. Most of our products are printed in the UK using responsibly sourced papers and boards. When we print overseas we ensure sustainable papers are used as measured by the Paper Chain Project grading system. We undertake an annual audit to monitor our sustainability.

**Library of Congress Control Number:** 2022949577

**British Library Cataloguing in Publication data**

A catalogue record for this book is available from the British Library

ISBN 978-1-5297-5296-0

ISBN 978-1-5297-5295-3 (pbk)

# Contents

# Introduction to Health Promotion and Health Education in Nursing

'Health Promotion and Health Education in Nursing' is a key textbook for nursing students, nurses and allied healthcare practitioners as well as those studying and practicing health promotion, health education, public health, health policy and health studies. This book complements and adds to the relatively small number of texts on health promotion and health education that are specific to nursing. Health promotion and health education are key parts of the nurse's role and yet are often confused or misunderstood in practice, or simply viewed as an optional addition to what nurses do. This book brings a fresh perspective on the nurse's role in health promotion and health education, drawing on health promotion across the lifespan and considering health promotion and health education in a range of different settings. Several authors from different countries have contributed to the writing of this book. These include Norway, Australia, Ghana, South Africa, Jamaica and Spain as well as the United Kingdom. This brings a wealth of context-specific knowledge and application to nursing practice which is unique to the field.

This book explores different aspects of health promotion and health education but, rather than having a narrow focus on individual behaviour change, it also considers important issues such as the social determinants of health, health-promoting settings, upstream approaches to promoting health, and key principles such as empowement and equity.

The book is divided into three sections. Section 1 highlights the underpinning theory and context of health promotion and health education. Section 2 identifies the core skills and processes of health promotion and health education, and Section 3 complements the first two sections by offering examples of health promotion and health education in practice across different stages of the lifespan and in a variety of nursing settings. Each section will be introduced in turn as we move through the book.

The book aims to simplify and contextualise complex concepts and ideas in health promotion and health education but also to provide a comprehensive view of contemporary health promotion and health education practice. Each chapter contains several key features designed to stimulate reflection on practice and enable engagement in the contents.

# List of Figures and Tables

## Figures

## Tables

# Key Features

*Learning outcomes* – each chapter provides learning outcomes to help the reader to identify what they will achieve by reading the chapter and engaging with its content.

*Key terms* – these detail the key concepts within each chapter and provide a quick and easy point of reference at the beginning of them.

*Tutorial Triggers* – these features present questions for consideration relating to the chapter content and often involve some sort of brief task for the reader to carry out to aid understanding and application.

*Points to Ponder* – these provide food for thought giving the reader a chance to pause and consider the issues raised during the chapter.

*Research in Brief* – relevant research is presented, where appropriate, in various chapters throughout the book which is intended to bring the content and theory to life and also to present evidence pertaining to the discussion within the chapter.

*Time to Reflect* – many chapters include this feature which invites the reader to reflect on a selected aspect of what they are reading about and think about how they might apply this to their own practice.

*Key Points* – each chapter ends with a list of the main points raised within it to help the reader to recap what has been covered.

The balance of these pedagogical features varies slightly from chapter to chapter depending on the content, however they are designed to support the reader in getting the most out of the book and to develop further understanding and appreciation of the nurse's role in health education and health promotion.

It is hoped that you will enjoy reading this book and that it will encourage and support you on your journey to promote health, not just for others but for yourself as well.

# About the Contributors

**Ruth Cross (Editor)** is the Course Director for Health Promotion at Leeds Beckett University. She teaches on a range of undergraduate and postgraduate modules within health promotion on subjects such as health communication, health psychology, critical public health and global health. Ruth worked as a Registered General Nurse for many years in England and overseas before moving into academia after completing an MSc in Health Promotion and Education. Ruth also has a PhD in Critical Health Psychology and was editor of the *International Journal of Health Promotion and Education* for six years. She has published widely in the health-promotion field including peer-viewed papers and several co-authored textbooks such as *The Essentials of Health Promotion* (2022), *Health Promotion: Global Principles and Practice* (2021), and *Health Promotion: Planning and Strategies* (2019).

**Navidad Canga Armayor, RN, MSc, PhD**, is a professor at the Nursing School of the University of Navarra, Spain. Her teaching experience has been developed in the field of Community Nursing, Epidemiology and Public Health. Her research focuses on Health Promotion and Education. Specifically, she has worked in clinical trials to help people to quit smoking and reduce alcohol consumption. Her current interests are related with the design and implementation of professional and peer-led interventions for reducing alcohol consumption among college students.

**Antoinette Barton-Gooden** is a Registered Nurse (RN) and a Certified Emergency Nurse (CEN) with 27 years' nursing experience. She has a BSc in Sociology and Public Administration (Majors), MScN (Education) and was awarded a PhD by the University of the West Indies, Mona Campus, Jamaica in March 2023. She taught adult nursing for eight years in the baccalaureate nursing programme. Currently she teaches in the MScN Leadership track, conducts clinical teaching and supervision with undergraduate nursing students in acute care settings. Antoinette's research focuses are Sickle Cell Disease, smoking cessation, patient safety and gender issues in nursing and chronic illnesses.

**María Pueyo Garrigues, RN, MSc, PhD,** is lecturer in Nursing in the School of Nursing at the University of Navarra, Spain. She has experience teaching in the Community Nursing field. Her research focuses on health promotion and health education areas, and psychometrics. Specifically, her current interests are related with the design and implementation of professional and peer-led interventions for reducing alcohol consumption among college students, and the development and validation of instruments for assessing nurses' health education competence. She is particularly interested in behaviour patterns issues regarding alcohol and tobacco among young people.

**María Lavilla Gracia, RN, MSc,** is research staff in training in the School of Nursing at the University of Navarra, Spain. She has experience in teaching in the Community Nursing and Public Health field. Her research is focused on health promotion and prevention. Specifically, she is investigating training nursing students in brief interventions to tackle unhealthy behaviours and evaluating the effectiveness of peer-led interventions for reducing alcohol consumption among university students. She is interested in peer-led and brief interventions to promote behaviour changes among young people.

**Firoza Haffejee** is Professor of Physiology and Epidemiology at Durban University of Technology in South Africa. She is an avid researcher in Public Health, with particular emphasis on HIV and Women's Health. Her special interest is on the social science aspects of disease prevention. She has published extensively on the risk factors for HIV acquisition and factors that impede prevention of HIV, particularly among young people and women. She is passionate about upliftment of women. This is evident from her community engagement work among impoverished communities at both Kenneth Gardens and the Dennis Hurley Centre in Durban, South Africa.

**Pandu Hailonga-van Dijk** is a public health expert in sexual and reproductive health, health and community systems strengthening. She has wide experience in the field including in sexual and reproductive health, gender, HIV/AIDS, orphans and vulnerable children, health systems strengthening and community development, and capacity development. She has a PhD in Development studies from the Netherlands and a master's degree in Health Education and Promotion from the UK. Pandu is interested in understanding the impact of structures on health and the intersectionality between gender equality and sexual reproductive health, especially adolescent health. Her professional career includes having worked for government, academic institutions, and international organisations. For more than 20 years Pandu has worked in project management, public health, sexual reproductive health and rights including HIV, safe motherhood, prevention of mother-to-child transmission of HIV, adolescent, youth, gender, community and health systems strengthening, capacity building, policy and programme development.

**Kari Ingstad** is a Professor of Sociology at The Faculty of Nursing and Health Sciences at Nord University, Norway. She received a B.N. in nursing in 1996 and M.S. in sociology in 2002 from the university of Oslo. She received her PhD in Sociology in 2011 from NTNU, Norway. She has edited three books, written two books, 15 scientific articles, and 22 book chapters. Her research interests fall within work, working conditions, innovation leadership. She is teaching students at bachelor, master and PhD level within sociology, methods, leadership and management at Nord University and OsloMet.

**Jed Montayre**, Associate Professor, is an internationally recognised researcher and has an exceptional research productivity. He has published over 76 papers in the last five years; secured competitive grants and is a recognised geriatric nursing researcher: – first in New Zealand; fourth in Australia and in the top 50 worldwide. Jed's research informed national policies in finding solutions to issues in accommodating the healthcare needs of an increasingly diverse ageing society. Jed led an international team commissioned by the World Health Organization (WHO) to review age-friendly interventions in rural and remote settings. This work informed WHO's work on age-friendly interventions as part of the United Nations Decade of Healthy Ageing initiative.

**Jasneth Mullings, PhD**, is a Social Epidemiologist in the Faculty of Medical Sciences, the University of the West Indies at Mona, Jamaica. She holds a masters of Public Health/Health Education and was the first PhD Epidemiology graduate of the University of the West Indies, Mona (2013). Her research interests span the arenas of mental health, urban health, community health and related interventions, with research focused on the mental health effects of neighbourhood structural and social processes. She currently serves as a strategic advisor to UrbanHealth360, global thought leaders in urban health and has held membership in the International Society for Urban Health.

**Paula Nersesian** is an Assistant Professor of Nursing at the University of Southern Maine in Portland, Maine, United States of America. She earned her PhD and MPH at the Johns Hopkins University and her BSN at the University of Michigan. She is the co-author of the International Family Nursing Association's Position Statement on Planetary Health and Family Health and has authored several blogs and presentations on planetary health. Her research focuses on loneliness.

**Tiffany Northall** has significant teaching experience gained during her employment as a clinical nurse specialist and as a teacher at TAFE and university. Tiffany has worked clinically in acute care since graduating in 1995. Her experience has been gained in a range of fields including palliative care, high dependency, patient flow, medical, surgical, emergency and primary health care. Tiffany has completed the Bachelor of Nursing degree, Masters of Nursing Research and Doctorate of Philosophy at Western Sydney University and has also completed a Graduate Certificate in Clinical Education.

**Ivy O'Neil** is former Principal Lecturer/Professional Lead for the Health Promotion team in Leeds Beckett. Her background is in nursing (Registered General Nurse, Registered Midwife, Registered Sick Children's Nurse and Registered Health Visitor). Her MSc by Research, was primarily research into the health needs of ethnic minority families. She is a Registered Practice Educator with a post-graduate Diploma (with Merit) in Education and was Course Leader for the MSc Public Health – Health Promotion course, and led and developed the Distance Learning version of the course. Her interests are in health needs assessment, public health workforce development and digital health communication. She is co-author of *"Health Communication – theoretical and critical perspectives"* (2017), *Health Promotion Global Principles and Practice*, 2nd Edition (2021) and author of *Digital Health Promotion – A Critical Introduction* (2019).

**Ebenezer Owusu-Addo** is the Director of the Bureau of Integrated Rural Development, Kwame Nkrumah University of Science and Technology, Ghana. He has a PhD in Health Promotion (Programme Evaluation) and over 16 years of work experience in the health and social sectors. He is a leading figure in health promotion research and evaluation, more specifically through his work on the role of public policies and intersectoral actions in addressing the social determinants of health and health inequity. His research interests are in the social determinants of health, health equity, social protection, and the interface between public health and town planning.

**Julian David Pillay** is a Professor in the Faculty of Health Sciences at Durban University of Technology, South Africa. His teaching and academic management is aligned to the basic medical sciences in allied health programmes and is further involved in research that integrates public health and health sciences. Much of this research involves engaging in qualitative and quantitative methods, structured experimental components and large-scale public health measurement, surveillance, and intervention studies. He leads several international collaborations as the South African representative/lead researcher and currently leads the Global Health and Sustainability Research Focus Area at the university.

**Lindsay Smith** started a nursing career in the 1980s supporting families across the lifespan and moved into university education in 1992, receiving two major teaching awards for outstanding contributions to nursing education. Lindsay is an elected Director for the International Family Nursing Association and Deputy Chair for the Tasmanian Human Research Ethics Committee. Lindsay developed the Australian Family Strengths Nursing Assessment conversation guide to help advance child and family participation in health care, which is recommended in the Queensland Royal Children's Hospital and Community Child Health Services (2020) Child and Youth Health Practice Manual. In 2021 Lindsay was appointed to the Tasmanian Department of Premier and Cabinet Community Consultative Group for Child & Youth Wellbeing Strategy where her passion is to help government policy and services optimise child, youth and family health and well-being.

**Susan R. Thompson, RGN, MPH, PGHCE, FHEA, MIHPE** has worked in the field of public health and health promotion for over 30 years within nursing, health promotion services and academia. She has been an academic since 2006 and has published a range of articles, delivered international conference presentations and workshops and written a seminal book, *The Essential Guide to Public Health and Health Promotion*, shortly to be published by Routledge in a second edition.

**Louise Warwick-Booth** is a Reader and Associate Director of the Centre for Health Promotion Research. Louise teaches on a range of modules including sociology, health policy, research methods, community health and global health. She leads a range of diverse research and evaluation projects within the voluntary and statutory sector. Her expertise relates to the evaluation of health-promotion interventions with vulnerable populations, including women experiencing domestic abuse. Louise has published several textbooks such as *Social Inequality* 3rd Edition (2022), *Creating Participatory Research* (2021 with colleagues), and *Contemporary Health Studies: An Introduction* 2nd Edition (2021).

**Dean Whitehead** has a national/international reputation in his specialist fields of health promotion and health education theory and practice – both within and outside the nursing disciplines. He is an active researcher and publisher where his main focus lies within health promotion and health education theory and practice, health policy, public health and primary health care. He has close to 200 peer-reviewed theoretical/research publications in these fields which enjoy high impact and citation in the health promotion/health education research and professional community.

**Trude Wille** earned a Bachelor's degree in nursing in 1999. She has a Master's degree in Health-sciences NTNU, Norway from 2007. She is also a trained Supervisor. Trude has taught at the Faculty of Nursing and Health Sciences at Nord University, Norway from 2009–2021. She has participated by writing two research articles and two chapters in textbooks. Trude is at the moment working as a nurse in the municipal health service.

**James Woodall** is a Reader in Health Promotion and also departmental lead at Leeds Beckett University. He teaches on a range of undergraduate and postgraduate modules within health promotion and supervises a number of doctoral students. He is currently Editor-in-Chief of the journal *Health Education*. James has published widely on a range of health promotion issues; he has also been involved in publishing several textbooks such as *The Essentials of Health Promotion* (2022), *Practical Health Promotion* (2020) and *Health Promotion: Planning and Strategies* (2019).

**Cloudina Venaani** is a gender expert, with an interest in adolescent girls and young women, sexual and reproductive health, HIV, and gender-based violence. Her professional career of over 18 years includes having worked as a project manager, and advisor and coordinator in the private sector, government, non-governmental organisations and international organisations, including the United Nations. Cloudina is currently the National Coordinator for Adolescent Girls and Young Women with the Ministry of Health and Social Services in Namibia. She is also in the process of completing her Masters in Gender Studies at the University of Free State in South Africa. Cloudina is interested in understanding how social-economic factors affect adolescent girls and young people's well-being, and the role of governments and communities in addressing these challenges.

# Acknowledgements

Acknowledgements and sincere thanks go to the following people for their role in the creation of this book from start to finish:

Dean Whitehead proposed the original idea for this book and played a key role in the early development of it by contributing Chapter 6 and the pedagogical features in Chapter 1.

Much gratitude to the team at SAGE for the encouragement and support along the way, particularly to Sahar Jamfar and Laura Walmsley for the final push in the latter stages of the project.

Huge thanks to the chapter contributors from around the world who have given up their valuable time to share their expertise and their passion for their subject areas. Their efforts and contributions are greatly appreciated and are an asset to the book.

# Introduction to Section 1

# What is Health, Health Promotion and Health Education?

This first part of *Health Education and Health Promotion for Nurses* sets the scene for the book and introduces a range of underpinning theory and context that frames the discussion in the subsequent chapters. Section 1 begins with Chapter 1 which discusses the nature of health and what influences health experience and outcomes. It considers several different dimensions of health and explores a range of health concepts including biomedical perspectives and a chronic care model of health. The social model of health is presented alongside discussion of the social determinants of health which opens up a discussion of health inequalities. Chapter 2 provides a detailed discussion about the nature of health promotion and health education, drawing careful distinctions between the two in terms of approaches aimed at the individual and structural levels. Detailing the nuances between the use and application of the two, this chapter provides an in-depth exploration of the characteristics of health education and health promotion including at what level these both operate. The chapter closes by considering the potential barriers that nurses might encounter when trying to promote health in different contexts. Chapter 3 outlines a history of health promotion and health education, detailing the key role that the World Health Organization has played in the development of health promotion as a global concern as well as cataloguing how health promotion has emerged as a field in its own right. The chapter also explores how health promotion coheres with related fields of practice such as public health, primary health care, community health, population health and environmental health. Chapter 4 then goes into finer detail about several different approaches to promoting health and explicates a range of relevant theory and models that can offer useful frameworks for health promoting practice. Finally, in this section, Chapter 5 specifically focuses on two of the key strategies of the seminal World Health Organization's Ottawa Charter for Health Promotion – reorienting health services and developing personal skills specifically considering these under a positive health paradigm. It considers each of these in detail in relation to the nurses' role in promoting health, ending with an emphasis on the importance of active engagement.

# 1

# Health and its Determinants

## Ruth Cross and Dean Whitehead

## Introduction

This chapter discusses the concept of health and outlines the importance of understanding its nuances to underpin effective health promotion and health education efforts. The chapter starts by considering various dimensions of health and each will be explored. These include physical, mental, emotional, social, sexual, spiritual and ecological health. It then moves on to explore and explain a range of health concepts such as biomedical perspectives and a chronic care model of health. The chapter will describe aspects of disease and illness and align these to more positive concepts of health such as prevention, wellness and well-being. The social model of health will be presented, drawing on the understandings of the social determinants of health which will also be explicated. The chapter ends by exploring and explaining why individuals and communities have different health experiences related to health care and health service access, quality and equity, and critiques the resulting differences in mortality and morbidity rates. It also critically discusses why, in some areas, inequalities in health have widened rather than reduced.

By the end of this chapter the reader will be able to:

1. Understand the complexity of 'health' as it relates to international, population and individual health contexts.
2. Appreciate and describe different dimensions of health.
3. Understand the biomedical and social models of health, recognising the importance of lay perspectives of health.
4. Describe social determinants of health and recognise the impact that these have on health experience and health equity.

## Key terms

Biomedical health, social model of health, social determinants of health, well-being, health inequalities

## Health – a complex phenomenon

It might seem strange to have such a relatively large section devoted to discussing what health is given that we use the word so frequently in everyday conversation and take it for granted most of the time. However, as pointed out by Wills (2023: 2) the term can 'embody a huge range of meanings, from the narrowly technical to the all-embracing moral or philosophical'. Aside from the classic definition of health offered by the constitution of the World Health Organization (see Box 1.1) there are numerous ways of defining and understanding what health is. As such, it has been argued that health means different things to different people at different times (Green et al., 2019). Health is also understood to be a complex, contested and multidimensional concept that is difficult to define and often highly individual or subjective (Cross, 2020; Svalastog et al., 2017). There is no doubt that our health experience influences how we think about health as do other things such as our age, our culture, our values, our life experience, and our position in the social hierarchy (Warwick-Booth et al., 2021). Whilst the World Health Organization's definition has been criticised on a number of counts such as being unattainable, unrealistic and impractical (Bickenbach, 2017) one of its strengths is its *holistic* nature and, indeed, it has largely stood the test of time as a consequence of how the WHO's agenda around health (and health promotion) has developed over the past few decades (Warwick-Booth et al., 2021). This will be discussed in more detail in Chapter 3: A history of health promotion and health education.

**Box 1.1**

## The World Health Organization's definition of health (WHO, 1946)

'Health is a state of complete physical, mental and social well-being and not merely the absence of disease or infirmity.'

Definitions of health encompass several different things. Health can be defined in positive or negative ways and lay perspectives on health (that is 'non-professional' views) draw on various understandings of what health is (Cross et al., 2021). Our ideas about what health is differ according to several things including our gender, socio-economic status, our experiences through the lifecycle, our culture, ethnicity, educational journey and upbringing (Evans et al., 2017). For example, research in South Africa shows that the notion of freedom is very important in young adults' ideas of health. This can be better appreciated in the context of the country's apartheid history (De Jong et al., 2019). Charlier et al. (2017) cite the example of the Mathias Colomb First Nation community in Canada who talk about being healthy in terms of 'having a good relationship with the land, having access to good food, but also having access to traditional culture' (p. 36). Such ideas are common in many indigenous peoples' perspectives on health. Of course, there are also basic human needs that have to be met in order for health to be achieved, such as shelter, food and water (Capone et al., 2018). In addition, as Raworth (2017) points out, access to health care, education and having personal security and political voice should also be viewed as basic necessities for health.

So, health can also be viewed positively or negatively (Warwick-Booth et al., 2021) or, as Antonovsky (1986) theorised, as existing on a continuum whereby we constantly slide or move between ill-health and full-health. The concept of health is essential to nursing practice (Cross, 2020). In nursing it has long been standard practice to embrace the idea that pain is what the patient says it is, the point being that pain is 'whatever the experiencing person says it is, existing whenever the experiencing person says it does' (McCaffery, 1968, cited in Bernhofer, 2012). Perhaps we should also be saying that 'health is what the person says it is' – that health is whatever the experiencing person says it is, existing (or not) *when*ever and *how*ever the experiencing person says it does.

Evans et al. (2017) summarises research into lay people's ideas about health over the past 50 years in terms of some recurring, common perspectives:

- in terms of not being ill
- in the context of physical fitness
- in terms of risk and control
- in terms of having a health problem that interferes with daily life

- in the context of social relationships
- as psychosocial well-being.

This illustrates the diversity of people's concepts of health and the meanings that are ascribed to feeling or being healthy.

---

### Tutorial Trigger 1.1

As identified, people's 'interpretation' of their health status (positive and negative states) varies over time and depends on a whole range of factors.

Draw a health timeline for your last 5 years. Identify your notable health 'peaks/positives and troughs/negative'. What do you notice about them? More peaks than troughs perhaps? What types of health status are they i.e., bio-psycho-social? Do you see any sort of patterns? The following 'dimensions of health' content may assist your timeline in identifying different broad categories of health.

---

## Dimensions of health

### Physical health

This dimension of health is often the one that we first think about which is not surprising given that we live out, and move through, our lives via our physical bodies. A lot of research points to the high value that we place on physical health in terms of being able to *function* and adapt, that is, to do what we want and need to do, and in terms of being independent (Blaxter, 2010; Yang et al., 2018). As we grow older, being able to function independently becomes more of a central concern about what it means to be healthy; some older people frame this as not wanting to be a burden on others. Of course, when we are young, we are more likely to take physical health and vitality for granted. In addition, those with caring responsibilities (such as mothers) often refer to health as functionality in terms of being able to look after their family and do what needs to be done (Yang et al., 2018). Similarly, for some people, being healthy is about being about to work and earn money to support yourself and others; or maintaining physical fitness (Linsley and Roll, 2020). Without a degree of physical health and ability all of these aspects of life become more challenging. Interestingly, it is often at the point of physical inconvenience or distress that people will seek help and support with their health – that is, when someone is not able to carry out the activities of daily living that they normally can, or when a symptom interferes with what they want to do (for example, a painful joint causing inconvenience and discomfort when trying to carry out a much-loved leisure activity). For people in less wealthy circumstances or who are living in absolute or relative poverty, physical health is of paramount importance as it is often key to day-to-day survival. In addition, for those who do not have access to healthcare services (either through not being able to afford them or a lack of availability), maintaining a good degree of physical health is crucial.

## Social health

The social dimension of health is reflected in definitions of health that consider our connection with others and with the concept of community. The various lockdowns that took place in different countries across the world during 2020 and 2021 because of the global Covid-19 pandemic, brought into sharp focus the importance of the social dimension of health. Many people suffered from lack of social interaction causing isolation, loneliness, anxiety and depression (Wong and Kohler, 2020). Social health is about having a sense of being supported by other people such as friends and family and having people to talk to and do things with (Wills, 2023). For some cultures, such as Māori and Native Alaskans for example, ideas about health are closely entwined with concepts of community, wider social systems, belonging and sharing (Bradley et al., 2017; Rolleston et al., 2016). Social health is about being able to form and sustain relationships with others (Wills and Jackson, 2014). Collectivist societies tend to value social health over other dimensions of health as they appreciate the importance of social health to the human experience. Social health is about how we get along with other people, it is also concerned with how we manage, adapt to and cope in social situations. The quality of our relationships with others makes a big difference to our overall quality of life. Trust, reciprocity and having someone to talk to or rely on when life is hard are all important features of our social health (Wong and Kohler, 2020). People who have healthy relationships with others tend to report a higher level of subjective well-being and also live longer. Huber et al. (2011) cited in Dröes et al. (2016: 4) therefore describe three dimensions of social health as follows:

1. Capacity to fulfil potential obligations
2. Ability to manage life with some degree of independence
3. Participation in social activities

## Mental health

Mental health is receiving more and more attention in popular and academic circles and is increasingly recognised as an important, if not crucial, dimension of health (and human) experience. Mental health is often closely associated with 'well-being' (Gu et al., 2015), a concept that will be discussed in more detail later in this chapter. Like *health* there are several definitions of mental health and there is not the space here to discuss these in any detail; suffice to say that mental health is concerned with our mental or psychological well-being. It is about having a 'positive sense of purpose and an underlying belief in one's own worth e.g., feeling good, feeling able to cope' (Wills, 2023: 3). Mental health is about being able to think clearly, being able to make decisions, being able to cope and adapt, and is concerned with having resilience (Wills and Jackson, 2014). 'Mental health refers to a person's emotional, social and psychological well-being. Good mental health includes the ability to control and manage emotions, concentrate on what you are doing, use memory and express emotion' (Linsley and Roll, 2020: 8). It is also about an individual's perceptions of their own value and well-being (Gottman and Goodman-Brown, 2012). Mental health is closely associated with emotional and social health (Scriven, 2017), both of which are discussed in this chapter. In summary, having good or positive mental health is about being able to cope with what life throws at us and being able to adapt to it at the same time. However, it is important to be aware that often, when we use the term 'mental health', we are actually referring to mental *ill*-health.

## Emotional health

In some ways emotional health is closely associated with mental health but for the purposes of this chapter we will consider this dimension of health in its own right as it is not the same as mental health (Lamothe, 2019). Emotional health is concerned with the expression of emotions (Wills and Jackson, 2014), being able to recognise, understand and manage how we feel whether those emotions are positive ones (such as joy) or negative (such as fear and grief) (Scriven, 2017). Emotional health is about being able to cope with our emotions (Evans et al., 2017) and being able to manage feelings of stress, anxiety and anger for example. Emotional health is also concerned with developing and sustaining relationships 'for example, feeling loved' (Wills, 2023: 3). So, it is not about always feeling happy or being 'okay' – rather emotional health is about having the necessary skills and resources to cope with the ups and downs of everyday life (Lamothe, 2019). Research into emotional health tends to try to measure things like perceived energy levels, and how anxious, irritable or depressed someone reports to be as well as trying to determine the extent to which emotional problems might interfere with everyday life or activities (McKerrow, 2020). Good emotional health includes being aware of distressing emotions as they occur, being aware of our own self-judgements, and being curious about our thoughts and feelings and why they might occur at different times, or in response to different things (Lamothe, 2019). Good emotional health results in having greater resilience to stress, being able to develop deeper more meaningful relationships, having better self-esteem, and having more energy (Ibid.). So, the importance of the emotional dimension of health to overall health is clear.

## Sexual health

Sexual health is another important dimension of health, and it overlaps with other dimensions of health such as physical health and emotional health. Healthy relationships are an important feature of sexual health which also coheres with social health. As Cooper and Thorogood (2013) point out, sexual practices and behaviours are located within social, personal and cultural meanings that 'often have little to do with health … but [are] frequently influenced by discourses such as those pertaining to desire, intimacy, trust, morality, and danger' (p. 23). Being able to negotiate safer sex within a healthy relationship is vital to sexual health but not always possible due to issues of power for example, the subjugation of women in some societies. Sexual health means having 'the ability and freedom to establish intimate, loving relationships as well as the choice and ability to procreate' (Evans et al. (2017) : 8) and Wills (2023) defines sexual health as 'the acceptance and ability to achieve a satisfactory expression of one's sexuality' (p. 3). Clearly this can be impacted upon in many ways – largely through our interactions with other people and whether they are accepting of who we are (or not). Sexual health is an integral part of life and has a physical and psychological dimension so physical difficulties in sexual function or a lack of ability to express ourselves sexually can affect our overall quality of life and, likewise, impact on our emotional and mental well-being (Vajrala et al., 2019).

---

### Point to Ponder 1.1

We often refer to the established 'bio-psycho-social' model of health when looking at the overall health status of individuals. The 'risk' of this is that it separates out aspects of health into 'compartments/silos' – when many aspects of an individual's general health are closely related and intertwined. Take sexual health for instance. There are aspects of 'biomedical' health – such as prevention and treatment of sexually transmitted infections; there are also aspects of 'psychological' health – such as emotional health related to sexuality and sexual well-being – and, finally, there are aspects of 'social' health – such as the establishment of sexual relationships. For any given individual these aspects may be 'in play' at any given time each closely influencing and impacting the other.

---

## Spiritual health

Alborzi et al. (2019) argue that spiritual health is a significant dimension of health. Spiritual health is viewed by some people as a relatively neglected dimension of health but in recent years we have seen this dimension of health gaining increasing recognition (Nunes et al., 2018). Chirico (2016), among others, has called for the World Health Organization to include spiritual health in its classic definition, however this has not explicitly happened yet although, in 2014, the World Health Organization did confirm that spirituality was encompassed in the definition of health. Spiritual health is concerned with having purpose, being at peace with ourselves and finding calm (Wills and Jackson, 2014), and also being 'able to achieve peace of mind or being at peace with your own self' (Evans et al., 2017). Spiritual health is not simply about religion or being religious however, it is concerned with *spirituality* which can be achieved by other means such as meditation and certain behavioural and mindful practices. Having said that 'being able to recognize, express and practice (our) core beliefs i.e., religious views, morals and values' (Gottwald and Goodman-Brown, 2012:16) is a vital part of spiritual health, as is having a sense of connection with others, and a sense of meaning (Alborzi *et al.,* 2019). For some people it might also be about the feeling of having a higher purpose in life (Wills, 2023) or centred on a firm belief in a higher or transcendent being/power. Such beliefs can bring huge comfort to people in times of stress, ill-health and trauma and enable people to achieve a sense of meaning from their experiences and life itself.

## Ecological health

Ecological or planetary health has gained more and more attention over recent decades. Wills (2023) refer to this as 'global health' which, in their view, involves 'caring for the planet and ensuring its sustainability for the future' (p. 3). Whilst debates about climate change rage on we are left in no doubt about the impact that humanity has on the earth in which we live. For those living on the margins of society, or in relative or severe deprivation or disadvantage, this dimension of health might seem much less personally relevant in a context where just trying to survive is the main goal. However, ecological health is vital to our survival as a species. Kate Raworth's (2017) book 'Doughnut Economics' maps out a model for optimum conditions for humans and our planet to thrive. The model looks like a circle with a hole in it, hence the 'doughnut' analogy. There are two key concepts within the model – the *social foundation* and the *ecological ceiling*. Between the two boundaries depicted in the model lies a space of optimum conditions for human and planetary survival – 'an ecologically safe and socially just space' (Raworth, 2017: 45). The social foundation part of the model lays out twelve basics for human life – food; water and sanitation; access to energy; education; health care; good housing; a minimum income and employment; and access to networks of information and social support. In addition, gender equality; social equity; political voice; and peace and justice are also considered vital basics. When we overshoot the ecological ceiling, we move further away from the ecologically safe space – think things like climate change, air pollution, freshwater contamination etc. Raworth's model inextricably links human health to the health of our planet highlighting the interconnectedness of the complex socio-ecological system that we are all part of.

## Biomedical perspectives

According to biomedical perspectives, health is defined in opposition to disease and illness and this understanding is firmly rooted in the biological sciences (Bicken-bach, 2017). This is where the (bio) medical model of health dominates and it often (necessarily) forms the basis of healthcare services which, ironically, tend to be more like 'sick'-care services, caring for people when they are ill or injured (Cross et al., 2021). A biomedical view of health locates health within the individual and defines it in a relatively narrow or simple way, typically as the absence of disease, illness or injury (Hubley et al., 2021). The broader influences on health (those outside of the physical body) tend not to be considered. The biomedical perspective is heavily influenced by scientific and expert (professional) knowledge which is given high value and privilege over other types of knowledge, for example lay (non-expert) knowledge (Wills, 2023). This can result in an imbalance of power whereby the pro-fessional is viewed as the expert and someone who is in authority whilst the 'patient' is viewed as passive and dependent (Evans et al., 2017). In the biomedical model of health individual responsibility for health is emphasised (Friesen, 2017). The focus is therefore on educating people to change their behaviour to reduce individual risk factors and prevent ill-health. Another assumption underpinning biomedical perspectives is that individuals have the freedom to choose whether to engage with, or access, healthcare services (Horrill et al., 2018). The biomedical model underpins many healthcare systems in so-called 'Western' countries and elsewhere. Despite the criticisms levelled at biomedical perspectives, particularly in relation to the narrow conceptualisation of health, they do have a valuable and significant contribution to make in terms of health improvement for example, treatment and cure (Evans et al., 2017). As Horrill et al. (2018: 2) state, 'biomedical research is responsible for many medical discoveries and has played a significant role in the discovery and advance-ment of treatments for both acute and chronic diseases'.

---

## Point to Ponder 1.2

It is noted that health professionals (especially nurses) often wear 'two hats' in their health-related professional encounters with clients/patients. These two hats are a 'social' hat i.e., personal health beliefs related to our own personal social experiences and a 'professional' hat i.e., what we have learnt as part of our professional education/training. Sometimes these can be complementary – and other times not. For instance, we may bring personal 'empathy' to our clinical encounters that is based on our own personal experiences e.g., 'I can appreciate that it is difficult to change health-related lifestyle behaviours.' Alter-natively, we may adopt a less complementary professional approach i.e., this is what the evidence states or 'do as I say – rather than as I do'. It is important to go into these encoun-ters with the insight of 'which hat am I wearing – and is it an appropriate hat?'

## The chronic care model

The nature of our contemporary environments and associated lifestyles has led to an increased burden of chronic conditions, not just in more wealthy contexts but within the emerging middle classes of low- and middle-income countries (Davy et al., 2015). The Chronic Care Model (CCM) was developed by Wagner and colleagues in the 1990s in response to increasing recognition that people were presenting more and more frequently with chronic conditions that needed to be managed within a primary care setting where an emphasis on acute care was not as relevant or appropriate (Boehmer et al., 2018). The model was developed to support the redesign of the delivery of care for people living with chronic conditions in primary care (Kadu and Stolee, 2015). Wagner et al.'s CCM comprised six key areas: self-management support, decision support, delivery system design, clinical information systems, healthcare organisation, and community resources (Coleman et al., 2009). The original CCM has evolved since its inception and been applied differently in various scenarios (Davy et al., 2015) yet the emphasis on delivering evidence-based care, mobilising community resources and empowering individual patients remains (Kadu and Stolee, 2015). Since the 1990s it has been recognised that people with coexisting multiple chronic conditions (or multimorbidity) present a challenge to the CCM which does not necessarily consider how to address multiple conditions at the same time (Boehmer et al., 2018).

### Research in Brief 1.1

The aim of this study by Padilha et al. (2018) was to propose nursing-related clinical practice changes to improve the development of patient self-management of Chronic Obstructive Airways Disease clients. Control of the disease's progression, the preservation of autonomy in self-care, and maintenance of quality of life are extremely challenging for patients to execute in their daily living. A participatory action research study was performed in a medical in-patient department and the outpatient unit of a Portuguese hospital. The sample comprised 52 nurses and 99 patients and collected data using interviews, participant observation and content analysis. The main elements of nursing clinical practice that were identified as a focus for improvement measures were the healthcare model (Chronic Care Model), the organisation of health care and the documentation of support decision-making processes, designed to improve the development of self-management skills related to the awareness of the need for 'change', hope, involvement, knowledge and abilities. The overall conclusion and recommendations of the study promote the involvement and participation of nurses and patients in the conceptualisation, implementation and evaluation of practice/ policy change to improve the quality of nursing care and clinical outcomes for those with existing chronic health conditions.

Padilha, J.M., de Sousa, P.A.F. and Pereira, F.M.S. (2018). Nursing clinical practice changes to improve self-management in chronic obstructive pulmonary disease. *International Nursing Review* 65, 122–30.

## Tutorial Trigger 1.2

For many, the 'Chronic Care Model' view of health is the 'link/bridge' between the biomedical model of health and the social model of health.

Draw a two-column table. In one column identify what you consider the biomedical aspects of the CCM i.e., treatment. In the other column identify what you consider to be the social aspects i.e., self-care/management. At the same time, consider which aspects you think 'cross-over' into each column.

## Prevention, wellness and well-being

Prevention is an important part of health promotion. Essentially it is about stopping people getting ill in the first place or at least slowing down the progression of disease and helping people to avoid injury. The prevention of ill-health sits well with a social model of health although there are aspects of medicine that are about prevention, certainly the prevention of worsening of conditions in the event of a diagnosis, or preventing disease through a vaccination programme.

Wellness is, of course, a state we might describe ourselves in if we are free from illness, disease, stress and trauma. It could be argued that wellness tends to be something that we take for granted. Like health, wellness is often conceptualised as being multidimensional. The Global Wellness Institute recognises that wellness is about more than being physically okay; it is about thriving, being able to maintain and improve health, prevention of ill-health, and an essential part of life. Please see Box 1.2 for more information.

---

**┌ Box 1.2 ┐**

## Wellness as defined by the Global Wellness Institute

The active pursuit of activities, choices and lifestyles that lead to a state of holistic health.

There are two important aspects to this definition:

1. Wellness is not a passive or static state but rather an 'active pursuit' that is associated with intentions, choices and actions as we work toward an optimal state of health and wellbeing.
2. Wellness is linked to holistic health – that is, it extends beyond physical health and incorporates many different dimensions that should work in harmony.

*Source*: <globalwellnessinstitute.org>

---

There has been a general trend towards recognition of health as a more fluid, flexing concept and an encompassing of a range of different ideas such as resilience, adaptability, coping and connecting with much more of an emphasis on the positive nature of health (Scriven, 2017).

Wellness connects to well-being. It is not easy to define well-being – another term that is in common parlance yet defies a common definition. However, well-being suggests a sense of wholeness and is usually associated with good mental and social health as well as being able to achieve what we want to, i.e., feeling in control of what happens to us (Johnson et al., 2016). It is broadly connected with what makes a good life (Wills, 2023) and therefore serves to widen understandings of health beyond merely the absence of disease or injury. For example, 'in Maori culture, the concept of well-being combines spiritual, ecological, kinship and economic well-being interwoven as interdependent dimensions' (Raworth, 2017: 54).

Well-being is a concept that has received increasing attention over the past couple of decades and many countries now factor subjective well-being into how they measure or assess how their populations are faring. So, there has been a change in focus from simply measuring indicators of ill-health or disease, to considering well-being (Scriven, 2017). Well-being indicators include, for example, things like work-life balance, subjective well-being, and social connections as well as the consideration of factors such as inequalities between and within different groups of people, and the resources that people have available to them (OECD, 2016).

Health, happiness and well-being are inextricably linked. Box 1.3 illustrates the similarities between well-being and happiness.

─── Box 1.3 ───────────────────────────────────

## Wellbeing and Happiness

- both relate to a perception of a state of being
- both have a prominent mental/emotional dimension
- people associate both of these with feelings of satisfaction and a sense of fulfilment
- both are in common use in contemporary governmental policy in many contexts
- both are useful for measuring individual welfare.

*Source*: <globalwellnessinstitute.org>

## The social model of health

The social model of health is a central concept for health promotion and makes a significant contribution to our understanding of what health is. Many aspects of the social model of health stand in direct contrast to the biomedical perspective discussed earlier. The social model of health allows for the complexity of health and considers lay perspectives, subjective experiences and individual views about what health is rather than prescribing a narrow medical definition of health on people (Warwick-Booth et al., 2021). What's more, it recognises that everyone is the expert of their own lives and experiences (Warwick-Booth and Cross, 2018). The social model of health also takes the social determinants of health into account (these are discussed in more detail in the next section of this chapter). It views health in a more holistic way and emphasises collective (or social) rather than individual responsibility for health. The social model of health views ill-health as caused by social structures and conditions (such as poverty and inequality) not just disease processes. It considers the different dimensions of health (as discussed earlier in this chapter) not just physical health and tends to form the basis of traditional or 'alternative' healthcare systems (Cross et al., 2021). So, the social model of health offers a more holistic definition of health in recognition that health is not solely understood by medicine or science (Yuill et al., 2010).

The social model of health 'embraces all aspects of human experience and places health fully in the dynamic interplay of social structures and embodied human agency' (Yuill et al., 2010). As Wills (2023) points out, it draws on sociological ideas to make sense of health and illness and therefore considers health (and any type of ill-health) to be a result of social (mal)functioning. The key elements of the social model of health are, according to Yuill et al. (2010):

- individual health is enabled or inhibited by social context
- the body is simultaneously social, psychological and biological
- health is cultural
- biomedical and medical science is something – but not everything
- health is political.

## Social determinants of health

Exploring the social model of health naturally leads us to consider the wider, social determinants of health. It is sometimes easy to forget the influence of these on health experience especially when one works in an acute, medically led setting; however, in terms of health promotion it is crucial that we take social determinants into account. By the social determinants of health we mean, as defined by Cross et al. (2021: 1), 'those factors that enable people to live healthy and productive lives – these factors include […] decent housing, access to education, employment opportunities, nourishing food, well-functioning and accessible healthcare, cohesive communities, good systems of government and peaceful nation-states'. The social determinants of health can either create the conditions for people to thrive and be healthy or mitigate against this.

A classic model of determinants of health is Dahlgren and Whitehead's (1991) rainbow model (see Figure 1.1). As can be seen from Figure 1.1 this model starts, at the centre, with the individual and factors that affect our health which can't be altered, such as our age and our genetic inheritance. The next layer of the rainbow represents our actions and behaviour (individual lifestyle factors) which are, in turn, influenced by social and community factors and then the many aspects of life that constitute our living and working conditions, such as education, housing, healthcare services, employment, water and sanitation, and agriculture and food production. In the outermost layer of the rainbow model our general socioeconomic, cultural and environmental conditions are taken into account.

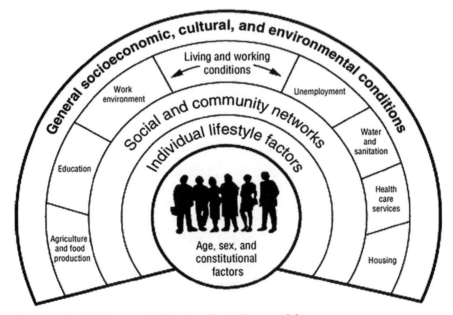

**Figure 1.1**   Dahlgren and Whitehead's rainbow model

Dahlgren and Whitehead's model is over 30 years old now, however it offers a very helpful way to understand determinants of health clearly illustrating the importance of the relationships between the different factors that influence our health experience and health outcomes, and it is still widely used. Nevertheless, the model has limitations and there are determinants of health that are not accounted for within it. A subsequent adaptation of the rainbow by Barton and Grant (2006) resulted in a 'health map' in which the model was adapted and extended to include consideration of political, global and market influences on health as well as factors within the ecosystem such as climate change, biodiversity and sustainability (see Figure 1.2). This model highlights the influence of our environment as a key determinant of health and forefronts the ecological dimension of health discussed earlier.

Another, more complex way of understanding social determinants of health was later developed by Solar and Irwin (2010) – see Figure 1.3. This framework came out of work on the social determinants of health led by the World Health Organization and was intended to make sense of the complex range of factors that influence, impact on and determine health (Warwick-Booth and Cross, 2018). As you will see from Figure 1.3 the framework distinguishes between *structural* determinants of health such as the socioeconomic and political context, and our socioeconomic position, and *intermediary* determinants of health such as our material circumstances, behavioural, biological and psychosocial factors. It is much more complex than Dahlgren and Whitehead's (1991) model offering a more nuanced understanding of the social determinants of health yet the similarities between the main components are clear.

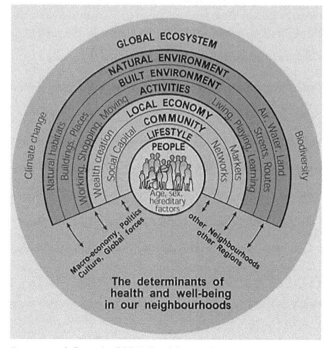

**Figure 1.2**   Barton and Grant's (2006) 'health map'

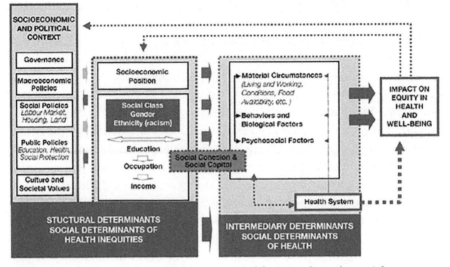

**Figure 1.3**   Solar and Irwin's (2010) conceptual framework on the social determinants of health

Whilst we have considered three different models of social determinants of health, none of these constitute a perfect representation of their complexities. For example, none of the models really consider the influence of our virtual techno-logical world as a determinant of health which is changing rapidly all the time. Each model has its strengths and limitations but it would be difficult to establish a fully comprehensive theoretical account given the magnitude of factors that influence and determine our health. Suffice to say, it is clear that our health is socially determined in a myriad of ways and that these different factors all combine to create or reduce opportunities for maximum health whether at an individual, community, society or even global level. Hence, the importance of the social determinants of health to health promotion – 'while health status is influenced by individual characteristics and behaviour, it continues to be significantly determined by the different social, economic, and environmental circumstances of individuals and populations' (Morgan and Cragg, 2013: 111).

———— Time to Reflect 1.1 ————————————————————

Social determinants of health (SDH) are an integral part of what determines an individual's health status, both positively and negatively. The nature of SDH means that some aspects can be managed 'internally' (internal drivers) such as the motivation to access local parks for exercise and recreation. However, what if such parks are quite a distance to get to and there is a lack of public transport (external drivers)? Think about your local community or the geographical area that you live in. What SDH-type factors determine to what extent you view it as healthy or not?

## Health inequalities

Health inequalities are reflected in early deaths, the unequal distribution of certain illnesses and diseases, and the unequal experience of ill-health, injury and disease. Inequalities in health exist between, and within, countries. A simple indication of health inequalities is life expectancy. In wealthier countries average life expectancy is significantly higher than in poorer countries. Other indicators of health and well-being also reveal disparities. In countries where there is a greater gap between the most well-off and the least-well off there is more obesity, mental ill-health and individual-level violence (Wilkinson and Pickett, 2009; Pickett and Wilkinson, 2018). See Box 1.4 for some examples.

---

### Box 1.4

### Examples of health inequalities

#### Life expectancy

In Switzerland the average life expectancy for a man is 81.9 years and 85.7 years for a woman. In contrast, in Chad the average life expectancy for a man is 52.6 years and 55.4 years for a woman.

*Source*: <www.worlddata.info/life-expectanct.php>

#### Rates of obesity

In 2016, 36 per cent of adults in the United States of America were obese compared with 3.9 per cent of adults in India.

*Source*: <www.ourworldindata.org/obesity>

#### Intentional homicide

In 2017 there were 61.8 deaths by intentional homicide per 100,000 people in El Salvador and in the same year in Austria there was less than 1 death per 100,000 people.

*Source*: <indexmundi.com/facts/indicators>

#### Deaths by road traffic accidents

In 2018 there were 61.90 deaths by road traffic accident per 100,000 people in Zimbabwe compared with 2.31 per 100,000 people in Sweden.

*Source*: <www.worldlifeexpectancy.com/cause-of-death/road-traffic-accidents>

---

There are many complex reasons for the disparities seen in the examples given in Box 1.4; however, the vast majority of these can be attributed to the social determinants of health discussed earlier in this chapter. This includes access to healthcare services and the distribution and quality of those services. A simple measure of this is the number of physicians per 1,000 people per country. In 2018 there were 1.7 physicians per 1,000 people in Algeria compared with 8.4 per 1,000 people in Cuba (World Bank, 2021). Infrastructure and transport also play a huge part in access to healthcare services and people living in rural areas tend to fare worse. 'As nursing professionals, we believe access to health care is fundamental to health and that it is a determinant of health' (Horrill et al., 2018: 1).

Politics and the distribution of power have a lot to do with this. As the World Health Organization constitution states, 'governments have a responsibility for the health of their peoples which can be fulfilled only by the provision of adequate health and social measures' (WHO, 1946).

Health inequalities exist for many different reasons. Typically, minority ethnic or marginalised groups suffer worse health than majority populations on a range of measures including, for example, life expectancy, substance misuse, access to healthcare services, multiple material disadvantages, and discrimination (Crisp, 2016). Income inequality has a detrimental social and psychological impact on people. In countries where there is a larger gap between the most well-off and the least well-off everyone fares worse on a range of indicators including, for example, mental illness, crime, unplanned teenage pregnancy and the number of people in prison (Pickett and Wilkinson, 2018; Wilkinson and Pickett, 2009).

Whilst many measures of health have improved over recent decades, such as average life expectancy and infant mortality, in some instances inequalities in health have widened rather than reduced. In England for example, we have seen things worsen over the past decade, not get better. In 2010 'Fair Society, Healthy Lives: A Strategic Review of Health Inequalities in England' was published which highlighted the health inequalities of the time and reinforced the existence of a social gradient in health whereby 'the lower a person's social position, the worse his or her health' (Marmot et al., 2010). The review set out six key policy objectives as follows:

1.  Give every child the best start in life.
2.  Enable all children, young people and adults to maximise their capabilities and have control over their lives.
3.  Create fair employment and good work for all.
4.  Ensure a healthy standard of living for all.
5.  Create and develop healthy and sustainable places and communities.
6.  Strengthen the role and impact of ill-health prevention.

Notably, none of these policy recommendations are specifically concerned with the provision of healthcare services, they are all to do with the social determinants of health. In 2020, ten years later Marmot and colleagues carried out another review which resulted in the publication of *Health Equity in England: The Marmot Review*

*10 years on* (Marmot et al., 2020a). The review concluded that life expectancy (a key measure of health) had stalled and that inequalities in life expectancy had increased as had the amount of time that people spend in poor health (Marmot et al., 2020a). This decline is largely attributed to the imposition of austerity measures and funding cuts. The review noted a significant difference in the levels of health between people living in deprived areas in the north of England and people living in the relatively affluent south of the country. The coronavirus pandemic has shone another spotlight on health inequalities in England in several ways. As Bambra et al. (2020) point out, the inequalities in coronavirus-related morbidity and mortality rates reflect inequalities in chronic (non-communicable) disease more generally, and of the social determinants of health. People in lower paid jobs, living in relative poverty, with existing health conditions, in positions of socio-economic disadvantage and people in minority ethnic groups all have a greater risk of becoming seriously ill with coronavirus (Ibid.). *Build Back Fairer: The COVID-19 Marmot Review* further illustrated the harm to health and well-being caused by social, environmental and economic inequality (Marmot et al., 2020b).

After defining health (see Box 1.1) the constitution of the World Health Organization goes on to state that 'the enjoyment of the highest attainable standard of health is one of the fundamental rights of every human being without distinction of race, religion, political belief, economic or social condition' (WHO, 1946). The continued existence of health inequalities at any level illustrates how much further we have to go in creating a fairer and more socially justice world for everyone.

## Research in Brief 1.2

Strategies for addressing discrimination against multiple and intersecting social identities in the practice setting are lacking, and interlocking systems of privilege and oppression continue to sustain health inequalities (Bowleg, 2012). The intersectionality found within the Two-Spirit, Lesbian, Gay, Bisexual, Transgender, and Queer (2SLGBTQ) communities can be used to investigate for a broad understanding of discrimination in healthcare. Research as such could produce findings that address a broad range of social issues that influence individual health practices (Ibid.). The health disparities that are disproportionately found within 2SLGBTQ patient populations can be understood as symptoms with social causes; they are adverse outcomes of structural inequalities. This makes the 2SLGBTQ communities a key group for health research that seeks to understand how systems of privilege and oppression sustain health inequalities.

Lane, J. (2020). Intersectionality and investigating systems of privilege and oppression in nursing and health research. *Canadian Journal of Nursing Research* *52*(4), 243-5.

## Summary

This chapter has explored different dimensions of health and highlighted the wider, social determinants of health. In doing so it provides an important foundation for the rest of this book because we need to appreciate what health *is* before we can seek to promote it (Cross et al., 2021). The dimensions and determinants of health are complex (Fleming, 2020). As Scriven (2017) argues, it is important to understand how people think about health because their understanding will influence their experiences of health as well as their beliefs and behaviours. As such, this chapter has outlined several different dimensions of health and discussed the importance of the social model of health in terms of understanding health more broadly beyond the mere absence of illness. Understanding the social determinants of health is also vital to understanding how health might be promoted, created and sustained.

────── Key Points ────────────────────────────────────

Many factors influence and determine an individual's (and overall community) health. These range from medical through to social perspectives and, in particular, the social determinants of health (SDH). These factors determine the 'health status' of individuals – both positively and negatively.

Health promotion privileges the social model of health and therefore lay perspectives are key to understanding health experience.

A focus on health inequalities is a central concern for promoting health for everyone. Healthy public policy has a huge role to play in this.

## References

Alborzi, S., Movahed, M., Ahmadi, A. and Tabiee, M. (2019). Sociological study of spiritual health in young adults with an emphasis on social and cultural capital. *Health Spiritual Medical Ethics* 6(4), 36–42.

Antonovsky, A. (1986). The salutogenic model as a theory to guide health promotion. *Health Promotion International* 11, 11–18.

Bambra, C., Riordan, R., Ford, J. and Matthews, F. (2020). The COVID-10 pandemic and health inequalities. *Journal of Epidemiology and Community Health* 74(11), 964–8.

Barton, H. and Grant, M. (2006). *The Determinants of Health and Well-Being in our Neighbourhoods*. The Health Impacts of the Built Environment. Institute of Public Health in Ireland.

Bernhofer, E. (2012). Ethics: Ethics and pain management in hospitalized patients. *The Online Journal of Issues in Nursing* 17(1), doi: 10.3912/OJIN.Vol17No01EthCol01

Bickenbach, J. (2017). WHO's definition of health: Philosophical analysis. In T. Schramme and S. Edwards (Eds), *Handbook of the Philosophy of Medicine* (pp. 1–14). London: Springer.

Bowleg, L. (2012). The problem with the phrase Women and Minorities: Intersectionality – an Important Theoretical Framework for Public Health. *American Journal of Public Health 102*(7), 1267–73.

Blaxter, M. (2010). *Health.* 2nd Ed. Cambridge: Polity.

Boehmer, K.R., Dabrh, A.M.A., Giofriddo, M.R., Erwin, P. and Montori, V.M. (2018). Does the chronic care model meet the emerging needs of people living with multi-morbidity? A systematic review and thematic synthesis. *PLoS One 13*(2), e0910852.

Bradley, P.V., Hall, L.J., Hannigan, G.G. and Wood, F.B. (2017). Native voices: Native people's concepts of health and illness in New Mexico: opening a local conversation by hosting a national traveling exhibit. *Journal of the Medical Library Association 105*(3), 243–8.

Capone, D., Ferguson, A., Gribble, M. and Brown, J. (2018). Open defecation sites, unmet sanitation needs, and potential sanitary risks in Atlanta, Georgia, 2017–2018. *American Journal of Public Health 108*(9), 1238–40.

Charlier, P., Coppens, Y., Malaurie, J., Brun, L., Kepanga, M., Hoang-Opermann, V., ... Hervé, C. (2017). A new definition of health? An open letter of autochthonous peoples and medical anthropologists to the WHO. *European Journal of Internal Medicine 37*, 3–7.

Chirico, F. (2016). Spiritual well-being in the 21st century: It's time to review the current WHO's health definition? *Journal of Health and Social Sciences 1*(1), 11–16.

Coleman, K., Austin, B.T., Brach, C. and Wagner, E.H. (2009). Evidence on the chronic care model in the new millennium. *Health Aff (Millwood) 28*(1), 75–85.

Cooper, S. and Thorogood, N. (2013). Social construction of health and health promotion. In L. Cragg, M. Davis and W. Macdowall, W. (Eds), *Health Promotion Theory,* 2nd Ed. (pp. 20–34). Maidenhead: Open University Press.

Crisp, N. (2016). One World Health: An Overview of Global Health. London: CRC Press.

Cross, R. (2020). Understanding an individual's concept of health. *Nursing Standard,* doi: 10.7748/ns.2020.e11539

Cross, R., Rowlands, S. and Foster, S. (2021). The Foundations of Health Promotion. In R. Cross, L. Warwick-Booth, S. Rowlands, J. Woodall, I. O'Neil, and S. Foster, *Global Principles and Practice,* 2nd Ed. (pp. 1–40). Wallingford: CABI.

Dahlgren, G. and Whitehead, M. (1991). *Policies and Strategies for Promoting Social Equity in Health.* Stockholm: Institute of Futures Studies.

Davy, C., Bleasel, J., Liu, H., Tchan, M., Ponniah, S. and Brown, A. (2015). Effectiveness of chronic care models: opportunities for improving healthcare practice and health outcomes: a systematic review. *BMC Health Services Research 15,* 194. doi: 10.1186/s/121913-015-0854-8

De Jong, M., Collins, A. and Plüg, S. (2019). 'To be healthy to me is to be free': how discourses of freedom are used to construct healthiness among young South African adults. *International Journal of Qualitative Studies on Health and Well-being 14*(1), 1603518 doi: 10.1080/17482631.2019.1603518.

Dröes, R.M., Chattat, R., Diaz, A., Gove., M., Graff, M., Murphy, K., ... Charras, K. (2016). Social health and dementia: a European consensus on the operationalization of the concept and directions for research and practice. *Ageing and Mental Health 21*(S1), 4–17.

Evans, D., Coutsaftiki, D. and Fathers, C.P. (2017). *Health Promotion and Public Health for Nursing Students,* 3rd Ed. London: Sage.

Fleming, M. (2020). The importance of health promotion principles and practices. In M. Fleming and L. Baldwin, *Health Promotion in the 21st Century: New approaches to achieving health for all* (pp. 1–14). London: Allen & Unwin.

Friesen, P. (2017). Personal responsibility within health policy: Unethical and ineffective. *Journal of Medical Ethics 44*(1). doi: 10.1136/medethics-2016-103478

Gottwald, M. and Goodman-Brown, J. (2012). *A Guide to Practical Health Promotion.* Maidenhead: Open University Press.

Green, J., Cross, R., Woodall, J. and Tones, K. (2019). *Health Promotion: Planning and Strategies,* 4th Ed. London: Sage.

Gu, J., Strauss, C., Bond, R. and Cavanagh, K. (2015). How do mindfulness-based cognitive therapy and mindfulness-based reduction improve mental health and well-being? A systematic review and meta-analysis of meditation studies. *Clinical Psychology Review 37*, 1–12.

Horrill, T., McMillan, D.E., Schultz, A.S.H. and Thompson, G. (2018). Understanding access to healthcare among Indigenous peoples: A comparative analysis of biomedical and postcolonial perspectives. *Nursing Inquiry 25*: e12237.

Hubley, J., Copeman, J. and Woodall, J. (2021). *Practical Health Promotion,* 3rd Ed. Cambridge: Polity.

Johnson, D., Deterding, S., Kuhn, K., Staneva, A., Stoyna, S. and Hides, S. (2016). Gamification for health and wellbeing: a systematic review of the literature. *Internet Interventions 6*, 89–106.

Kadu, M.K. and Stolee, P. (2015). Facilitators and Barriers of Implementing the Chronic Care Model in Primary Care: A Systematic Review. *BMC Family Practice 16*, 12. https://dx/doi.org/10.1186/s13875-014-0219-0

Lamothe, C. (2019). *How to Build Good Emotional Health.* [Internet] Available at: <healthline.com/health/emotional-health> Accessed 6 February 2021.

Linsley, P. and Roll, C. (2020). *Health Promotion for Nursing Students.* London: Sage.

Marmot, M., Goldblatt, P. and Allen, J. (2010). *Fair Society, Healthy Lives.* Executive Summary. [Internet] Available at: <www.instituteofhealthequity.org> Accessed 20 February 2021.

Marmot, M., Allen, J., Boyce, T., Goldblatt, P. and Morrison, J. (2020a). *Health Equity in England: The Marmot Review 10 Years On.* Executive Summary. [Internet] Available at: <www.instituteofhealthequity.org> Accessed 20 February 2021.

Marmot, M., Allen, J., Goldblatt, P., Herd, E. and Morrison, J. (2020b). *Build Back Fairer: The COVID-19 Marmot Review.* Executive Summary. [Internet] Available at: <www.instituteofhealthequity.org> Accessed 20 February 2021.

McKerrow, I., Carney, P.A., Caretta-Weyer, H., Furnari, M. and Juve, A.M. (2020). Trends in medical students' stress, physical, and emotional health throughout training. *Medical Education Online 25*. doi: 10.1080/10872981.2019.1709278

Morgan, A. and Cragg, L. (2013). The determinants of health. In L. Cragg, M. Davis and W. Macdowall (Eds), *Health Promotion Theory,* 2nd Ed. (pp. 98–113). Maidenhead: Open University Press.

Nunes, S.A.N., Fernandes, H.M., Fisher, J.W. and Fernandes, M.G. (2018). Psychometric properties of the Brazilian version of the lived experience component of the Spiritual Health and Life-Orientation Measure (SHALOM). *Psicologia:Reflexão e Crítica 31*(2). doi: 10.1186/s41155-018-0083-2

Office for Economic Co-operation and Development (OECD) (2016). *Measuring well-being and progress: well-being research.* [Internet] Available at: <oecd.org/statistics/measuring-well-being-and-progress.htm> Accessed 6 February 2021.

Pickett, K. and Wilkinson, R. (2018). The Inner Level: How More Equal Societies Reduce Stress, Restore Sanity and Improve Everyone's Well-Being. London: Penguin.

Raworth, K. (2017). Doughnut Economics: Seven Ways to Think Like a 21*st* Century Economist. London: Random House Publishing.

Rolleston, A.K., Doughty, R. and Poppe, K. (2016). Integration of kaupapa Māori concepts in health research: a way forward for Māori cardiovascular health? *Journal of Primary Healthcare 8*(1), 60–6.

Scriven, A. (2017). Ewles and Simnett's Promoting Health: A Practical Guide. 7th Ed. London: Elsevier.

Solar, O. and Irwin, A. (2010). A conceptual framework for action on the social determinants of health. *Social Determinants of Health Discussion Paper 2 (Policy and Practice).* Geneva: World Health Organization.

Svalastog, A.L., Donev, D., Kristoffersen, J. and Gajovíc, S. (2017). Concepts and definitions of health and health-related values in the knowledge landscapes of the digital society. *Croatian Medical Journal 58,* 431–5.

Vajrala, K.R., Potturi, G. and Agarwal, A. (2019). A pilot study of randomized clinical controlled trial on role of physiotherapy on physical and psychological dimensions of sexual health in post stroke patients. *Indian Journal of Physiotherapy & Occupational Therapy, 13*(4), 73–7.

Warwick-Booth, L. and Cross, R. (2018). *Global Health Studies: A Social Determinants Perspective.* Cambridge: Polity.

Warwick-Booth, L., Cross, R. and Lowcock, D. (2021). *Contemporary Health Studies: An Introduction.* 2nd Ed. Cambridge, Polity.

WHO (1946). *Constitution of the World Health Organization.* [Internet] Available at: who.int/about/who-we-are/constitution. Accessed 16 January 2021.

Wilkinson, R. and Pickett, K. (2009). *The Spirit Level: Why Equality is Better for Everyone.* London: Penguin.

Wills, J. and Jackson, L. (2014). Health and Health Promotion. In J. Wills (Ed.), *Fundamentals of Health Promotion for Nurses.* 2nd Ed. (pp. 4–21). Chichester: John Wiley & Sons.

Wills, J. (2023). *Foundations for Health Promotion.* 5th Ed. London: Elsevier.

Wong, S.Y. and Kohler, J.C. (2020). Social capital and public health: responding to the COVID-19 pandemic. *Globalization and Health 16*(88) doi: 10.1186/s12992-020-00615-x

World Bank (2021). *Physicians (per 1,000 people).* [Internet] Available at: <www.data.worldbank.org> Accessed 20 February 2021.

Yang, Y., Bekemeier, B. and Choi, J. (2018). A cultural and contextual analysis of health concepts and needs of women in a rural district of Nepal. *Global Health Promotion 25*(1), 15–22.

Yuill, C., Crinson, I. and Duncan, E. (2010). *Key Concepts in Health Studies.* London: Sage.

# 2

# Defining Health Promotion and Health Education

María Pueyo Garrigues and
Navidad Canga Armayor

## Introduction

This chapter discusses the concepts of health promotion and health education and highlights the importance of understanding their nuances in order to underpin their effective and sustainable implementation in both clinical and community settings. The chapter starts by considering a brief and general overview of the main differences between both terms as well as their interaction. It then moves on to a deeper definition and explanation of the characteristics of health promotion and health education, and to a synthesis of what is needed for their successful application and their main outcomes, providing also specific examples facilitating their operationalisation. The chapter continues expounding a range of related concepts such as counselling, health coaching or health communication for its theoretical differentiation, facilitating the exact language use and its application to clinical practice and other health arenas. It then provides an overview about the different levels where health promotion and health education operate (micro, meso and macro). The chapter ends by exploring possible barriers that nurses may encounter when trying to engage in health-promoting practice in different contexts and gives suggestions for overcoming these.

By the end of this chapter the reader will be able to:

1. Understand the complexity of health promotion, recognising the importance of working among different sectors for promoting citizen health.
2. Identify and describe what health education consists of, and the role of nurses for its performance.
3. Appreciate and describe the main differences between related terms used in the health promotion and education field.
4. Recognise the most common barriers for health-promoting practices and the current health focus predominating in the clinical and community fields and appreciate the impact that these might have on nurses' potential application of health education and health promotion.

### Key terms

Health promotion, health education, counselling, health coaching, health communication

## Differentiating Health Promotion and Health Education - A General Overview

The concepts of health promotion and health education are complex and ever evolving. While they complement each other and are interrelated, there are differences between them (Whitehead, 2018). It is important to make a conceptual distinction between health promotion and health education in order to allow a clear foundation from which nurses can define their work and identify and evaluate their roles (Whitehead and Irvine, 2010). Douglas et al. (2007) provides a useful distinction between structuralist and individual approaches in the health promotion and education field, suggesting that structuralist approaches focus on efforts to change the wider determinants of health – such as the physical, social and economic environment – whereas individual approaches focus on encouraging and empowering people to change their behaviour and adopt healthy lifestyles. Thus, it could be stated that health promotion falls into the structuralist approach, and health education is concerned with the individual one (Whitehead and Irvine, 2010).

Box 2.1

**Key difference between health promotion and health education**

Health promotion is based on a structuralist approach focused on efforts to change the wider determinants of health. Health education is based on an individual approach focused on encouraging people to change their behaviour and adopt a healthy lifestyle. Health promotion activities support health education.

Sassen (2018) defines health promotion as an overarching concept that includes health education, being traditionally drafted as an 'umbrella term'. Health education implies an orientation on individuals' lifestyle and health behaviour; and health promotion, in addition to this lifestyle-oriented approach, is supported by an environment-oriented approach.

Under the socio-ecological approach, health promotion is focused not only on intrapersonal behavioural factors but also on the multiple-level factors that influence the specific behaviour in question (Stokols, 1996), encompassing a broad process aimed at providing people with the means to improve their health and exercise greater control over their health, limiting as far as possible negative influences (Cross, 2005). Therefore, health promotion comprises not only actions aimed at increasing people's skills and capabilities, but also those aimed at changing the social, environmental and economic conditions that impact on public health (Whitehead, 2004). In support of health education, health promotion offers structural measures – (healthcare) facilities, laws and regulations – used with the goal of achieving a better effect on people's healthier behaviour and on changing lifestyles (Sassen, 2018).

Both health promotion and health education can coexist since their common focus is health. This accounts for the established position that health education and health promotion can be different in their nature, although they directly complement and mutually reinforce each other (Gelius and Rütten, 2018). Whitehead (2018) identifies health education as a component of wider health promotion, but not the other way around. In this line, it is recognised that effective health education programmes are those that are conducted in the context of overall health planning and in conjunction with a range of health promotion activities (Pueyo-Garrigues et al., 2019; Whitehead, 2003). So then, individual health education interventions may complement, but do not constitute, the collective action that underpins health promotion. In this way, social action may involve elements of education, but it is essentially a 'radical' political process (Whitehead, 2004).

In summary, health education is a strategy to act at the individual level through an interpersonal relationship to increase individual control over one's health while health promotion has a population/community health orientation. Although health promotion can also encompass a set of actions at the individual level to promote healthy lifestyles, it is mainly a global socio-political process at the inter-sectoral level aimed at influencing social, political, environmental and economic determinants to increase the health of people (WHO, 2012).

## What is Health Promotion?

Health promotion is a broad field encompassing educational, social, economic and political efforts to improve the health of a population. Kickbusch (1986) stated that health promotion is positive and dynamic. It opens up the field of health to become an inclusive social, rather than an exclusive professional activity. It is applied in a wide variety of settings – such as schools, workplaces, organisations, and health-care facilities – by workers of different backgrounds and occupations such as, for example, nurses, physicians, nutritionists, or social workers (Burtler, 2001). Given that the major socio-economic determinants of health are often outside individual or even collective control, health promotion aims to empower people to have more control over aspects of their lives that affect their health (Scriven, 2017).

Despite health promotion as a concept with a long trajectory, it is often con-fused with other approaches such as disease prevention. The difference between prevention and promotion can be explained based on the work of Antonovsky (1987), who argued that most of the attention to increased health has focused on understanding the origins of disease (pathogenic/disease prevention) rather than on understanding the origins of health (salutogenics/health promotion) (Miedema, Lindahlnd, and Elf, 2019).

---

### Box 2.2

**Two common definitions of health promotion**

The process of enabling people to increase control over the determinants of health, and thereby improve their health ... a commitment to handle the challenges of decreasing inequities and helping individuals to cope with their circumstances ... creating environments and conditions conducive to health (WHO, 1986)

'Any planned combination of educational, political, regulatory and organisational supports for actions and conditions of living conducive to the health of individuals, groups or communities'. (Green & Kreuter, 1991, p. 432)

---

Health promotion, under the socio-ecological approach, represents 'a mediating strategy between people and their environments, synthesising personal choice and social responsibility in health' (WHO, 1984, p.2). Focusing on the characteristics of health promotion, the Working Group on Concepts and Principles in Health Promotion (WHO, 1984) listed five basic features:

1. *Health promotion involves the population as a whole in the context of their everyday life*, rather than focusing on people at risk for specific disease. Thus, the first feature is enabling people to take control over, and responsibility for, their health as an important component of everyday life – both as spontaneous and organised actions for health.
2. *Health promotion is directed towards action on the determinants or causes of health*. So then, the second characteristic is requiring the close cooperation of sectors beyond the health services; it means working between the health care sector and other sectors in society, reflecting in this way the diversity of conditions that influence health.
3. The third feature is *combining diverse, but complementary, methods or approaches*, including communication, education, legislation, fiscal measures, organisational changes, community development and spontaneous local activities against health hazards.
4. The fourth characteristic is *encouraging effective public participation*, encompassing the development of individual and collective problem-solving and decision-making skills. It implies that the needs of the target group have to be the starting point for intervention development, and that these needs play an important role in the solution of the health problem in communities.
5. Finally, *involving health professionals* for working towards developing their special contributions in education and health advocacy.

---

## Tutorial Trigger 2.1

A key feature of health promotion is intersectoral collaboration; nurses alone cannot address all the determinants of health and promote population health.

Despite this, nurses in both clinical and community settings can make clients aware of the community resources available to them so that they can make use of them. What social resources can you identify in your own neighbourhood/city?

---

In 1986 the World Health Organization drew up the Ottawa Charter for Health Promotion (WHO, 1986) which formally defined health promotion, being the most influential global movement for defining and refining health promotion reform. Five main action areas are delimited: create supportive environments; strengthen

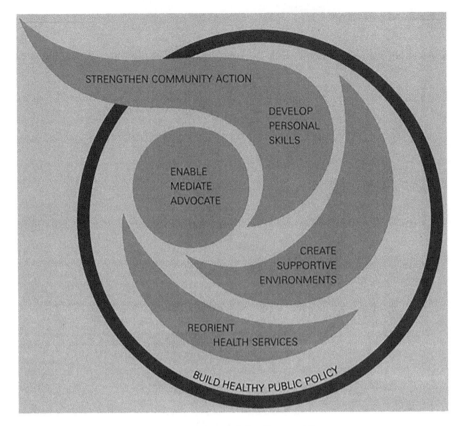

**Figure 2.1**  The health promotion logo of the Ottawa Charter

community action; develop personal skills; reorient health services, and build healthy public policy. Further, this Charter outlines three strategies for health promotion, which are essential to the achievement of the above action areas: enablement, mediation and advocacy (see Box 2.3, and Figure 2.1, the health promotion logo). These health promotion actions and strategies focus on preventing the 'causes of the causes' of ill-health; in recognition that it is not sufficient to only focus on treatment once individuals have become ill (Phillips, 2019).

─── Box 2.3 ───────────────────────────────────────────

### Health promotion actions and strategies

Five health promotion actions in the Ottawa Charter for Health Promotion are:

1  BUILD HEALTHY PUBLIC POLICY

Putting health on the agenda of all policies in all sectors and at multi-levels.

2 CREATE SUPPORTIVE ENVIRONMENTS

Creating living and working conditions that are safe, stimulating, satisfying and enjoyable.

3 STRENGTHEN COMMUNITY ACTION

Working to ensure that communities set priorities, make decisions, plan strategies and are able to implement them in order to achieve better health.

4 DEVELOP PERSONAL SKILLS

Providing people with information and education, enhancing life skills and enabling them to cope.

5 REORIENT HEALTH SERVICES

Develop healthcare services which focus on the total needs of the whole person and are sensitive to their cultural needs.

Three health promotion strategies to health promotion actions be achieved:

1 ENABLING

Taking action in partnership with individuals or groups to empower them, through the mobilisation of human and material resources, to promote and protect their health. Health promotion focuses on achieving equity in health. It aims at reducing differences in current health status and ensuring equal opportunities and resources to enable all people to achieve their fullest health potential. This includes a secure foundation in a supportive environment, access to information, life skills and opportunities for making healthy choices. People cannot achieve their fullest health potential unless they are able to take control of those things which determine their health.

2 MEDIATION

A process through which the different interests (personal, social, economic) of individuals and communities, and different sectors (public and private) are reconciled in ways that promote and protect health. Enhancing people's health cannot be ensured by the health sector alone. Governments, health, and other social sectors have a major responsibility to mediate in society for the pursuit of health.

3 ADVOCACY

A combination of individual and social actions designed to gain political commitment, policy support, social acceptance and systems support for a particular health goal or programme. Political, economic, social, cultural, environmental, behavioural and biological factors can all favour health or be harmful to it. Health promotion action aims at making these conditions favourable through advocacy for health.

(Adapted from Phillips, 2019, p.4)

---

Thus, health promotion attempts to promote adaptations and adjustments in individuals and communities to encourage maintenance and improvement of the health of whole populations, usually by applying wellness principles to organisations and institutions. Box 2.4 shows different activities that can be included under the umbrella of health promotion (Burtler, 2001).

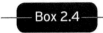
Box 2.4

**Examples of health promotion actions**

*Legislative interventions:*

- regulations aimed at reducing youth access to tobacco products and alcohol.
- regulations requiring companies to monitor air pollution and governmental actions to reduce it.
- professional advocacy for the social determinants of health to be a national priority in all countries.

*Political interventions:*

- development of smoking-free spaces in worksites and study places such as university campuses.
- development of support groups that provide services to people with different chronic diseases and disorders.
- defence access to health care and other social and economic services for the entire population, for equity and social justice.

*Community interventions:*

- creation of free air wellness centres
- formation of neighbourhood walking clubs encouraging individuals' participation in decision-making related to neighbourhood actions.

*Educational interventions:*

- sessions in school for children to develop skills to cope with peer pressure
- stress management classes for employees
- developing monthly workshops to improve patient self-management of type 2 diabetes mellitus.

## What is needed for effective health promotion practice?

The success of health promotion depends on the understanding that collective, rather than individual action, is needed together with an appreciation of the relationships between power and empowerment. As described above, health promotion is a dynamic process in which there is an acknowledgement of the necessity for collaboration and multi-agency involvement. If health promotion is to be successful, the issues of concern should be identified by the community (Whitehead and Irvine, 2010). Therefore, health promotion can be more effective when the target community is personally and actively involved (Sassen, 2018). Further, the capacity and capability of the community to engage in effective collective action is also paramount (Whitehead and Irvine, 2010). The current trend of people wanting to be involved and wanting to be empowered requires health promotion and health education to be focused on people individually. This focus on the individual and the encouragement of making their own (healthy) choices, increases the effectiveness of health promotion (Sassen, 2018). Thus, encouraging participation and empowering people from the target group are important success factors (Whitehead and Irvine, 2010).

Further, effective advocacy approaches are needed to promote a better understanding of health promotion and to communicate clearly its key purpose and functions and raise its visibility within public health, the health sector and in society more generally. In addition, it needs increasing leadership at the highest political level and intersectoral governance in adopting robust policies and action plans and ensuring that the necessary institutional capacity, funding and resources are made available for effective and sustained implementation of health promotion actions (Barry, 2021).

---

## Point to Ponder 2.1

Nursing is an appropriate profession to lead and coordinate health promotion strategies in different contexts. Health promotion is associated with common universal principles of nursing, being the most usual intervention in health education. Increasingly, nurses are participating more in planning, implementing and evaluating wider population-based interventions and projects. Important implications exist in nursing education based on the complex nature of these initiatives. Health promotion education consists of a variety of competencies, such as multidisciplinary knowledge (including knowledge of health in different age groups and epidemiology; or awareness of economic, social and cultural issues, and social and health policies), and skills-related competence (encompassing the application of the knowledge, and the ability to support behavioural changes, teamwork, time management, information gathering, and searching for information) (Kemppainen, Tossavainen and Turunen, 2013). Moreover, health-promotion practice by nurses can also require training in political competence to act as knowledge intermediaries in the field of health policies and general policy (Santillán-García, 2020), and to participate in the formulation and management of public policies. All these elements are the basis for nurses to adopt a proactive stance and act as an advocate achieving effective health promotion practice.

## Consequences of Health Promotion

Health promotion focuses on enabling people to take responsibility for their health, achieving their fullest health potential. People cannot attain this unless they are able to take control of those elements that determine their health, and this is very related with the strengthening of public participation. Thus, due to the nature of health promotion, its consequences are a raised level of community empowerment and the participation of empowered community members in collective political action. The attainment of outcomes that are usually sought by the community groups clusters around the desired achievement of necessary redistribution of resources, or decision-making and changes in policy to generate a positive influence on social determinants of health which, ultimately, bring about the improved health of the community (Whitehead and Irvine, 2010). Miedema, Lindahl and Elf (2019) also inform outcomes in terms of health equity such as enhancing accessibility.

### Research in Brief 2.1

The aim of the study by Basińska-Zych and Springer (2021) was to identify the outcomes for employers and employees related to workplace health promotion interventions (WHPIs). A systematic review (2000-2020) was performed, resulting in 29 empirical investigations included. The conducted analysis revealed that most of the outcomes refer to changes in the strategy and organisational culture, as well as the behaviour of employees, being confirmed by the majority of the studies. More rarely WHPIs led to savings or a reduction in costs resulting from sickness absenteeism, presentism, turnover, etc., and return on investment. The overall conclusion and recommendations of this work promotes the implementation of pro-health activities both for employees and organisations - comprehensive, multi-level and multicomponent interventions and policies - due to their greatest potential for effectiveness in creating healthier workplaces.

Basińska-Zych, A. and Springer, A. (2021). Organizational and Individual Outcomes of Health Promotion Strategies - A Review of Empirical Research. *International Journal of Environmental Research and Public Health* 18(2), 383. https://doi.org/10.3390/ijerph18020383

## What is Health Education?

Health education is considered one of the mechanisms of health promotion. Health education is aimed at the complementary social and political actions that will facilitate the necessary organisational, economic, and other environmental supports for the conversion of individuals' actions into health enhancements and quality-of-life gains (Green and Kreuter, 1999). Health education encompasses a series of planned activities affecting how people think, feel and act regarding their own health and the health of their communities. Since the health education concept first appeared, numerous definitions have emerged, and they are increasingly comprehensive. Some of these definitions are listed below in Box 2.5.

---

**Box 2.5**

## Evolution of definitions of health education

'Health education is any planned combination of learning experiences designed to predispose, enable, and reinforce voluntary behaviour conducive to health in individuals, groups, or communities' (Green & Kreuter, 1991: p. 432).

'Health education is an activity that seeks to inform the individual on the nature and causes of health/illness and that individual's personal level of risk associated with their lifestyle-related behaviour. Health education seeks to motivate the individual to accept a process of behavioural-change through directly influencing their value, belief and attitude systems, where it is deemed that the individual is particularly at risk or has already been affected by illness/disease or disability' (Whitehead, 2004: 313).

'Health education is a continuous, dynamic, complex and planned teaching-learning process throughout the lifespan and in different settings that is implemented through an equitable and negotiated client and health professional "partnership" to facilitate and empower the person to promote/initiate lifestyle-related behavioural changes that promote positive health status outcomes. Health education takes into account individuals'/groups' internal and external factors that influence their health status through potentially improving their knowledge, skills, attitudes and beliefs in relation to their health-related needs and behaviour, within a positive health paradigm' (Pueyo-Garrigues et al., 2019: 133).

---

What all the definitions have in common is the notion of health education as a process. It is a planned process that usually combines a variety of educational experiences and facilitates voluntary adaptations or establishment of behaviour conducive to health. Health educators provide information (often value-laden) that helps individuals understand all the relevant alternatives, and their implications and consequences, in an effort to encourage voluntary behaviour choices. They also help people to enhance their motivation to achieve healthier habits through change, and to acquire the necessary skills to carry out their chosen behaviours

(Burtler, 2001). Furthermore, health education may advocate changes in the environment that will facilitate healthy living conditions and healthy behaviour.

The work of Pueyo-Garrigues et al. (2019) identified five main features of health education:

- *Health education is a learning-teaching process*: it is characterised by its complexity and dynamism – it encompasses the interaction of physical, psychological and social dimensions to generate positive changes throughout the individual's life course. The educational input for learning to take place, is a planned and intentional process facilitating the active participation of the person in their health-related learning.
- *Health education is health-focused*: it is based on the positive definition of health. Aligned with this, a health-focused trajectory is supported by the notion of health as a dynamic and fluid continuum of health-related peaks and troughs that fluctuate throughout the normal process of the lifespan. Therefore, health-focused health education acknowledges the person's health journey along a fluctuating timeline, including healthy and unhealthy transition periods.
- *Health education is multidimensional*: health education activities take into account personal/social behaviour-influencing factors that are indispensable for building and enhancing people's ability to deal with different situations (barriers and enablers) related to their health status. Intrapersonal factors include biological aspects; knowledge and cognitive abilities; emotional encompassing beliefs, attitudes, values and feelings; and personal aptitude related to social abilities, resilience and personal capacity. Other related external factors include a close social environment and resource and support structures.
- *Health education is person-centred*: health education works 'from where each person is' and adapts to what the individual perceives as their health needs aligned to their experiences and abilities. Health education is aimed at careful consideration of an individual's own available behavioural alternatives, focusing on the advantages and disadvantages that are personally relevant to her/him. If the health educator starts from the needs and demands of the patient, it is desirable for the patient to be invited to play an active and participatory role with nurses.
- *Health education is partnership*: health education implies an active and collaborative nurse–person relationship process, underpinned by the principles of respect and autonomy. Also, the voluntary principle is important, which implies that the person has a high degree of choice in respect of the particular behaviour. Health education allows patients to choose the desired health behaviour voluntarily, but also to choose not to change the behaviour.

**Tutorial Trigger 2.2**

As identified, health education practice is characterised by five main attributes (learning process, health-oriented, multidimensional, person-centred and partnership).

Draw up a list with each of the five attributes. Think of the three last times you provided health education in your workplace. Identify the basic elements presented in the cases. What do you notice about the attributes of health education? Do you appreciate any similarity? Are they examples of health education or really of any other related terms such as health information or counselling? What would you change (if any) to enhance your given health education?

Focusing on the operationalisation of health education covers a broad range of educational interventions that nurses can use. Whitehead and Irvine (2010) provide a useful distinction between health education as information-giving, as self-empowering and behaviour change depending on the individual's health needs, and consequently the desired outcomes to achieve.

1. *Health education as information-giving.* Under this form, health education moves beyond imparting information and advice, to develop a bidirectional and cooperative process between the professional and the person. It is focused especially on increasing an individual's knowledge, and also can involve clarifying values, exploring attitudes and enabling processes. The nurse educator uses communication, together with educational and counselling methods, to motivate individuals to bring about health-related change. Brief advice together with pamphlets, brochures or websites are the most frequent strategies/interventions (see Box 2.4). When effective, these strategies can help to reduce people's risk of ill-health, but their nature means that the effect is limited (Whitehead and Irvine, 2010).

    i. As Burtler (2001) said, improving knowledge rarely leads to behaviour change, especially the kind that is sustainable in the long term. We now know conveying information does not necessarily change attitudes, nor are attitudes always consistent with behaviour. For example, when a patient with multiple risk factors for cardiovascular diseases and type 2 diabetes receives a booklet containing background information on high cholesterol levels and obesity, this can lead to an increase in knowledge. If the booklet also informs about the beneficial effect that an improvement in physical activity may have, nurses should not expect the patient to change her/his lifestyle and start moving (Sassen, 2018). A second example is when a nurse advises a patient about the importance of attending to a colon cancer screening, properly using in this way healthcare facilities, and the patient does not want to be checked. In both previous cases, although giving knowledge was important, patients need to go beyond information for promoting a behaviour change, healthier lifestyle and proper use of healthcare resources.

2. *Health education as self-empowerment.* Health education can also aim to empower individuals, that means to encourage personal growth, by focusing on people's ability to develop skills, understanding and awareness. Self-empowerment requires both intrapersonal aspects – such as self-esteem and self-efficacy – and interpersonal aspects – such as involving sharing, helping and partnerships, assertiveness – that enable people to make autonomous decisions about their health. Thus, health education as self-empowerment facilitates individuals to use personal resources to maximise their chances of developing healthy life-styles (Whitehead and Irvine, 2010). The motivational interview is the most used strategy for motivating and empowering individuals for behaviour change (See Box 2.5).

3. *Health education as behaviour change.* Under this form, health education implies achieving the establishment or modification of a behaviour. It could be said that this is a result of the combination of both previous interventions as most of the health-related learning processes must go beyond giving information imparted by the nurse, and including empowerment education. The health educator ensures a conscious change in the person's knowledge, attitude, and behaviour. It is always the patient's own choice whether she/he wants to change her/his lifestyle or health behaviour, and the way they handle her/his health (Sassen, 2018).

## What is Needed for Effective Health Education Practice?

In order to be an effective health educator, nurses need the health education competence so that they practice in line with the underlying principles of health education (Haugan and Eriksson, 2021). This implies nurses need sound knowledge of what health education consists of and what interventions can be effectively adopted, sound personal, social and pedagogical skills, and possessing motivation and personal commitment for health education's daily application (Sassen, 2018). The effectiveness of health education is also determined by the individual's willingness and motivation to act as well as the extent to which the patient understands that health 'partly' depends on lifestyle and behaviour (Buchbinder et al., 2014; Sassen, 2018). Other factors such as resources and time support will also need to be present to enable nurses to engage effectively in health education (Whitehead, 2004; Whyte et al., 2006).

## Consequences of health education

Health education should lead to the improvement of the health of individuals. However, it is likely that this aim will be achieved incrementally and will be determined by the outcomes of health education related to knowledge and health literacy gain, awareness-raising, individual motivation and empowerment, and behaviour change (Guzys et al., 2017; Whitehead and Irvine, 2010). Examples of positive health outcomes are increasing self-confidence, better coping with ongoing disease/disability, improved decision-making, perceived better well-being related to place and community and the efficient use of (healthcare) facilities (Glanz et al., 2008; Pueyo-Garrigues et al., 2019). Furthermore, health education contributes to health promotion. Increasing individual capability and empowerment could promote better control of social situations and surroundings, and a greater awareness in terms of making informed health choices enhancing community health and empowerment (Ibid.). As a result of all of this, health education can lead to a positive social/economic impact through a reduction of 'acute' services related to issues such as hospital admission, lower use of medications, comorbidities, etc. (Glanz et al., 2008; Pueyo-Garrigues et al., 2016). Finally, it is important to note that if health education fails in recognising and incorporating the preferences and priorities of individuals and groups, it runs a very high risk of being ineffective (Whitehead, 2004).

## Related Terms in the Health Promotion and Education Field

As it will be expounded in Chapter 3, the concepts of health promotion and health education have evolved over time and, in addition to the new emerging terms in the health-promotion and education field, this contributes to nurses misunderstanding of their proper use (Guzys et al., 2017; Whitehead and Russell, 2004). This fact hinders its operationalisation at the theoretical level and, consequently, impacts the potential benefits at the clinical interface. Explicit conceptualisation helps to move towards a more precise meaning and role clarity (Whitehead, 2004, 2011). The main related terms, some of them used interchangeably, are health information, counselling, patient education, health coaching, and health communication. Each will now be briefly defined in turn.

*Health information* refers to the unidirectional knowledge provided to patients about their health conditions, its impact on their lifestyle, and options to manage perceived and actual health threats (Wagner and Bear, 2009).

*Counselling* concerns a purposeful partnership that empowers individuals to achieve a satisfactory resolution of 'problems in living' and to accomplish mental health, wellness, education and career goals. It involves resolving problems that are not necessarily related to health but that are the person's felt needs (McLeod, 2013).

*Patient education* is defined as a planned process designed to enable those with existing illness, disease and disability to improve knowledge, attitudes and skills to restore, maintain or improve their existing condition through their active and voluntary participation. In contrast with health education, patient education does not adopt a health focus, but rather the emphasis is on illness, acute or chronic conditions (Piredda, 2004).

*Health coaching* is explained as a goal-oriented, client-centred partnership that is health-focused and occurs through a process of individual enlightenment and empowerment. Its main objective is to activate a patient's own motivation for resolving their ambivalence about health behaviour change and for achieving objectives that enhance quality of life and health (Olsen, 2014).

Finally, *health communication* includes those interpersonal or mass communication strategies and activities to inform and influence decisions and actions for improving the health of individuals and populations (Ishikawa and Kiuchi, 2010).

## Point to Ponder 2.2

The only way health professionals can be seen to be credible within the wider health promotion community, is if we all fully use the exact language and context of health promotion and health education and apply this to clinical practice and other health arenas.

### Research in Brief 2.2

The aim of the study by Pardavila-Belio et al. (2015) was to evaluate the efficacy of a nursing intervention aimed at helping university student smokers to quit smoking. A pragmatic randomised controlled trial comparing a multicomponent intervention, tailored to university students, with a brief counselling session with a 6-month follow-up was conducted. The sample consisted of 255 university student smokers, and data were collected by means of questionnaires and biochemical validation (urine cotinine).

The main elements identified as key in increasing smoking cessation and reducing the number of cigarettes per day among participants were the theoretical basis of the programme (Triadic Influence Theory), the combination of various strategies (such as a 50-minute motivational interview, self-help material, reinforcement messages and group therapy), the implementation of face-to-face strategies and the profile of the educator (a nurse trained in motivational interviewing procedures, who followed a specific protocol adapted to the characteristics of the young people). The overall conclusion of the study promotes the involvement of nurses in the design and implementation of smoking cessation programmes on university campuses.

Pardavila-Belio, M.I., García-Vivar, C., Pimenta, A.M., Canga-Armayor, A., Pueyo-Garrigues, S. and Canga-Armayor, N. (2015). Intervention study for smoking cessation in Spanish college students: pragmatic randomized controlled trial. *Addiction* *110*(10), 1676-83. https://doi.org/10.1111/add.13009

## Health Promotion and Health Education Operating Levels

When we talk about health, we tend to focus on health care and everything that is organised around it (hospital resources and health centres, health professionals, treatments, etc.). However, in recent decades, there has been growing evidence of the influence on health of the social, political and economic structure in which people live, as well as the importance of community networks and educational, social and work-related factors. Taking this into account, and under the socio-ecological view of health promotion previously explained, health promotion and health education should operate at the three levels: individual (micro), community (meso) and national/international/global (macro).

At the individual (micro) level, health education implementation is what pre-dominates. It comprises, specially, the healthcare setting, the most cited level in the literature – this setting includes both primary and specialised/hospital care (Perea, 2009; Salci et al., 2013). These contexts make it possible to have person-centred encounters with clients, which is a defining characteristic of health educa-tion. Furthermore, they are a source of important health experiences that enhance the development of health-promoting interventions aimed at the active participa-tion of people to protect, promote or maintain health, reducing risky behaviours, promoting self-care, and encouraging the use of available services and resources (WHO, 2012). However, it should be noted that this field, and more specifically the hospital context, is widely associated with illness, predominating practices under the biomedical paradigm (Pueyo-Garrigues et al., 2019).

In addition, it is important to mention that a large body of literature uses the term 'behavioural health-promotion' referring to the more individualistic approach of telling people what to do to change their unhealthy lifestyles, when the term behavioural is more commonly associated with health education (Whitehead, 2018). This is why at this operating level, health education and behavioural health-promotion can coexist. However, the shift from person-centred to community-oriented and socio-ecological-based health promotion is increasingly taking place.

At the community (meso) and the national/global (macro) levels, what takes place is the operation of health promotion. At the community level, it could include, among others, the school/university environment, the workplace and neighbourhoods, which are both naturally conducive to health promotion (Glanz et al., 2008). Health education can be also present at this level, promoting indi-vidual or group citizens' active participation to increase their health and promoting healthy and safe habits and practices as well as environments that facilitate healthy decision-making (Perea, 2009; WHO, 2012). Regarding the macro level, health pro-motion is conductive mainly through collaborative intersectoral actions and public policies that incorporate a health lens into decision-making, considering the health implications of decisions in all sectors.

As health promotion and education operate on different levels, and are present in different settings, it is not strange that both are embedded in the multidisciplinary framework of health professionals such as physicians, nutritionists, psychologists and other workers. This is coherent with the socio-ecological perspective which is inherently interdisciplinary. Ecological analyses integrate the community-wide, preventive strategies of public health and epidemiology with the individual-level, therapeutic and curative strategies of medicine. Determinants of health problems – environment, medical care, personal lifestyle – often are discovered in the public health realm. The ecological perspective also encompasses the behavioural and social sciences' emphases on the active role played by persons and groups in modifying their own health behaviour; and the development and testing of theoretical models describing people–environment transactions (Burtler, 2001; Stokols, 1996). Finally, education science (the study and practice of teaching and learning) plays a role in the development of health education. Learning theory, educational psychology, human development, pedagogy are all rooted in the education literature (Burtler, 2001). Specifically, the literature identifies nurses as the best positioned (Glanz et al., 2008; WHO, 2012), both in hospital and community settings. But most nursing practice remains within the primary focus of health education instead of more global health promotion practices (Whitehead, 2008).

## Barriers to Developing a Health-Promoting Practice

A number of areas of concern have been noted in the literature as barriers to working in a health-promoting way. One of the most repeated barriers is the lack of competence in health promotion and education fields, that is related with less positive thoughts about ones capability and confidence for health-promoting interventions. Specifically, a lack of effective education and training in health promotion and education is the biggest necessity identified by nurses, as most report they had never received training in their educational role (Chang et al., 2020; Forbes et al., 2021; Whitehead, 2018). Further, Whitehead and Irvine (2010) describe workplace influence in nurses' performance of health promotion and health education. As they stated, healthcare settings can be physically and mentally demanding because of long hours, heavy workloads, staffing problems, insufficient resources, and emotional burden. Coping with all this can affect the quality of nurse–patient relationships and job satisfaction, and can even result in illness on the part of the nurse. The organisational environment results also in social and physical barriers to nurses developing health-promoting practice such as lack of time, inadequate and scarce resources and equipment, disease/task orientation, lack of authority in decision-making, poor interpersonal relationships (Casey, 2007; Phillips, 2019).

It is important not to neglect to mention that currently most health professionals across all primary, secondary and tertiary care settings still conduct their core business aligned to a biomedical paradigm, that is focused on health problems rather than health potential (Salci et al., 2013). Some authors have been critical of the healthcare facility setting for health promotion practices because they are often associated with medicalisation, individualisation, and institutionalisation rather than health empowerment among groups and communities. It therefore remains difficult to implement health promotion initiatives (Miedema, Lindahl and Elf, 2019). The achievement of the paradigm shift in healthcare settings will require radical changes both to pre-registration curricula and continued professional development, emphasising training in health promotion/education competence within a framework of public health using participatory pedagogical methods such as video-tapping, and *in vivo* supervisions will be needed for increasing nurses' knowledge, skills and favourable attitudes. Pre-registration nursing programmes are quite varied in their health education and health promotion content (Whitehead and Irvine, 2010).

Finally, centring attention on more social-environmental health-promoting practices, there is a tendency to focus health promotion actions on individual lifestyles and campaigns targeting risky behaviour. Embedded in the rationale of neoliberalism, the focus is set on individual responsibility to take a healthy path in the numerous health-promotion strategies and initiatives (Jelsøe et al., 2018). This tendency is proposed by Jelsøe et al. (2018) to be contested through health promotion because it seeks to understand health practices as initiatives that must be directed towards people's scope for action in relation to structures and societal conditions in different settings such as schools, local communities, workplaces and so on. Political commitment also is key to addressing institutional barriers at a policy and political level and bringing a clear focus on the promotion of population health and health equity (Barry, 2021).

---

## Tutorial Trigger 2.3

List the main barriers to health-promoting practice that you encounter in your role as a nurse, and consider how these might be overcome. Think about what would need to change, and who would need to be involved.

---

## Summary

This chapter has explored nuanced elements of health promotion and health education. As Pueyo-Garrigues et al. (2019) argues, establishing a benchmark around how health promotion and education are conceptualised is essential to facilitate its practical application in nursing care. As such this chapter provides an important foundation to understand and reorient nursing practice. It also has outlined several different terms related to the health promotion and education field, highlighting the main differences, and discussed the main factors that hinder their implementation. Being aware of these aspects is essential to understanding how health professionals behave, and the way we have to retake for a suitable practice reorientation. The only way nurses can be seen to be credible with the wider health promotion community is if we all fully use the exact language and context of health promotion and health education.

────── Key Points ──────────────────────────────────────────

- Health promotion is a broad concept that encompasses educational, social, economic and political efforts to improve peoples' health. It is applied in a wide variety of settings by different professionals.
- Health education is complementary to health promotion and is a planned process that usually combines a variety of educational experiences and that facilitates voluntary adaptations or establishment of behaviour conducive to health.
- Health education is a strategy to act at the individual level through an interpersonal relationship to increase individual control over one's health, while health promotion has a population/community health orientation.
- Main barriers to effective health-promoting practice are health professionals' lack of competence in the health promotion and education field, the persistence of the biomedical paradigm and initiatives focused mainly on individual lifestyles and risk behaviours, and organisational characteristics and environment of the workplace.
- Health education contributes to health promotion. Increasing individual capability and empowerment could promote better control of social situations and surroundings, and a greater awareness in terms of making informed health choices enhancing community health and empowerment.

## References

Antonovsky, A. (1987). *Unravelling the Mystery of Health*. San Francisco: Jossey-Bass.

Barry, M.M. (2021). Transformative health promotion: what is needed to advance progress? *Global Health Promotion*. doi:10.1177/17579759211013766

Buchbinder, M., Wilbur, R., Zuskov, D., McLean, S. and Sleath, B. (2014). Teachable moments and missed opportunities for smoking cessation counseling in a hospital emergency department: a mixed-methods study of patient-provider communication. *BMC Health Services Research 14*, 651. doi:10.1186/s12913-014-0651-9

Burtler, J.T. (2001). *Principles of Health Education and Health Promotion.* 3rd Ed. Wadsworth.

Casey, D. (2007). Nurses' percections, understanding, and experiences of health promotion. *Journal of Clinical Nursing 16*, 1039–49.

Chang, Y.W., Li, T.C., Chen, Y.C., Lee, J.H., Chang, M.C. and Huang, L.C. (2020). Exploring knowledge and experience of health literacy for Chinese-speaking nurses in Taiwan: A cross-sectional study. *International Journal of Environmental Research and Public Health 17*(20), 1–14. doi:10.3390/ijerph17207609

Cross, R. (2005). Accident and Emergency nurses' attitudes towards health promotion. *Journal of Advanced Nursing 51*(5), 47–83

Douglas, J., Earle, S., Handsley, S., Jones, L., Lloyd, C.E. and Spurr, S. (2007). *A Reader in Promoting Public Health: Challenge and Controversy.* London: SAGE Publications.

Forbes, R., Clasper, B., Ilango, A., Kan, H., Peng, J. and Mandrusiak, A. (2021). Effectiveness of patient education training on health professional student performance: A systematic review. *Patient Education and Counseling,* S0738-3991(21), 00139-7. doi:10.1016/j.pec.2021.02.039

Gelius, P. and Rütten, A. (2018). Conceptualizing structural change in health promotion: why we still need to know more about theory. *Health Promotion International 33*(4), 657–64. doi:10.1093/heapro/dax006

Glanz, K., Rimer, B.K. and Viswanath, K. (2008). *Health Behavior and Health Education, Theory, Research and Practice.* 4th Ed. San Francisco: John Wiley & Sons.

Green, L.W. and Kreuter, M.W. (1991). *Health Promotion Planning: An Educational and Environmental Approach.* Mountain View: Mayfield.

Green, L.W. and Kreuter, M.W. (1999). *Health Promotion Planning: An Educational and Ecological Approach.* 3rd Ed. Mountain Veiw: Mayfield.

Guzys, D., Brown, R., Halcomb, E. and Whitehead, D. (2017). *An Introduction to Community and Primary Health Care.* 2nd Ed. Cambridge: Cambridge University Press.

Haugan, G. and Eriksson, M. (2021). *Health Promotion in Health Care – Vital Theories and Research. Springer.* doi:10.1007/978-3-030-63135-2

Ishikawa, H. and Kiuchi, T. (2010). Health literacy and health communication. *BioPsychoSocial 4*(18). doi:10.1186/1751-0759-4-18

Jelsøe, E., Thualagant, N., Holm, J., Kjærgård, B., Andersen, H.M., From, D.-M., Land, B. and Pedersen, K.B. (2018). A future task for health-promotion research: Integration of health promotion and sustainable development. *Scandinavian Journal of Public Health 46*(20 suppl.), 99–106, doi:10.1177/1403494817744126

Kemppainen, V., Tossavainen, K. and Turunen, H. (2013). Nurses' roles in health promotion practice: an integrative review. *Health Promotion International 28*(4), 490–501. https://doi.org/10.1093/heapro/das034

Kickbusch, I. (1986). Introduction to the journal. *Health Promotion International 1*(1), 3–4. doi:10.1093/heapro/1.1.3

McLeod, J. (2013). *An Introduction to Counselling.* 5th Ed. New York: McGraw-Hill.

Miedema, E., Lindahl, G. and Elf, M. (2019). Conceptualizing health promotion in relation to outpatient healthcare building design – a Scoping review. *Health Environments Research & Design Journal 12*(1), 69–86. doi:10.1177/1937586718796651

Olsen, J.M. (2014). Health coaching: A concept analysis. *Nursing Forum 49*(1), 18–29. doi:10.1111/nuf.12042

Perea, R. (2009). *Health Promotion and Education: Innovative Trends.* 2nd Ed. Madrid: Díaz de Santos D.L.

Phillips, A. (2019). Effective approaches to health promotion in nursing practice. *Nursing Standard 34*(4), 43–50. doi:10.7748/ns.2019.e11312

Piredda, M. (2004). Patient education: a concept analysis. *International Nursing Perspective 4*(2), 63–71.

Pueyo-Garrigues, M., San Martín Loyola, Á., Caparrós Leal, M.C. and Jiménez Muñoz, C. (2016). [Health education in transplant patients and their families in an intensive care unit]. *Enfermería intensiva 27*(1), 31–9. doi:0.1016/j.enfi.2015.11.002

Pueyo-Garrigues, M., Whitehead, D., Pardavila-Belio, M.I., Canga-Armayor, A., Pueyo-Garrigues, S. and Canga-Armayor, N. (2019). Health education: A Rogerian concept analysis. *International Journal of Nursing Studies, 94,* 131–8. doi:10.1016/j.ijnurstu.2019.03.005

Santillán-García, A. (2020). [Proposals for the political participation of Spanish nurses]. *Tesela 28.* e13147

Sassen, B. (2018). *Nursing: Health Education and Improving Patient Self-Management.* New York: Springer.

Salci, M.A., Maceno, P., Rozza, S.G., Vieira da Silva, D.M.G., Boehs, A.E. and Heidemann, I.T.S.B. (2013). Health education and its theoretical perspectives: a few reflections. *Florianópolis 22*(1), 224–30.

Scriven, A. (2017). *Promoting Health: A Practical Guide. 7th* Ed. Elsevier.

Stokols, D. (1996). Translating socio-ecological theory into guidelines for community health promotion. *American Journal of Health Promotion 10*(4), 282–98. doi:10.4278/0890-1171-10.4.282

Wagner, D. and Bear, M. (2009). Patient satisfaction with nursing care: a concept analysis within a nursing framework. *Journal of Advanced Nursing 65*(3), 692–701. doi:10.1111/j.1365-2648.2008.04866.x

Whitehead, D. (2003). Health promotion and health education viewed as symbiotic paradigms: bridging the theory and practice gap between them. *Journal of Clinical Nursing 12*(6), 796–805.

Whitehead, D. (2004). Health promotion and health education: advancing the concepts. *Journal of Advanced Nursing 47*(3), 311–20.

Whitehead, D. (2008). An international Delphi study examining health promotion and health education in nursing practice, education and policy. *Journal of Clinical Nursing 17*(7), 891–900. doi: 10.1111/j.1365-2702.2007.02079.x

Whitehead, D. (2011). Before the cradle and beyond the grave: a lifespan/settings-based framework for health promotion. *Journal of Clinical Nursing 20*(15–16), 2183–94. doi: 10.1111/j.1365-2702.2010.03674.x

Whitehead, D. (2018). Exploring health promotion and health education in nursing. *Nursing Standard 33*(8), 38–44. doi: 10.7748/ns.2018.e11220

Whitehead, D. and Irvine, F. (2010). *Health Promotion & Health Education in Nursing: A Framework for Practice.* Palgrave Macmillan.

Whitehead, D. and Russell, G. (2004). How effective are health education programmes – resistance, reactance, rationality and risk? Recommendations for effective practice. *International Journal of Nursing Studies 41*(2), 163–72.

Whyte, R.E., Watson, H.E. and McIntosh, J. (2006). Nurses' opportunistic interventions with patients in relation to smoking. *Journal of Advanced Nursing 55*(5), 568–77.

World Health Organization. Regional Office for Europe. (1984). *Health promotion: a discussion document on the concept and principles: summary report of the Working Group on Concept and Principles of Health Promotion, Copenhagen, 9-13 July 1984*. Copenhagen: WHO Regional Office for Europe. https://apps.who.int/iris/handle/10665/107835

World Health Organization. (1986). The Ottawa Charter for health promotion. *Health Promotion 1*(1), iii–v.

World Health Organization. (2012). *Health Education: Theoretical Concepts, Effective Strategies and Core Competencies*. World Health Organization, Cairo. Retrieved from http://applications.emro.who.int/dsaf/EMRPUB_2012_EN_1362.pdf

# 3

# A History of Health Promotion and Health Education

## Ruth Cross and James Woodall

## Introduction

This chapter presents a brief history of health promotion and health education which frames contemporary understanding of what these are about. It considers how health promotion has emerged as a field in its own right, detailing how the rise of health promotion in the 1980s and early 1990s occurred in reaction to the focus on addressing existing 'lifestyle-related' diseases, illness and disability. Instead, health promotion turned attention back to the need to tackle underlying social issues and the significance of the wider (social) determinants of health. The chapter focuses particularly on the World Health Organization's role in the development of global health promotion and introduces a cornerstone document, The Ottawa Charter (WHO, 1986), alongside other key global documents and milestones in the chronicles of health education and health promotion. The chapter will then out-line where health promotion is today. The manner in which health promotion has and does align and overlap with other fields such as public health, primary health care, community health, population health and environmental health will also be discussed. This chapter is complemented by the discussions that will take place in

Chapter 5 – *The Ottawa Charter- Re-orienting health services and developing personal skills*, and Chapter 11 – *The future of health promotion and health education for health professionals*.

By the end of this chapter the reader will be able to:

1.  Appreciate how health promotion has evolved as a distinct field of practice.
2.  Appreciate the influential role of the World Health Organization in the development of health promotion.
3.  Understand and describe key milestones in health promotion over the past four decades with reference to the major WHO conferences and documents.
4.  Describe and discuss key distinctions between health promotion and other related fields of practice.

## Key terms

Health promotion, health education, World Health Organization, Ottawa Charter, public health, primary health care, community health, population health, environmental health, health promotion and health education

────── Time to Reflect 3.1 ──────────────────────────────

Before you read any further take some time to think about what the terms 'health education' and 'health promotion' mean to you.

Health promotion and health education are often viewed as being the same, however they are distinct. One of the earliest influences on the development of health promotion as a field was the Lalonde Report (Lalonde, 1974). This report, published in Canada, called for a new way to think about health and deconstructed ideas about health as being solely the responsibility of healthcare services; instead, it emphasised the need for a much broader approach to tackling the health issues including considering lifestyles and the role of the environment, in short, a focus on prevention (Cross et al., 2021). However, this different emphasis on promoting health through broader means challenged received wisdom about traditional health education which tended to focus more on telling people what to do as a means of improving health behaviour. For many people the mention of health promotion brings to mind giving someone an information leaflet or providing advice about a health issue (Wills, 2023). Yet, as we point out in this book (please see Chapter 2: *Defining health promotion and health education*), it is so much more than that. As Wild and McGrath (2019, p. 31) argue, 'health education at the simplest level is provision of information and knowledge about health and how to maintain it'. Health education therefore tends to aim to persuade people to change their behaviour in some way, the purpose of which is to improve their health (Green et al., 2019). This assumes that giving information will lead to increased knowledge which will lead to a change in attitude which, in turn, will lead to a change in behaviour which will, ultimately, lead to better health outcomes (Cross and O'Neil, 2021). This set of assumptions is problematic because behaviour change is more multifaceted and far less linear than this (Tapper, 2021). So, unfortunately, it is not that simple and such an approach can lead to victim-blaming because it tends not to take into account the wider contexts that health behaviour takes place in. As demonstrated in Chapter 1: *Health and its determinants*, things are much more complex than that.

Green et al. (2019: 343) define health education as 'a planned process designed to achieve health- and illness-related learning' whilst the World Health Organization has consistently defined health education as 'comprising of consciously constructed opportunities for learning involving some form of communication designed to improve health literacy, including improving health knowledge, and developing life skills' (WHO, 1998 cited in Scriven, 2017: 21). The nurse has a large part to play in this as it is an important facet of their role. Whatever context nurses practise in there will be many opportunities to provide tailored health education whether formally, informally or simply opportunistically. Please see Box 3.1 for an example of opportunistic health education in recent practice from the United Kingdom.

---

### Box 3.1

**Making every contact count**

Making Every Contact Count (MECC) was an approach to behaviour change and population health that was introduced by Health Education England, which is the part of the National Health Service that plans, recruits, educates and trains the health and social care workforce. MECC is designed to make the most of the millions of everyday encounters that health and social care staff have with people.

> *The Making Every Contact Count approach encourages health and social care staff to use the opportunities arising during their routine interactions with patients to have conversations about how they might make positive improvements to their health or wellbeing.*

In practice this means, for example, a person might attend their GP about a specific issue and the GP would then take the opportunity to talk to them about their general health and health behaviour perhaps bringing up things like stopping smoking, improving their diet, being less sedentary, losing weight, managing stress, reducing alcohol - whatever is relevant to that particular person at that particular time - and signpost them to further support as necessary.

For further information please see <www.makingeverycontactcount.co.uk>

---

Health education is vital in the promotion of health but can be viewed as one way (of many others) in which health might be improved, hence the inclusion of the educational approach in Wills' (2023) five approaches to health promotion framework (alongside the medical, behaviour change, empowerment and social change approaches). Health literacy, which is specifically mentioned in the WHO's definition of health promotion, relates to understanding health information; it is not simply about being able to read and write but is concerned with a person being able to 'make sense of', and use, health information to improve their health (Wills and Jackson, 2014). The World Health Organization has identified health literacy as one of three key pillars of health promotion emphasising that people should have access to the knowledge and skills to enable them to make healthier choices (WHO, 2016). Whilst health education is an important part of promoting health it is rather narrow, focuses too much on behaviour change, and fails to address health inequalities (Hubley et al., 2021). Health promotion goes well beyond health education to address the wider, social determinants of health and to tackle inequalities in health. It 'encompasses a very broad range of activities that aim to facilitate people to achieve a full and healthy life, based on [a] broader view of health' (Evans et al., 2017: 13).

## Point to Ponder 3.1

Cross et al. (2021: 1) view health promotion as 'a social movement with the central aim of tackling the social determinants of health and so bringing about greater health and social justice'. By the 'social determinants of health' we mean those factors that enable people to live healthy and productive lives - these factors include the obvious ones of decent housing, access to education, employment opportunities, nourishing food, well-functioning and accessible health care, cohesive communities, good systems of government and peaceful, safe nation-states. The social determinants of health can either enable people and communities to flourish and do well, or not, depending on whether (or how) they create opportunities for better health.

---

Over time, health education has become encompassed within health promotion (WHO, 2012). In Tannahill's model of health promotion health education is one of three spheres comprising health promotion (alongside health protection and prevention) (Tannahill, 1985). However, it can also be considered more widely than this. Health education is not just about receiving health information or raising awareness, it is also about the development of motivation, skills, confidence and self-efficacy (WHO, 2012). Tones (1997) conceived of health promotion in the following way:

Health Promotion = Health Education + Healthy Public Policy

This formula recognises the important role that healthy public policy plays in providing environments in which behaviour change can be supported and sustained.

---

### Tutorial Trigger 3.1

- How do you think policy influences health and health outcomes? What role does/can policy play in creating environments in which health might flourish?
- Policy operates at many different levels – organisational/institutional, national, regional and global. What influence do you have on policy development and at what level?

---

## Health Promotion and the World Health Organization Agenda

The World Health Organization has been the key player in setting the global agenda for health promotion and has significantly influenced the development of health promotion over the past several decades. The most frequently used definition of health promotion originates from the Ottawa Charter (WHO, 1986) which came out of the first global conference on health promotion in Ottawa, Canada (see Box 3.2).

 Box 3.2

### The World Health Organization's definition of health promotion (WHO, 1986)

Health promotion is the process of enabling people to increase control over, and improve, their health. To reach a state of complete physical, mental and social well-being, an individual or group must be able to identify and to realise aspirations, to satisfy needs, and to change or cope with the environment. Health is, therefore, seen as a resource for everyday life, not the objective of living. Health is a positive concept emphasising social and personal resources, as well as physical capacities. Therefore, health promotion is not just the responsibility of the health sector but goes beyond healthy lifestyles to well-being.

The focus on policy and environmental solutions to tackling health in the Ottawa Charter represented a paradigm shift contrary to the prior focus on educating people to make them behave differently (Nutbeam, 2019). The Ottawa Charter has been described as a major milestone for health promotion (Scriven, 2017). The subsequent developments in the World Health Organization's agenda for health promotion have built on these early ideas and reinforced the position that health is not solely the domain of the individual but is influenced, and impacted on, by many different factors – the majority of which lie outside of a person's control.

Several common themes run through the documents on health promotion that have been produced by the World Health Organization over the years. These include an emphasis on a holistic view of health, the idea of health as fundamental human right, the need to acknowledge and tackle health inequalities and inequities between and within countries, health as a central social goal, the importance of social development to health, the need for cross-sectoral working and partnership, the centrality of education as a means of enabling meaningful community participation, and the rights and duty of people to engage in their own health

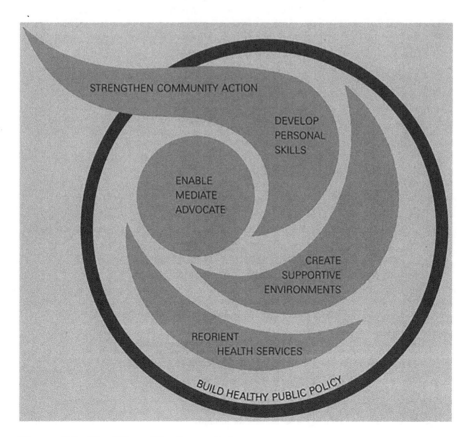

**Figure 3.1**  The Ottawa Charter symbol

care as individuals and communities (Green et al., 2019). In addition, the importance of policy has been highlighted throughout the different conferences with
considerable weight given to narrowing the health divide and achieving equity in
health care (Gottwald and Goodman-Brown, 2012). In more recent years issues of
sustainability and corporate responsibility have also loomed large on the agenda
in the context of climate change. The key values underpinning the WHO health
promotion agenda include what Green et al. (2019) refer to as the 'twin pillars of
health promotion' – *empowerment* and *equity*. The other emphasis in health promotion is that of *social justice* whereby everyone should be 'treated fairly and equita-
bly regardless of race age, gender of ethnicity' (Linsley and Roll, 2020). Table 3.1
outlines the key events and resulting charters or declarations that have occurred
in the World Health Organization-led agenda for health promotion over the past
several decades.

**Table 3.1**   Key historical milestones for health promotion in the WHO-led
agenda

| Date | Event | Associated Document and/or Key Outcomes |
|---|---|---|
| 1986 | The 1st International Conference on Health Promotion held in Ottawa, Canada | *The Ottawa Charter* (WHO, 1986)* <br> Identified three broad strategies for promotion of health: <br> • Advocacy <br> • Enabling <br> • Mediation <br> Listed five main areas for action: <br> • Build health public policy <br> • Create supportive environments <br> • Strengthen community action <br> • Develop personal skills <br> • Reorient health services <br> Recognition that health is created where people 'learn, work, play and love' started the 'settings approach' to health promotion (Green et al., 2019). |
| 1988 | The 2nd International Conference on Health Promotion held in Adelaide, Australia | Focused on health public policy (the first area of action from The Ottawa Charter) and laid out four areas for immediate action (WHO, 2009): <br> • Supporting the health of women <br> • Food and nutrition <br> • Tobacco and alcohol <br> • Creating supportive environments |
| 1991 | The 3rd International Conference on Health Promotion held in Sundsvall, Sweden | Focused on supportive environments for health (the second area of action from The Ottawa Charter) in terms of four main aspects: <br> • The social dimension <br> • The political dimension <br> • The economic dimension <br> • A gender dimension |

*(Continued)*

**Table 3.1**  Key historical milestones for health promotion in the WHO-led agenda (*Continued*)

| Date | Event | Associated Document and/or Key Outcomes |
|------|-------|------------------------------------------|
| 1997 | The 4th International Conference on Health Promotion, held in Jakarta, Indonesia | *The Jakarta Declaration on Leading Health Promotion into the 21st Century* (WHO, 1997)<br><br>Called for strong partnerships to promote health, including the private sector, and set out the following priorities for the 21st century:<br>• Promote social responsibility for health<br>• Increase investments for health development<br>• Consolidate and expand partnerships for health<br>• Increase community capacity and empower the individual<br>• Secure an infrastructure for health promotion |
| 2000 | The 5th International Conference on Health Promotion held in Mexico City, Mexico | Focused on bridging the inequity gap acknowledging that 'the promotion of health and social development is a central duty and responsibility of governments that all sectors of society share' and 'health promotion is a fundamental component of public policies and programmes in all countries in the pursuit of equity and health for all' (WHO, 2000). |
| 2005 | The 6th International Conference on Health Promotion held in Bangkok, Thailand | *The Bangkok Charter for Health Promotion in a Globalized World (WHO, 2005)*<br><br>Focused attention on increasing inequalities between countries, commercialisation, new patterns of consumption and communication, and environmental change and urbanisation.<br><br>The charter called for four major commitments to make health promotion:<br>• Central to the global development agenda<br>• A core responsibility for all of government<br>• A key focus for communities and civil society<br>• A requirement for good corporate practice |
| 2009 | The 7th International Conference on Health Promotion held in Nairobi, Kenya | *The Nairobi Call to Action (WHO, 2009)*<br><br>Addressed the need to close the implementation gap in health and development through health promotion (Catford, 2010) and called for the following (WHO, 2009):<br>• Strengthen leadership and workforces<br>• Mainstream health promotion<br>• Empower communities and individuals<br>• Enhance participatory processes<br>• Build and apply knowledge |
| 2013 | The 8th International Conference on Health Promotion held in Helsinki, Finland | *The Helsinki Statement on Health in All Policies (WHO, 2013)*<br><br>Highlighted the role of policy in the promotion of health and identified intersectoral action and healthy public policy as central requirements for the promotion of health emphasising the need for 'Health in All Policies' and calling for political will and cross-governmental working (WHO, 2013). |

*(Continued)*

**Table 3.1**   Key historical milestones for health promotion in the WHO-led agenda (*Continued*)

| Date | Event | Associated Document and/or Key Outcomes |
|------|-------|------------------------------------------|
| 2016 | The 9th International Conference on Health Promotion held in Shanghai, China | *The Shanghai Declaration (WHO, 2016)* |
| | | Focused on promoting health in the context of the 2030 Agenda for Sustainable Development in recognition that 'health and well-being are essential to achieving the [...] Sustainable Development Goals and reinforces the importance of structural factors and of the wider determinants of health' (WHO, 2016). |
| | | This latest conference resulted in the following call to action: |
| | | 'We recognize that health is a political choice and we will counteract interests detrimental to health and remove barriers to empowerment - especially for women and girls. We urge political leaders from different sectors and from different levels of governance, from the private sector and from civil society to join us in our determination to promote health and wellbeing in all the Sustainable Development Goals. Promoting health demands coordinated action by all concerned, it is a shared responsibility. With this Shanghai Declaration, we, the participants, pledge to accelerate the implementation of the SDGs through increased political commitment and financial investment in health promotion.' |
| 2021 | 10th Global Conference on Health Promotion held online and in Geneva, Switzerland | The title of this conference was 'Health Promotion: Well-being, Equity and Sustainable Development'. It marked the start of a global movement on the concept of well-being in societies and re-emphasised the need for different sectors to work together without destroying the planet (WHO, 2021). |
| | | The resulting Geneva Charter for Well-being outlined five key actions:<br>• Design an equitable economy that serves human development within planetary boundaries;<br>• Create public policy for the common good;<br>• Achieve universal health coverage;<br>• Address the digital transformation to counteract harm and disempowerment and to strengthen the benefits; and<br>• Value and preserve the planet |

*Please see more detail about The Ottawa Charter in Chapter 5

The conferences and resulting outputs detailed in Table 3.1 have had a significant impact on the trajectory of global health promotion since the inception of the Ottawa Charter. Through these the World Health Organization has led the development of health promotion. The definition of health promotion has remained core to this agenda but notably, after the Bangkok conference in 2005, the World Health

Organization refined its definition further to include an emphasis on the wider determinants of health as follows: 'health promotion is the process of enabling people to increase control over their health *and its determinants*, and thereby to improve their health' (WHO, 2005).

The conference in Shanghai in 2016 reiterated some of the key concerns of health promotion emphasising some of the things that were prominent in the Ottawa Charter three decades previously, such as the need for healthy public policy, and it built on some of the other themes that have emerged such as the importance of cross-sectoral working, collective approaches and working together in partnership to promote health. Crucially, the Shanghai Declaration also emphasised the importance of sustainability referring explicitly to the global sustainable development agenda as reflected by the commitment to the Sustainable Development Goals (SDGs). This emphasis highlights once again the importance of structural factors and the wider determinants of health (WHO, 2016) and acknowledges how health is integral to the achievement of many of the SDGs, not just Goal 3 (Ensure healthy lives and promote wellbeing for all at all ages) (Fleming, 2020). The world has changed a great deal since 1986. In some areas, such as technology and digital communication, this is beyond recognition compared to over 30 years ago yet the central concerns of the Ottawa Charter still resonate today (Ibid.). High level political will is still necessary to achieve a (global) commitment to promoting health (Cross et al., 2021) and this is particularly the case when it comes to issues such as development and sustainability (Wild and McGrath, 2019).

───── Time to Reflect 3.2 ──────────────────────────────────

Before you read any further take some time to think about the relationship between the following:

- health promotion and public health
- health promotion and primary health care
- health promotion and community care
- health promotion and population health
- health promotion and environmental health.

You may want to use the internet to help you with this if you are not quite sure what each term refers to. As you will see, each of these areas are distinct from, yet related to, health promotion. The next few sections of the chapter discuss each in turn.

────────────────────────────────────────────────────────────

## Health promotion and public health

As Green et al. (2019: 59) point out, 'for some [people], there is no distinction between health promotion and public health [...] however, for [others] health promotion and public health, although related, are not synonymous'. That is, they differ and are each distinct. For example, some people view public health as a broad area of activity under which health promotion falls (Hubley et al., 2021) or as an integral part of public health (Fleming et al., 2020). Others view public health as concerned with expert-led health protection and as centred on a medical model of health, whilst health promotion is viewed as being primarily concerned with community-led approaches to health improvement and centred on a social model of health. For still others, public health is seen as having a longer tradition than health promotion – public health efforts can be traced back hundreds of years whilst health promotion has emerged as a strategy in the past few decades (Wild and McGrath, 2019). In many ways public health was the forerunner of health promotion. The history of public health is long reaching. Concerns about public health efforts date back to the ancient Greeks who appreciated the importance of maintaining health and also the links between health, disease, the wider environment and human behaviour (Tountas, 2009). The Romans also adopted many public health measures to protect people's health including sanitation and the control of infectious disease. In fact, the term, public health (*medici publici*) has been traced back to ancient Rome (Karabatos et al., 2021). The medieval era brought with it an attendant focus on endemics, followed by a concern with disease prevalence in the eighteenth century whilst the industrial revolution turned attention to working conditions and the health of the workforce (Wild and McGrath, 2019). Great strides were made in the latter part of this period with much better appreciation of the links between sanitation and health, and poverty and ill-health and many attribute the development of modern day public health to this period – sometimes referred to as the 'sanitary movement' (McKee et al., 2011). This resulted in several social reforms designed to prevent ill-health and provide specific support for the poor. Subsequent scientific discovery of germs, bacteria and vaccines etc. paved the way for contemporary public health. Health promotion has emerged against this backdrop; however, it is not a term that is used consistently in different parts of the world; in some countries it is still very much at the forefront of health strategy, such as Canada and Australia. In others, such as the United Kingdom, the term 'public health' is often used rather than 'health promotion' to describe this facet of the nurse's role (Wills and Jackson, 2014). 'Health promotion' has, in general, become much less used in health strategy replaced by terms such as 'health improvement' and 'health protection'. Public health has been defined as 'the science and art of preventing disease, prolonging life, and promoting health through the organised efforts of society' (Acheson, 1988). As can be seen from the definition of health promotion provided in Box 3.1 there is a difference in emphasis between public health and health promotion and some argue that this is reflected in the difference in the underpinning values of both – health promotion being more concerned with empowerment and equity (Green et al., 2019).

## Health promotion and primary health care

The Declaration of Alma Ata (WHO, 1978) was followed the 30th World Health Assembly in 1977 at which the 'Health for All' movement began. This declaration forefronted primary health care as the way to improve health for all people. Primary health care was conceived as 'embracing all the services that impact on health, including, for example, education, housing and agriculture', as separate and distinct to primary medical care (Green et al., 2019: 21). The concept of primary health care adopted in the Declaration of Alma Ata focused on the importance of community participation (Hubley et al., 2021). Whilst health promotion also emphasises community participation it is the location of health services within the community that is central to primary healthcare efforts. Health centres, clinics and other primary healthcare settings provide a home for a range of primary healthcare practitioners (GPs, health visitors, practice nurses, community pharmacists, clinical officers etc). Health promotion can take place within primary care settings and may encompass many different things (see Box 3.3 for more information).

### Box 3.3

### Health promotion in primary care settings

- Educational work carried out with patients to assist in their treatment and recovery as well as with healthy persons accessing preventive services, such as family planning, antenatal care, child immunisation/child health clinics
- Well-person clinics that invite healthy persons to come for health promotion activities
- Outreach activities in the community through home visits
- Community-based activities working with schools, environment health services, social services, care institutions
- Community development working directly with neighbourhood and community groups

*Source*: Hubley et al. (2021: 215)

So, primary health care is an important function of health promotion and represents health promotion in practice or as 'process'. However, health promotion is much broader than primary health care. Notably primary health care is a vital provider of health promotion (and healthcare services) in resource-poor and rural settings across the world.

## Health promotion and community health

Community health has been described as 'the intersection of healthcare, economics and social interaction' (Brooks, 2019). It is a branch or subsection of public health that relates to a specific place or community and includes any efforts to enable the people of the community to achieve optimal health, to prevent disease and to prepare for, and manage, adversity and disaster. The focus in community health is on collective efforts to improve health and, not least, in this regard community health's values are closely aligned to health promotion. Community health encompasses the physical and social aspects of community life which include the geography of the area (for example access to green spaces, housing and infrastructure) and social cohesion (the lack of which might be manifest through high levels of crime or violence and low levels of trust among community members). Community health workers are an important feature of community health. These include, but are not limited to, general practitioners, community nurses, community pharmacists and community mental health workers. In relation to community mental health and in the context of American Indian/Alaskan Native communities in North America, O'Keefe et al. (2021) emphasise the importance of the role of Indigenous community health workers. They argue that, working alongside other Indigenous mental health professionals, this can 'create an ideal system in which tribal communities are empowered to restore balance and overall wellness, aligning with Native worldviews and healing traditions' (O'Keefe et al., 2021: 84). This is just one example of community health initiatives; there are many, and many more from different contexts and communities vary in nature and form. However, the key point here is that such community-level approaches are vital for tackling the health inequalities that are experienced by minority and marginalised communities. This is at the heart of health promotion as well, however, health promotion is broader still than community health.

## Health promotion and population health

Population health is a central feature of public health. As defined by The King's Fund (2018: 1), population health is 'an approach that aims to improve physical and mental health outcomes, promote wellbeing and reduce health inequalities across an entire population'. In practice it encompasses a range of approaches, all designed to improve, protect or maintain the health of whole populations through means that are focused at a population level rather than at an individual one. Population health interventions often need to be adapted to different contexts dependent on a range of factors such as culture and the specific demographics of the population concerned (Movsisyan et al., 2021). Such interventions might also take place at the policy (macro) level. Mass immunisation, i.e., through vaccination, is a good example of population health at work. Rolling out large-scale vaccination programmes is not without logistical challenges including supply and storage (AHC MEDIA, 2021). In addition, as seen in the case of the global coronavirus pandemic, vaccine hesitancy can be an issue. In

France, for example, around one in four people reported they would refuse to be vaccinated (Ward et al., 2020). Such population health approaches have proven to be extremely successful in tackling infectious diseases in the past, such as the eradication of smallpox in the 1970s (WHO, 2016a). A healthy population is crucial to the development and sustainability of specific countries and regions. For example, Immurana (2020) points out the links between population health and foreign investment in Ghana. They argue that a healthier population means a healthier workforce and better productivity/profitability which, in turn, increases demand for goods and services all of which lead to greater potential for foreign investment. Conversely, poor population health means a less healthy workforce. Of course, this is not specific to Ghana. Better population health is therefore a key aim for all nation states.

## Health promotion and environmental health

Health promotion and environmental health are linked but distinguishable from one another. Environmental health is a branch of public health that is concerned with the impact of our wider environment on our health. As we saw in Chapter 1: *Health and its determinants*, environment is a determinant of health. Factors such as air and water quality, sanitation and pollution are all obvious environmental health challenges that impact on human health and quality of life (Zhang and Lui, 2021). Traditionally, environmental health has focused on our physical surroundings; however, in recent decades it is recognised that other aspects such as our psychosocial and political environments are also key to health experience and health outcomes. We used Barton and Grant's health map in Chapter 1 to illustrate the wider determinants of health and it is also a very useful framework to draw on here to illustrate the complexities of our environment and its impact on health.

One of the key themes in the World Health Organization's agenda for health promotion earlier in this chapter was the necessity of creating supportive environments for health. This was laid out in the Ottawa Charter and carried through the key global conferences. Latterly the focus has shifted towards sustainability and planetary health as well. As Nuttman et al. (2020) argue in the context of food insecurity in Australia, we need to consider environmental challenges alongside the social and economic factors that impact on health. At the 2019 International Union of Health Promotion and Education Global Health Promotion Conference in Rotorua, New Zealand, the role of health promotion in planetary health and sustainable development was emphasised. Taking place against the backdrop of numerous ecological challenges and climate change the conference statements highlighted the necessity of addressing not only the health of people but also the well-being of the planet and its ecosystems at all levels (Tu'itahi et al., 2019).

---

**Point to Ponder 3.2**

Environmental and planetary health are increasingly on everyone's agenda in the light of climate change and the rise in extreme weather events. How might the nurse's role encompass actions that improve environmental and planetary health? What could you do in your own practice to make a positive difference?

---

**Tutorial Trigger 3.2**

Take some time out to look at the two legacy documents that resulted from the 2019 IUHPE Global Health Promotion Conference in Rotorua, New Zealand (see www.iuhpe2019.com):

- Rotorua Statement WAIORA: Promoting Planetary Health and Sustainable Development for All.
- Waiora - Indigenous Peoples' Statement for Planetary Health and Sustainable Development.

Consider these statements in the light of the global pandemic and in terms of how the world has changed since 2019. What are the implications of the statements for today's world?

---

## Where is health promotion today?

So far we have considered many areas allied to/closely aligned with health promotion and set out how and why we believe health promotion is distinct from these. From the discussion up until this point readers should now have a good appreciation of some of the complexities around defining health promotion and the associated concepts we have looked at. This brings us to the question 'Where is health promotion today?'. The answer to this question is not a simple one. In short, it depends on the context in which we are considering it. In some areas of the world health promotion is flourishing as a distinct disciplinary area of practice, whilst in others the term has taken more of a back seat to the more generic label of public health. For example, in the United Kingdom there was a very definite move away from using the term health promotion towards talking about things like health improvement and health protection; however, in early 2021, there was a renewed emphasis on health promotion with the government announcing a new Office for Health Promotion. This came about largely because of the Covid-19 pandemic and the new office promised to 'lead national efforts to improve and level up the health of the nation by tackling obesity, improving mental health and promoting physical activity' (Department of Health and Social Care, 2021). This was subsequently replaced by the Office for Health Improvement and Disparities (announced in September 2021) and 'health promotion' was abandoned along with the term 'health inequalities' which was replaced with 'health disparities' (Scally, 2021). Prior to this, discourse was much more concerned with public health than health promotion and it is no coincidence that there has not been a clear career path trajectory in this country for health promotion for some time either (Duncan, 2013; Warwick-Booth et al., 2018). Elsewhere in the world the situation is very different and health promotion remains at the forefront of efforts to improve peoples' health. In Canada and Australia, for example, health promotion remains a strong focus in policy and practice (Warwick-Booth et al., 2018). Singapore has a Health Promotion Board which was established by the Singapore Government in 2001 specifically to promote healthy living (for more information please see <www.hph.gov.sg>). In other countries, such as Ghana and The Gambia, governments have health promotion departments and directorates, a cadre of health promotion workers and a specific career development pathway. So, the answer to the question about where health promotion is today is not consistent. However, despite this situation, the key tenets of health promotion *are* consistent. The values and principles outlined in the World Health Organization's key themes can be seen in health promotion policy and practice across a range of global contexts and settings. Some people would argue that differences in terminology come down to semantics and that it doesn't matter what term we use if we are working to promote health in whatever guise. In terms of the nurse's role however, health promotion as we see it remains a central and necessary feature and to this end we subscribe to the definition of it as espoused by the Ottawa Charter (WHO, 1986) presented in Box 3.2 earlier in this chapter.

Health promotion and health education will likely always be around in some guise or other regardless of the terminology used to label them at various times and in various contexts. There will always be a requirement to promote health and to educate people about it. Nurses will continue to be vital to both endeavours wherever and however they operate. The future direction of health promotion and health education will depend on many factors and will likely be determined at different levels (regional, national and global). It is likely that the World Health Organization will continue to play a key part in the development of health promotion at a global level. Chapter 11, The future of health promotion and health education for health professionals, considers these issues in much more detail.

## Summary

This chapter has summarised the trajectory of health promotion over the past few decades and highlighted the role that the World Health Organization has played in shaping and defining the development of health promotion as a discrete field with a distinct character of its own. This is underpinned by a set of values and principles that run through this book (such as, for example, equity, empowerment and social justice). This chapter has considered the similarities and differences between health promotion other fields of practice such as public health, community health, population health, primary health care and environmental health, noting the synergies between them. Given the common but misleading assumption that health education *is* health promotion we have spent some time teasing out the differences between these two, concluding that health education is an important and necessary feature of health promotion but that health promotion is much more than simply telling someone what to do. All of this has implications for the nurse's role in supporting and enabling people to achieve optimal health experience.

─── **Key Points** ───────────────────────────────────

- Health promotion has often been equated with health education however, contemporary understandings of health promotion compass values and practice beyond health education.
- The World Health Organization has been pivotal in the development of the global health promotion agenda as evidenced in the series of international conferences that have taken place over the past few decades, and the declarations that have resulted from these events.
- Health promotion overlaps and coheres with several related fields of practice such as community health, environmental health, primary health care and population health.

# References

Acheson, D. (1988). *Public Health in England: The Report of the Committee of Enquiry into the Future Development to the Public Health Function.* London: DHSS.

AHC MEDIA (2021). How family planning providers can handle challenges of COVID-19 vaccine rollout: Issues with logistics, staff hesitancy. *Contraceptive Technology Update* 42(2), 1–4.

Brooks, A. (2019). *What Is Community Health and Why Is It Important?* [Internet] Available at: <www.rasmussen.edu> Accessed 29 March 2021.

Catford, J. (2010). Editorial: Implementing the Nairobi Call to Action: Africa's opportunity to light the way. *Health Promotion International* 25, 1–4.

Cross, R. and O'Neil, I. (2021). Health Communication. In R. Cross, L. Warwick-Booth, S. Rowlands, J. Woodall, I. O'Neil and S. Foster (Eds), *Health Promotion: Global Principles and Practice.* 2nd Ed. (pp. 106–47). Wallingford: CABI.

Cross, R., Rowlands, S. and Foster, S. (2021). The Foundations of Health Promotion. In R. Cross, L. Warwick-Booth, S. Rowlands, J. Woodall, I. O'Neil and S. Foster (Eds), *Health Promotion: Global Principles and Practice.* 2nd Ed. (pp. 1–40), Wallingford: CABI.

Department of Health and Social Care (2021). *New Office for Health Promotion to drive the improvement of nation's health: Press Release*. [Internet] Available at: <www.gov.uk> Accessed 14 April 2021.

Duncan, P. (2013). Failing to professionalise, struggling to specialise: The rise and fall of health promotion as a putative specialism in England, 1980–2000. *Medical History 57*(3), 377–96.

Evans, D., Coutsaftiki, D. and Fathers, C.P. (2017). Health Promotion and Public Health for Nursing Students. 3rd Ed. London, Sage.

Fleming, M. (2020). The importance of health promotion principles and practices. In M. Fleming and L. Baldwin (Eds.), *Health Promotion in the 21st Century: New approaches to achieving health for all* (pp. 1–14). London: Allen & Unwin.

Fleming, M., Parker, E. and Baldwin, L. (2020). The changing nature of health promotion. In M. Fleming and L. Baldwin, *Health Promotion in the 21st Century: New approaches to achieving health for all* (pp. 15–36). London: Allen & Unwin.

Gottwald, M. and Goodman-Brown, J. (2012). An Introduction to Why Health Promotion is Important. In M. Gottwald and J. Goodman-Brown (Eds), *A Guide to Practical Health Promotion* (pp. 7–25). Maidenhead: Open University Press.

Green, J., Cross. R., Woodall, J. and Tones, K. (2019). *Health Promotion: Planning and Strategies*, 4th Ed. London: Sage.

Hubley, J., Copeman, J. and Woodall, J. (2021). *Practical Health Promotion*. 3rd Ed. Cambridge: Polity.

Immurana, M. (2020). Does population health influence FDI inflows into Ghana? *International Journal of Social Economics 48*(2), 334–47.

Karabatos, I., Tsagkaris, C. and Kalachanis, K. (2021). All roads lead to Rome: Aspects of public health in ancient Rome. *Infections in the History of Medicine 3*, 488–91.

Lalonde, M. (1974). *A New Perspective on the Health of Canadians: A Working Document*. Ministry of National Health and Welfare: Ottawa.

Linsley, P. and Roll, C. (2020). *Health Promotion for Nursing Students*. London: Sage.

McKee, M., Sim, F. and Pomerleau, J. (2011). The emergence of public health and the centrality of values. In F. Sim and M. McKee (Eds), *Issues in Public Health*. 2nd Ed. (pp. 3–20). Maidenhead: Open University Press.

Movsisyan, A., Arnold, L., Copeland, L., Evans, R., Littlecott, H., Moore, G. et al. (2021). Adapting evidence-informed population health interventions for new contexts: a scoping review of current practice. *Health Research Policy and Systems 19*(13). doi: 10.1186/s12961-020-00668-9

Nutbeam, D. (2019). Health education and health promotion revisited. *Health Education Journal 78*(6), 705–9.

Nuttman, S., Patrick, R., Townsend, M. and Lawson, J. (2020). Health promotion and food insecurity: Exploring environmental sustainability principles to guide practice within Australia. *Health Promotion Journal of Australia 31*, 68–76.

O'Keefe, V.M., Cwik, M.F., Haroz, E.E. and Barlow, A. (2021). Increasing culturally responsive care and mental health equity with Indigenous community mental health workers. *Psychological Services 18*(1), 84–92.

Scally, G. (2021). England's new Office for Health Improvement and Disparities. *BMJ*, 374. doi: 10.1136/bmj.n2323

Scriven, A. (2017). *Ewles and Simnett's Promoting Health: A Practical Guide*. 7th Ed. London: Elsevier.

Tannahill, A. (1985). What is health promotion? *Health Education Journal 44*, 167–8.

Tapper, K. (2021). *Health Psychology and Behaviour Change*. London: Red Globe Press.

The King's Fund (2018). *A vision for population health: Towards a healthier future.* Available at: <www.kingsfund.org.uk/publications/vision-population-health>

Tones, K. (1997). Health education, behaviour change, and the public health. In R. Detels, W.W. Holland, J. McEwen and H. Tanaka (Eds), *Oxford Textbook of Public Health*. 3rd Ed. Oxford: Oxford University Press.

Tountas, Y. (2009). The historical origins of the basic concepts of health promotion and education: the role of ancient Greek philosophy and medicine. *Health Promotion International 24*(2), 185–92.

Tu'itahi, S., Stoneham, M., Ratima, M., Simpson, T., Signal, L. and Puloka, V. (2019). Timely and significant call for planetary health promotion. *Global Health Promotion 26*(4), 100–1.

Ward, J.K., Alleaume, C., Peretti-Watel, P. and the COCONEL Group (2020). The French public's attitudes to a future COVID-19 vaccine: The politicization of a public health issue. *Social Science & Medicine,* 265. doi: 10.1016/j.socscimed.2020.113414

Warwick-Booth, L., Woodall, J., Cross., R., Bagnall, A. and South, J. (2018). Health promotion education in changing and challenging times: reflections from the UK. *Health Education Journal 78*(6). doi: https://doi.org/10.1177/0017896918784072

WHO (1978). *Declaration of Alma Ata*. Geneva: World Health Organization.

WHO (1986). *The Ottawa Charter for Health Promotion*. Geneva: World Health Organization.

WHO (1997). *The Jakarta Declaration on Leading Health Promotion into the 21st Century*. Geneva: World Health Organization.

WHO (2000). *Mexico Ministerial Statement for the Promotion of Health: From Ideas to Action*. Geneva: World Health Organization.

WHO (2005). *The Bangkok Charter for Health Promotion*. Geneva: World Health Organization.

WHO (2009). *The Nairobi Call to Action*. Geneva: World Health Organization.

WHO (2012). *Health Education: Theoretical Concepts, Effective Strategies and Core Competencies*. Geneva: World Health Organization.

WHO (2013). *The Helsinki Statement on Health in All Policies*. Geneva: World Health Organization.

WHO (2016). *The Shanghai Declaration*. Geneva: World Health Organization.

WHO (2016a). *Smallpox Vaccines*. Available at: <www.who.org>

WHO (2021). *10th Global Conference on Health Promotion charters a path for creating 'well-being societies'*. <www.who.org>

Wild, K. and McGrath, M. (2019). *Public Health and Health Promotion for Nurses at a Glance*. Chichester: Wiley Blackwell.

Wills, J. and Jackson, L. (2014). Health and Health Promotion. In J. Wills (Ed.), *Fundamentals of Health Promotion for Nurses*. 2nd Ed. (pp. 4–21). Chichester: Wiley Blackwell.

Wills, J. (2023). *Foundations for Health Promotion*. 5th Ed. London: Elsevier.

Zhang, Z. and Liu, L. (2021). Environmental health and justice in a Chinese Environmental Model City. *Journal of Environmental Health 83*(6), 30–40.

# 4

# Health Promotion and Health Education Approaches

## James Woodall and Ruth Cross

## Introduction

Given the diversity of how health is conceived and, by extension, how health promotion is viewed and considered this chapter highlights a range of approaches, or ways, of doing health promotion and health education. Effective practice in health promotion not only depends on using evidence to make decisions but also on good theory (Caplan and Holland, 1990). This chapter will review several common approaches which can be applied to different contexts or health concerns. These health promotion approaches are generally theoretical and therefore they often provide a sanitised view of delivering health promotion interventions, but nonetheless provide useful ideas for practice. In reality, health promotion is complex and the practical application can be far removed from the theoretical ideal. To this end, a range of examples will be used to highlight how these approaches have been used in real-world situations.

By the end of this chapter the reader will be able to:

1.  Recognise the diversity of ways and means to promote health.
2.  Understand that health promotion models can operate at varying levels of practice, from individual approaches to community and national levels.
3.  Understand and describe several salient models of health promotion.
4.  Appreciate some of the main points of critique in relation to conceptual models used in health promotion.

> **Key terms**
>
> Health promotion, health education, models of health promotion, 'upstream', ecological models of health promotion

## A Diversity of Approaches

A salient point to make is that there is no universally agreed set of methods or approaches to undertaking health promotion. This is because there is no agreed definition of health and how it should be promoted. This has resulted in huge variance in the way in which health promotion is viewed, conceptualised, practised and in who is responsible for its delivery (Duncan, 2004). There are, however, a range of approaches that offer those working in health promotion and nursing a toolkit which they can apply in particular situations. The approaches and models discussed should not be viewed as being rigid and discrete, as there are lots of overlap and commonality and, in reality, practitioners rarely follow a very prescriptive formula. To confuse the matter further, commentators and academics talk about 'approaches', 'strategies', 'models', 'activities', 'principles' and 'typologies' in health promotion. Despite the semantics, they all very much try to outline a method for doing health promotion. Health promotion academics and practitioners have not always been good at clarifying what they do. Broad and fuzzy ideas about health promotion have continued to lead to increased confusion, creating an uncertain framework for practice (Woodall and Freeman, 2020).

## Levels of Health Promotion Practice

Identifying the 'level' of health promotion and where to intervene is very important, at least according to Hubley et al. (2021). Thinking about levels of intervention is important because it recognises that influences on our health can operate in different ways and that, accordingly, our health promotion activities need to be carried out at different levels. These include focusing at the level of the:

- individual
- family
- community
- district
- region
- national
- international

───── Time to Reflect 4.1 ─────────────────────────────────────

Take a health topic or concern of your choosing and consider how the health topic can be addressed using the various 'levels' of intervention. Alternatively, take road safety and/or reductions in road traffic accidents as an example and work through the different intervention levels considering what could be done to address the topic.

─────────────────────────────────────────────────────────────

This links to the issue as to whether our approaches in health promotion operate on an individual level or take a broader societal approach, or what we may refer to as the 'structural level'. By 'individual' we mean any activity that is aimed at the individual person (also referred to as 'individualist' or 'individualistic') and by structural approaches to promoting health we mean any activity that is aimed at changing the structures in society which in turn may improve health outcomes and health experiences for people (Woodall and Cross, 2021). Tension between individualistic and structural approaches remains a source of lively debate within current health promotion practice. A simple either/or polarisation of individualistic and structural approaches is useful but simplifies what are in fact a range of options for approaches to working with people and communities (Hubley et al., 2021). In almost all health contexts both approaches need to be combined, yet this is not always the case. That said, there are far more 'whole system' views of health (Bagnall et al., 2019) which recognise that successful approaches operate with individuals and communities and also at national and global levels. This type of holistic thinking is not novel. Tones (1986), for example, attempted to demonstrate the factors influencing health choices early in the development of health promotion. He argued that choices are based on both individual decision-making processes and structural forces – both of these need to be addressed. This is highlighted in Figure 4.1, where socio-political action and individually directed interventions are advocated to enable health choices to be made.

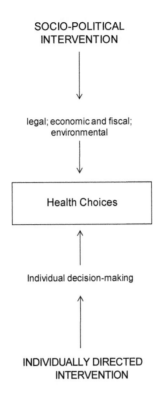

**Figure 4.1**   Factors influencing health choices

If health practitioners only consider the individual level *or* the structural level there are some real issues that emerge. If the focus is exclusively at the individual there is a danger of victim-blaming – which means a focus on the behaviour of individuals without a recognition of wider factors that may influence those decisions and choices. Crawford (1980) suggested that the notion of blaming the victim underplayed what he termed the 'assault' on health caused by structural and environmental forces. Individualising health fails to take into consideration the complex social factors and pressures that accompany behavioural choice and ignores the broader context in which personal behaviours are embedded. On the other hand however, focusing at the structural level can create a 'nanny state'. The nanny state is a term which is used to portray the state or governments overreaching into the lives of citizens. It is a term used to denote the influence on the state in what some see as private or personal decisions concerning health choices (Woodall and Cross, 2021).

## Tutorial Trigger 4.1

Think about the following and reflect on whether you feel governments are right to intervene to protect and promote the health of their citizens in these ways:

- banning junk food items
- banning e-cigarette use
- regulating the amount of sugary drinks you can buy in the supermarket
- insisting all restaurant menus publish the number of calories for each food item

## Common models

Well-cited models of health promotion have had significant longevity given that most are now in their third decade of existence. They are largely premised on whether people have their own free-will (agency) versus whether wider structures have a bigger influence. This links closely to the idea of 'upstream' and 'downstream' views in tackling health issues. This originates from a seminal idea from McKinlay (1979) who tells a story as follows:

> 'There I am standing by the shore of a swiftly flowing river and I hear the cry of a drowning man. So I jump into the river, put my arms around him, pull him to shore and apply artificial respiration. Just when he begins to breathe, there is another cry for help. So I jump into the river, reach him, pull him to shore, apply artificial respiration, and then just as he begins to breathe, another cry for help. So back in the river again, without end, goes the sequence. You know, I am so busy jumping in, pulling them to shore, applying artificial respiration, that I have no time to see who the hell is upstream pushing them all in.'

The upstream idea is very important in health promotion. It is about intervening early and recognising the 'causes of the causes'. By looking upstream, health promoters identify the wider, social determinants of health (or the factors that influence the decisions and choices people make). In contrast *downstream* approaches are concerned with action, treatment and cure once people are already sick or afflicted (Woodall and Cross, 2021). Within the following models and approaches in health promotion you will see influences of upstream and downstream thinking and some models combine these approaches to provide maximum effect. One such model is from Beattie (Beattie, 1991).

### Point to Ponder 4.1

Why is upstream thinking an important idea in health promotion? What benefits would an upstream approach provide? What are the challenges that practitioners might face in achieving upstream ways of working?

## Beattie's model

Beattie's model (Beattie, 1991) has become a consistent feature in many health promotion textbooks, providing an outlook that considers the mode of intervention – authoritative or more negotiated – and the focus, or level, of intervention – from individual to collective.

Beattie (1991) illustrated the breadth of health promotion approaches making the point that on many issues, a full range of actions (i.e., actions in each quadrant of Beattie's diagram 4.2) is required (Woodall and Rowlands, 2020). By tracing along each axis practitioners can locate their approach within one of four quadrants. Please see Box 4.1 for details.

---

### Box 4.1

**Beattie's Four Quadrants**

- *Health persuasion* is any activity that is authoritative or top-down in nature and is aimed more towards the individual; for example, telling someone to stop smoking.
- *Legislative action* is any activity that is authoritative or top-down in nature and is aimed at whole populations; for example, banning smoking in public places.
- *Personal counselling* is any activity that is aimed more towards the individual but that is negotiated in that the individual has more control over the process and isn't simply being told what to do or not to do; for example, using motivational interviewing to help someone identify whether and how they would like to become healthier.
- *Community development* is about activities that involve larger groups of people or whole populations and are more negotiated in that the community has more control or power.

*Source*: Woodall and Cross (2021)

---

The model has been adapted by Naidoo and Wills (2009) who have suggested that the methods used in health promotion imply different political perspectives (see Figure 4.2) which can influence the approach taken or the quadrant in which practice is located. These political ideologies and the methods associated with their approach can be summarised as follows:

> **Health persuasion techniques (Conservative):** This approach is expert-led and focused on the individual. It is concerned with individuals taking responsibility for their own health.
> **Personal counselling for health (New Right):** Neoliberalism focuses on the role of the individual in determining their own choice. However, a

more equal relationship between the health promoter and the individual is established.

**Community development for health (New Left):** This approach attempts to understand the processes which shape health outcomes and assists people to develop the competencies to challenge these processes. Participation and active involvement are stressed.

**Legislative action for health (Marxist, socialist):** Marxist and socialist political beliefs suggest that social class, determined by economic status, predicts life chances. The redistribution of power in favour of the disadvantaged is emphasised.

It is useful to focus on community approaches in health promotion as while this is one of four approaches outlined by Beattie, it is a common strategy in many health promotion programmes. A community development approach often means working with, not on, communities to encourage them to express their needs and for health promoters to support them in their collective action. It is about collective, rather than individual, responses to health challenges. A community development approach is about working with groups of people to identify their own health

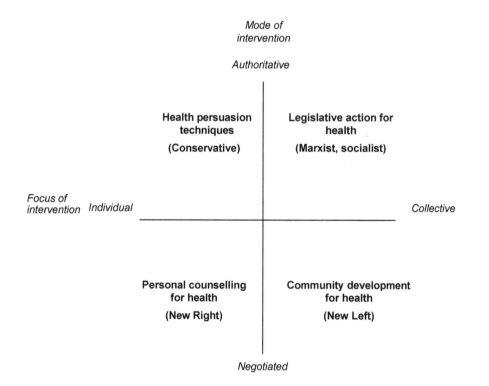

**Figure 4.2**　Strategies for health promotion: Beattie's typology

concerns and to take appropriate action, facilitated (not led) by health promoters (Scriven, 2017). As noted by Hubley et al. (2021), community development in health promotion works best when the community:

- are involved in the design, planning and evaluation of interventions
- identify the health issue to be tackled and determine what counts as success
- have a mechanism to give 'voice' to any concerns
- are able to communicate effectively with health workers and other paid employees
- are equal partners in decision-making, leadership and resource management with the professionals
- are members of the steering committee
- have confidence in the selection processes for any roles and membership of groups
- engage in regular dialogue and feedback about the progress
- are able to build relationships and trust in the 'outsiders'
- see the longer-term benefits in capacity building and self-confidence.

─────── Time to Reflect 4.2 ───────────────────────────────

Take a health issue that is of importance to you and use Beattie's model to try and identify activities that could be mapped in each of the quadrants. Consider which quadrants are 'easier' to locate than others - consider why that may be the case. Also try to think about which of the quadrants are more commonly used in health promotion - again consider the reason why that may be.

## Naidoo and Wills' typology

A typology is a very useful way of classifying health promotion approaches and one of the most popular typologies in this regard is from Naidoo and Wills (2016). This divides health promotion practice into five ways as outlined below in Box 4.2. It is useful in capturing the spectrum of activity and moreover making clear distinctions between individual and structural approaches and top-down directed approaches and more bottom-up, community-driven strategies. Some of the approaches here map directly against Beattie's model – there are clear commonalities between an educational approach and health persuasion techniques. Similarly, Beattie's community development quadrant shares similar characteristics and attributes to the empowerment approach in Naidoo and Wills' (2016) typology.

| Approach | Examples |
|---|---|
| **Medical or Preventative**<br>Activity that aims to reduce illness, disability and deaths targeted at whole populations or high-risk groups using medical intervention. | • Assessing body mass index<br>• Immunization<br>• Pharmaceutical interventions |
| **Behaviour Change**<br>Activity that encourages people to behave in more healthy ways. | • Weight-loss programmes<br>• Exercise on prescription |
| **Educational**<br>Activity that provides knowledge, information and the skills needed to make an informed, healthier choice. | • Providing information leaflets<br>• One-to-one counselling<br>• Internet campaigns |
| **Empowerment**<br>Activity that enables people to take control over their health and lives. | • Client-centred approaches<br>• Community development |
| **Social Change**<br>Activity that focuses on the socio-environmental or policy level (sometimes also called 'radical health promotion'). | • Developing healthy public policy<br>• Providing sustainable transport systems |

*Adapted from Naidoo and Wills (2016: 76-81)*

Box 4.2

## Naidoo and Wills' typology

- **Programme:** delineates the area that is being addressed. This is an umbrella term that includes all the activities involved in developing and running, for example, a coronary heart disease programme or a community development programme.
- **Strategy:** the preferred course of action for achieving immediate or longer-term goals. It is selected tactically on the basis of evidence, theory or experience. The term can be used at all levels - for example, an 'overall programme strategy' or an 'implementation strategy'.
- **Plan:** an outline of all the various components and how they relate to each other.
- **Aim:** a broad statement of what is intended to be achieved. Aims can be developed at different levels - for example, overall programme aims, educational aims, policy aims.
- **Objective:** precise and detailed statements of the intended outcomes that will contribute to the overall aim.
- **Intervention:** the activities or collection of activities that will contribute directly to the desired change.
- **Method:** specific approaches or techniques used.

## Caplan and Hollands' model

Observers will note how Caplan and Hollands' (1990) model looks very similar to Beattie's model in that both share two-axis creating quadrants for activities. Despite their visual similarity, they are quite different in conceptualising health promotion approaches. Caplan and Hollands' model was first developed in relation to mental health but has since been expanded to encompass a range of issues and topics. The y-axis represents the nature of society and positions two opposing viewpoints. *Radical change* is concerned with challenging structural oppression, such as racism, poverty etc., to create conditions which no longer disadvantage some sections of society:

> 'Radical change is thus concerned with the dynamics of change best described in such terms as emancipation realised through the potential of deprived classes and groups to transform the social, economic-political and cultural conditions which sustain their deprivation.' (Caplan and Holland, 1990: 11)

In contrast *social regulation* takes the position that society is organised and harmonious and that society has organised itself into various institutions which serve to satisfy the needs of individuals. Changes are therefore made by individuals to 'fit-in' with the societal structures and regimes.

The x-axis focuses on the nature of knowledge. Objective knowledge, at the one end, is measurable and quantifiable whilst subjective knowledge, at the other end, is not (Woodall and Cross, 2021). In relation to depression, objective knowledge would consider the condition as being a manifestation of bodily functions and processes and could be measured using scales and assessment tools. Subjective knowledge, on the other hand, would suggest that depression is socially constructed and variable and set in a context that is time-bound and dynamic (rather than fixed). Like Beattie's model, four quadrants are created by the axis. These are listed in Table 4.1.

## Ecological model of health promotion

Bronfenbrenner (1977) proposed an ecological theory of development which has been relevant to the design of ecological models applied in health promotion. In this framework, behaviour is viewed as being affected by, and effecting, multiple levels of influence (McLeroy et al., 1988). Bronfenbrenner describes these multiple levels as the micro-, meso-, exo- and macrosystem levels. The microsystem refers to face-to-face influences in specific settings, for example, the home, school or workplace. The mesosystem is the system of microsystems and pertains to the interrelations among the various settings in which the individual is involved (Ibid.). The exosystem refers to forces within the larger social system in which the individual is embedded. Finally, the macrosystem refers to the overarching institutional

**Table 4.1**  Caplan and Hollands' (1990) four perspectives on health promotion

| | |
|---|---|
| Humanist | Health is defined by experts but subjective experience is acknowledged. Interventions would include working with people to enable them to understand what they can do for themselves and equipping them with the skills/knowledge needed to change. |
| Traditional | Health is objective and related to biomedical knowledge. Interventions are expert-led and would include telling people what to do (education) or doing things to them in order to improve their health (biomedical intervention). |
| Radical Humanist | Health is subjectively experienced and the individual determines, in dialogue with an 'expert', how they might want to change. |
| Radical Structuralist | Health is objectively measured but created by socio-economic and environmental factors such as inequalities. The nature of society needs to change in order to improve health. |

*Source*: Adapted from Warwick-Booth et al. (2021).

patterns of the culture or subculture that influence both the microsystem and the mesosystem (Bronfenbrenner, 1977).

McLeroy et al. (1988) have proposed an ecological model for health promotion, where behaviour is seen as being determined by intrapersonal factors, interpersonal processes and primary groups, institutional factors, community factors and public policy (see Table 4.2). This model draws on the work by Bronfenbrenner (1977) and is underpinned by an assumption that a comprehensive, multifaceted approach is more effective than a single level approach (Sallis and Owen, 1997).

# Health Promotion Models Specific to Nursing and Midwifery

Two models of health promotion have been developed and applied specifically with nursing and midwifery in mind, both of which are worth consideration in the context of this chapter. These are, for nursing, Pender's Health Promotion Model (Pender, 1982; Pender et al., 2006) and, for midwifery, Piper's Model of Health Promotion (Piper, 2000, 2005).

## Pender's health promotion model

Pender's Health Promotion Model (Pender, 1982; Pender et al., 2006) incorporates both behavioural science (psychology) and nursing perspectives to consider what factors influence health and illness behaviour. The model reflects a holistic

**Table 4.2**  An ecological model for health promotion

| Level of influence | Approach | Example |
|---|---|---|
| Intrapersonal factors | Efforts to modify individuals' knowledge, attitudes, skills etc. Interventions at this level suggest that behavioural change lies with the individual rather than the social environment. | Educational programmes. |
| Interpersonal processes and primary groups | Focuses on changing individuals through social influences (family, friends, social networks). This approach aims to modify the interpersonal social influences which serve to encourage, support and maintain undesirable behaviours. | Family support programmes. |
| Institutional factors | Creating organisational change (in a workplace, school, hospital, prison etc.) to support individual health. Organisations should be encouraged to be supportive of health issues and develop an ethos which is aligned to health promotion's philosophy. | Organisational policy directed to enable individuals to adopt healthy behaviours in settings. |
| Community factors | Strengthening community structures. | Delivering health promotion through already established community venues and networks. |
| Public policy | Large scale efforts enabling the healthy choice to be the easy choice for societies. | Healthy public policy at a national level. |

*Source*: McLeroy et al. (1988, p. 355).

appreciation of human functioning and draws on some assumptions from behavioural science that people weigh up the pros and cons of taking action (i.e., give it careful thought) whilst also taking into account wider influences on behaviour such as the environment and socio-economic factors. When it was first developed, the model initially had seven cognitive-perceptual factors and five modifying factors that were assumed to impact on behaviour change but subsequently, based on research, it was revised to include three more factors (see Box 4.3). The model is referred to as a model of health promotion but has more in common with other behaviour change models such as the Health Belief Model (Cross, 2010; Piper, 2009) thus many of the criticisms levelled at models of behaviour change might also be applied to Pender's model of health promotion. Nevertheless, it has been widely used in the literature in the global north where it was first developed and many of the variables within the model have been empirically tested resulting in evidence that supports the theoretical underpinnings of it.

---
Box 4.3

**Pender's Health Promotion Model - Factors**

*Cognitive-perceptual factors*

- the importance of health
- perceived control of health
- definition of health
- perceived health status
- perceived self-efficacy
- perceived benefits
- perceived barriers

*Modifying factors*

- demographic characteristics
- biological characteristics
- interpersonal characteristics
- situation influences
- behavioural influences

*Additional factors*

- activity-related effect
- commitment to a plan of action
- immediate competing demands and preferences

*Adapted from Cross (2010)*

---

Pender's model of health promotion has health-promoting behaviour as its end-point (or action outcome) and considers the factors that contribute to the process of behaviour change and has therefore been criticised as reflecting [a] 'narrow agenda of the [...] nurse as a behaviour change agent' (Piper, 2009: 89), an image we are keen to move away from in recognition that health promotion, and the nurse's role within it, is much broader and more complex than this. Pender's model is predicated on four assumptions. First, that people monitor and try to change their behaviour; second, that people interact with their environment and their environment impacts on them; third, that nurses are often a part of the environment that influences people at various times during their lifetimes; and finally, that 'self-initiated reconfiguration of the person-environment interactive patterns is essential to changing behaviour' (Petiprin, 2020). Petiprin (2020) also details 13 theoretical statements that come from Pender's model – please see Box 4.4 for details.

**Box 4.4**

## Theoretical statements from Pender's model of health promotion (Petiprin, 2020)

1   Prior behaviour and inherited and acquired characteristics influence beliefs, affect, and enactment of health-promoting behaviour.
2   Persons commit to engaging in behaviours from which they anticipate deriving personally valued benefits.
3   Perceived barriers can constrain commitment to action (a mediator of behaviour) as well as actual behaviour.
4   Perceived competence or self-efficacy to execute a given behaviour increases the likelihood of commitment to action and actual performance of the behaviour.
5   Greater perceived self-efficacy results in fewer perceived barriers to a specific health behaviour.
6   Positive affect towards a behaviour results in greater perceived self-efficacy, which can in turn, result in increased positive affect.
7   When positive emotions or affect are associated with a behaviour, the probability of commitment and action is increased.
8   People are more likely to commit to and engage in health-promoting behaviours when significant others model the behaviour, expect the behaviour to occur, and provide assistance and support to enable the behaviour.
9   Families, peers, and healthcare providers are important sources of interpersonal influence that can increase or decrease commitment to and engagement in health-promoting behaviour.
10  Situational influences in the external environment can increase or decrease commitment to or participation in health-promoting behaviour.
11  The greater the commitments to a specific plan of action, the more likely health-promotion behaviour are to be maintained over time.
12  Commitment to a plan of action is less likely to result in the desired behaviour when competing demands over which people have little control require immediate attention.
13  People can modify cognitions, affect, and the interpersonal and physical environment to create incentives for health actions.

*Source:* <nursing-theory.org/theories-and-models/pender-health-promotion-model.php>

Developed in the global north within the context of a specific healthcare system the model may not resonate in other situations quite as well; however, it does provide a way to take into account the different variables that impact on behavioural outcomes including past behaviour and a consideration of how committed a person might be to changing their behaviour. The model also takes into account the social context that behaviour takes place in, acknowledging this as a major influence on health that can either create opportunities for health and well-being or might miltitate against it. Interestingly, Pender also holds the opinion that nurses should model healthy lifestyles to their patients and clients (Piper, 2009).

## Piper's model of health promotion

Piper's model of health promotion (Piper, 2000, 2005) is a modification of Beattie's model of health promotion that has been developed specifically for midwifery. The model incorporates top-down and bottom-up approaches resulting in four quadrants whereby each was initially (re)presented as patient information, patient empowerment, structural change and collective action (Piper and Brown, 1998). The latter two were subsequently re-labelled as strategy and development, and patient action (Piper, 2000). There are two axes running through the centre of the model. The horizontal axis separates the individual from the population whilst the vertical axis separates subjective and objective knowledge. Each of the four quadrants is referred to as separate and distinct models that, together, form a comprehensive framework for health promotion interventions (Piper, 2009). According to the model the midwife can be identified as a behaviour change agent, an empowerment facilitator, a strategic health promotion practitioner and a collective empowerment facilitator depending on which area (quadrant) of the model their work falls into (Bowden, 2017). See Box 4.5 for further information.

---

### Box 4.5

**Piper's model of health promotion applied to practice**

*Behaviour Change Agent*

Perhaps more aligned with more traditional approaches to health promotion (health education) the midwife holds the power and the aim is to encourage the woman to change their behaviour through increasing knowledge and awareness.

*Empowerment Facilitator*

Here the woman holds the power and the midwife is a facilitator of the process enabling the woman to identify her own needs and make her own decision about how these might be addressed thereby increasing self-esteem and confidence.

*Strategic Practitioner*

Here the midwife will be much more involved in the wider issues that impact on women's experience of pregnancy and childbirth such as tackling socio-economic inequalities, improving healthcare provision, and influencing policy and legislation but from a position of relative power.

*Collective Empowerment Facilitator*

In contrast to the above the midwife will work in a bottom-up way with groups of women and support/encourage the expression of health needs, and the development of social networks leading to communal action.

*Adapted from Bowden (2017)*

---

### Tutorial Trigger 4.2

Think about your own practice and experience and consider whether Pender or Piper's models resonate with your experiences. Do they apply well to your practice, or would another model (presented earlier in the chapter) be more appropriate?

---

## Critical perspectives

Theory and approaches to 'doing' health promotion are important, but they should never be applied or used uncritically. Many of the models presented here are decades old and much has changed during this period of time. It is perhaps timely to re-engage in conceptual discussion about where health promotion is and where it may be going and even to suggest new forms of conceptualising delivery (Woodall and Freeman, 2020). Recent analysis, for example, suggests that health promotion has lost focus and is 'going in all directions' (Lindström, 2018: 97).

At the beginning of the 1990s, it was anticipated that there would be rich theoretical discussion about the purpose of health promotion which would steer practice and policy into the twenty-first century (Bunton and Macdonald, 1992). On reflection, this was a utopian vision and one that was never fulfilled. Perhaps it is timely to engage in further analysis, given that there are concerns about the further decline of health promotion as a discipline and practice across several parts of the world (White and Wills, 2011). Clarifying models and approaches is one way of achieving this.

---

### Point to Ponder 4.2

One of the key criticisms of many approaches and models is their lack of empirical testing. In effect, these models remain largely theoretical and have not been fully researched or applied in a range of contexts. In addition, many of the models in health promotion have been derived from high-income countries with contributions less forthcoming from middle- and low-income countries. This may suggest that there is significant scope to broaden or redefine health promotion approaches to be more aligned to these specific contexts.

## Summary

This chapter has presented several models of health promotion and health education describing the features of each of these in some detail. It has shown a diversity of approaches and views on health promotion and how it is conceptualised. The chapter has also shown how some of the models can be applied in practice and described two specific models related to nursing and midwifery.

─────── **Key Points** ───────────────────────────

- There are a range of approaches, or ways, of doing health promotion.
- Models of health promotion can provide a useful 'blueprint' to aid practitioners working towards health improvement outcomes with individuals and communities.
- No single model can adequately conceptualise health promotion, although some models have become seminal and applied consistently in practice. Rarely have these models been empirically tested - they remain largely theoretical.
- There continues to be an opportunity to broaden or redefine health promotion approaches to reflect contemporary issues and global perspectives.

## References

Bagnall, A-M., Radley, D., Jones, R. et al. (2019). Whole systems approaches to obesity and other complex public health challenges: a systematic review. *BMC Public Health 19*(1), 8.

Beattie, A. (1991). Knowledge and control in health promotion: a test case for social policy and social theory. In J. Gabe, M. Calnan and M. Bury (Eds), *The Sociology of the Health Service*. (pp. 162–202). London: Routledge.

Bowden, J. (2017). Using health promotion models and approaches in midwifery. In J. Bowden and V. Manning (Eds), *Health Promotion in Midwifery: Principles and practice*. (pp. 47–61). London: CRC Press.

Bronfenbrenner, U. (1977). Toward an experimental ecology of human development. *American Psychologist 32*, 513–31.

Bunton, R. and Macdonald, G. (1992). *Health Promotion. Disciplines and diversity*. London: Routledge.

Caplan, R. and Holland, R. (1990). Rethinking health education theory. *Health Education Journal 49*(1), 10–12.

Crawford, R. (1980). Healthism and the medicalization of everyday life. *International Journal of Health Services 10*(3), 365–88.

Cross, R. (2010). Health promotion theory: models and approaches. In D. Whitehead and F. Irvine (Eds), *Health Promotion and Health Education in Nursing: A framework for practice*. (pp. 22–44). Basingstoke: Palgrave Macmillan.

Duncan, P. (2004). Dispute, dissent and the place of health promotion in a 'disrupted tradition' of health improvement. *Public Understanding of Science 13*(2), 177–90.

Hubley, J., Copeman, J. and Woodall, J. (2021). *Practical Health Promotion.* Cambridge: Polity Press.

Lindström, B. (2018). Workshop salutogenesis and the future of health promotion and public health. *Scandinavian Journal of Public Health 46*(20_suppl.), 94–8.

McKinlay, J.B. (1979). A case for refocusing upstream: the political economy of illness. In E.G. Jaco (Ed.), *Patients, Physicians, and Illness.* 3rd ed. (pp. 9–25). New York: The Free Press.

McLeroy, K.R., Bibeau, D., Steckler, A. et al. (1988). An ecological perspective on health promotion programs. *Health Education Quarterly 15*(4), 351–77.

Naidoo, J. and Wills, J. (2009). *Foundations for Health Promotion.* London: Bailliere Tindall.

Naidoo, J. and Wills, J. (2016). *Foundations for Health Promotion.* London: Elsevier.

Pender, N.J. (1982). *Health Promotion in Nursing Practice.* Norwalk: Appleton-Century-Crofts.

Pender, N.J., Murdaugh, C.L. and Parsons, M.A. (2006). *Health Promotion in Nursing Practice.* New Jersey: Pearson Prentice Hall.

Petiprin, A. (2020). *Pender's Health Promotion Model.* [Internet] Available at: <nursing-theory.org/theories-and-models/pender-health-promotion-model.php>

Piper, S. (2000). Promoting health. *Nursing Management 7*(4), 8–11.

Piper, S. (2005). Health promotion as a practice framework for midwives. *British Journal of Midwifery 13*(5), 284–8.

Piper, S. (2009). *Health Promotion for Nurses: Theory and practice.* Abingdon: Routledge.

Piper, S.M. and Brown, P.A. (1998). The theory and practice of health education applied to nursing: a bipolar approach. *Journal of Advanced Nursing 27*, 383–9.

Sallis, J.F. and Owen, N. (1997). Ecological models. In K. Glanz, F.M. Lewis and B.K. Rimer (Eds), *Health Behavior and Health Education.* (pp. 403–24). San Francisco: Jossey-Bass.

Scriven, A. (2017). *Promoting Health: A practical guide.* London: Bailliere Tindall.

Tones, B.K. (1986). Health education and the ideology of health promotion: a review of alternative approaches. *Health Education Research 1*(1), 3–12.

Warwick-Booth, L., Cross, R. and Lowcock, D. (2021). *Contemporary Health Studies: An introduction.* Cambridge: Polity Press.

White, J. and Wills, J. (2011). What's the future for health promotion in England? The views of practitioners. *Perspectives in Public Health 131*(1), 44–7.

Woodall, J. and Cross, R. (2021). *Essentials of Health Promotion.* London: Sage.

Woodall, J. and Freeman, C. (2020). Where have we been and where are we going? The state of contemporary health promotion. *Health Education Journal.* Available at: https://doi.org/10.1177/0017896919899970.

Woodall, J. and Rowlands, S. (2020). Professional Practice. In R. Cross, S. Foster, I. O'Neil et al. (Eds), *Health Promotion: Global principles and practice.* London: CABI.

# 5

# The Ottawa Charter - Reorienting Health Services and Developing Personal Skills

María Pueyo Garrigues, María Lavilla Gracia and Navidad Canga Armayor

## Introduction

This chapter discusses the relevance of the Ottawa Charter for public health, putting the focus especially on two of the five core strategies for health promotion action: reorienting health services and developing personal skills. The chapter starts by considering what the Ottawa Charter is and its contribution, describing its five core strategies for enabling people to increase control over, and to improve, their health. It then moves on to a critical discussion about the current status of both cited actions implementation, exploring the main challenges such as the persistence of biomedical-pathogenic perspectives or economical facts. The chapter will describe what might be the future direction for reorienting health services and developing personal skills under a positive health paradigm. The chapter ends by exploring and explaining why and how the nursing profession across the health care and health services must be actively involved and engaged in both.

By the end of this chapter the reader will have:

1. An overview of the main lines of action of the Ottawa Charter that have been developed so far.
2. An appreciation of how the reorientation of health services and personal skills development has grown so far, and the main barriers that hinder the translation of these actions within the ecological health paradigm as well as different routes to promote their integration.
3. Identification of the contribution of nurses as essential to lead the change towards more positive health paradigms.

## Key terms

Ottawa Charter, reorienting health services, developing personal skills, biomedical paradigm, ecological paradigm

## The Ottawa Charter - a general overview

At the first World Conference on Health Promotion, held in Ottawa in 1986, health was seen as a resource of everyday life, and it was defined as a positive concept emphasising social and personal resources, as well as physical capacities (WHO, 1986). As described in Chapter 2: *Defining health promotion and health education*, it is at this time that the World Health Organization drew up the Ottawa Charter (WHO, 1986) which formally defined health promotion, and the three basic principles for health promotion work (advocate, enable and mediate).

The Ottawa Charter clearly stated that the major aim of health promotion is to achieve equity in health by enabling all people to achieve their fullest health potential. To achieve this goal, five core strategies for health promotion action were identified: (1) Building a healthy public policy, (2) Creating supportive environments, (3) Strengthening community action, (4) Developing personal skills, and (5) Reorienting health services (WHO, 1986). Please see Chapter 2 for details.

Subsequent world conferences on Health Promotion, held in Adelaide (1988), Sundsvall (1991), Jakarta (1997), Mexico (2000), Bangkok (2005), Nairobi (2009), Helsinki (2013) and Shanghai (2016), have promoted a framework for action based on these five lines of action (López-Dicastillo et al., 2017). Please see Chapter 3: *A history of health promotion and health education*, for details. The principles of the Ottawa Charter have stood the test of time, and the first four actions are, in general, developing well. However, the principle of 'reorienting health services' has, until recently, been given less attention (Haugan and Eriksson, 2021). Even 'developing personal skills', despite the fact that it has been worked on during the past few decades, is limited in its full potential as it has been mainly focused on ill people, or just giving information.

## Reorienting Health Services - Challenges

The Ottawa Charter has contributed to shifting the rhetoric and discourse upstream away from merely focusing on individuals who are at risk of developing ill-health and towards organisations, systems and environments that can be used to prevent ill-health and promote good health (Thompson et al., 2018). Ottawa's principles have been widely applauded, and conceptual development in the area of health promotion has attempted to establish them; nevertheless opportunities to transfer these principles into the radical changes and practical solutions needed globally to improve health have been missed (Haugan and Eriksson, 2021; López-Dicastillo et al., 2017).

Available evidence guiding the healthcare services into a more health-promoting direction is still scarce. Reorienting health services refers to making sure health promotion becomes more embedded in mainstream health care services (Thompson et al., 2018). According to the Ottawa Charter (WHO, 1986), it means that the responsibility for health promotion in healthcare services is shared among individuals, community groups, health professionals, health service institutions and governments. They must work together towards a healthcare system which contributes to the pursuit of health. Health services should support the needs of individuals and communities for a healthier life and open channels between the health sector and broader social, political, economic and physical environmental components.

Thirty-six years after the Ottawa conference there had been slow progress in making health promotion a core business for health services, and there is a need to reframe, reposition and renew efforts. And now is the time, more than ever, due to the current global health issues, including the economic crisis, climate change and the wide range of public health threats, that pose new challenges as well as new opportunities (Ziglio, 2011).

Box 5.1

## Definition of 'Reorienting health services' action of the Ottawa Charter for Health Promotion

Individuals, community groups, health professionals, health service institutions and governments must work together towards a healthcare system which contributes to the pursuit of health. The role of the health sector must move increasingly in a health promotion direction, being sensitive and respecting cultural needs. This mandate should support the needs for a healthier life, and open channels between the health sector and broader social, political, economic and physical environmental components.

Some reasons for this somewhat lethargic progress are widely described by different authors internationally. Ziglio (2011) stated that the field of health systems and related policy development is still dominated by the provision of tertiary services and often those who work at this level. Within this, there is an increasing imperative for health services to demonstrate their clinical and cost-effectiveness. Alami et al. (2017) add that in the current economic situation, interventions that have already proven their effectiveness are favoured, which implies financial flows mainly for curative purposes – such as the share of health expenditure allocated to the consumption of health products (such as medicines, technologies and medical devices) or to the management of health crises. This trend could also be explained by the fact that the population is more 'sensitive' to issues of 'life-saving' urgency as opposed to long-term health issues (e.g., support for prevention or promotion campaigns).

Another reason is the presence of the biomedical approach in the entire social framework, which influences the organisation of the health system, the way professionals work, the approach to policies, users and, transversally, the methods, strategies and forms of evaluation (please see Chapter 10: Global health for more discussion on this). As a consequence, there is a lack of structural support and opportunities to promote health from a psychosocial perspective, which is paradoxical considering the relevance of the benefits attributed to it (López-Dicastillo et al., 2017).

Alami et al. (2017) point out that the training of health professionals, mostly focused on the individual clinical and biological dimensions of health, has been a major contributor. The way of proceeding under this umbrella is not adapted to the complexity of interventions, based on population-based approaches promoted by health promotion, which partly explains the difficulties in gaining the support of decision-makers and thus in implementing them. In this regard, Thompson et al. (2018) concluded that, in general, health services continue to pursue medical model interventions, including assessment and management of coronary heart disease risk factors, screening services and immunisations, but, in England, action on other areas of prevention and the wider determinants of health has become the responsibility of local public health departments. Further, within the field of health promotion we frequently focus on making the case for action on the social determinants. So much so that we often downplay the role and contribution that health systems can make (Ziglio et al., 2011).

The latter is a prevailing debate today. Has the health system ever opened up to health promotion, and is health promotion interested in the health system? Some authors consider that the current health promotion agenda makes any attempt to reorient services impossible. Alami et al. (2017) attribute this to the fact that health promotion advocates have focused their efforts on basing their actions on the social determinants of health, with the risk of minimising the role and contribution of health systems in improving population health.

## Which measures should be taken for promoting the needed radical change?

There is a growing consensus worldwide that contemporary patterns of health service development and expenditure are simply unsustainable (Catford, 2014). The current emphasis of health systems investment in tertiary level curative and clinical services cannot be maintained. They are becoming unaffordable and it is important to take measures for health systems to be not only more effective but also sustainable (Ziglio et al., 2011). Because of this, Catford (2014) claimed that it is time the healthcare sector moved increasingly in a health promotion direction, beyond its responsibility for providing clinical and curative services focused on the health problem. Maintaining this balance is critical to the success of this mission, which requires complementarity and synergy between the two approaches in order to aim for greater health equity (Alami et al., 2017).

---

### Tutorial Trigger 5.1

It is time to recognise that we cannot leave our health and individuals' health and well-being entirely in the hands of the healthcare system. A system that was created to provide an answer to the old picture, infectious diseases, and that today cannot respond alone to many of today's major health problems such as loneliness, stress, obesity, mental illness or addictions. What measures can you identify that would transform our healthcare systems?

---

Nigel Crisp, co-chair of the Nursing Now campaign, points out in his book *Health is made at home: hospitals are for repairs* (Crisp, 2020), that the public has the major role in creating and keeping good health, and in tackling many of today's major health and social challenges including communicable and non-communicable disease, mental health, loneliness, poverty and substance use disorders. In this, healthcare systems play a major role in 'creating health' and dealing with many of the underlying causes of poor health (International Council of Nurses, 2021).

——— Time to Reflect 5.1 ———————————————————————————

If the health system plays a fundamental role in 'creating health', as nursing professionals constitute the backbone of the health industry, we also have a part in it.

Are we, as nurses, aware of this?

Are we willing to take our share of responsibility? If so, how would our practice change?

Today's health challenges require transforming our healthcare system, moving towards more efficient and positive models of care. Thus, one proposal is to focus on reorienting the system itself – not just the delivery of services – by health promotion leaders engaging more actively in system development (Ziglio et al., 2011). The vision for future health care also calls for a partnership between the health system, other sectors (e.g., education, transport, housing etc.), government and the public to work together (Crisp, 2020). This means that all parties will be responsible for building the conditions in which people can be healthy throughout the life course as the Ottawa Charter stated. This sharing of responsibility and 'leadership' will give all actors the feeling that they are part of the same dynamics of change and, in this case, of improving the health of the population. The importance of developing other ways of doing things, by favouring transdisciplinary approaches and intersectoral actions, and by insisting on the concentration of the different actors, has already been demonstrated (Alami et al., 2017). Enhancing intersectoral action is key given the strong links between education, health outcomes and inequalities (Ziglio et al., 2011).

## Point to Ponder 5.1

Nursing is a suitable profession to lead intersectoral work. To facilitate its development, it would be an essential step to promote it in the university education of future nursing professionals. An initiative to promote such learning is through intersectoral subjects or optional modules, in which nursing students work first-hand with people from other disciplines. In the literature, there are few studies that include the development of skills to carry out intersectoral work in nursing curricula. Zeydani et al. (2021), for example, evaluated the effect of community-based education on undergraduate nursing students' skills. During the learning, students were in the community setting working with nursing educators, community members and representatives from other sectors. They found that, after the community-based education, students improve nurses´ skills such as communication, critical thinking and teamwork (Zeydani et al., 2021).

It is known that collaborative practice in interprofessional teams is essential to achieve quality health care. An example could be found in the report entitled 'Multisectoral and intersectoral action for improved health and well-being for all: mapping of the WHO European Region' (WHO, 2018). In it shows how in Romania they worked on a project to integrate community-based services with a collaborative perspective. Professions such as community nurses were incorporated into the system to work together with the line ministries, local government, civil society and development partners.

---

Reorienting health services requires changes in professional education and training. It should focus more on the total needs of individuals and populations as a whole, in order to change the attitude and organisation of health services towards a vision of health promotion (Haugan and Eriksson, 2021).

Finally, reorienting health services requires stronger attention to health research (Haugan and Eriksson, 2021). It is necessary to create outcome indicators in health promotion to complement the existing ones focused on 'disease', 'problem', 'deficit', 'risk', 'disability', 'morbidity' and 'mortality', evaluating other dimensions that take into account personal and social development, as well as the environmental factors that condition it (López-Dicastillo et al., 2017). Methodologies need to take into account the complex and changing nature of health promotion interventions and the time they require. It is also important that all professionals in the health system are committed. This role is clearly mentioned in the Ottawa Charter, which states that health promotion requires the concerted action of all actors (Alami et al., 2017).

In sum, we need to be ready to lead, deliver, research and educate on the adventure ahead. Our principal challenge is to ensure that the strategic shifts that are coming to health systems are designed through a health promotion lens (Catford, 2014). These include:

- from 'downstream' acute repair – to 'upstream' health improvement

- from individual response – to population focus and accountability

- from single episode transactions – to care continuum management

- from working alone – to working in partnership with other sectors

- from patient compliance – to consumer control and centredness

These conditions, once met, could enable the different actors to easily identify with this discourse and better place themselves in perspective. The reorientation of services will thus aim to integrate all activities aimed at promoting, restoring and maintaining the health of individuals and populations.

## Developing Personal Skills – Challenges and Future Directions

Developing personal skills is another of the five key action areas for health promotion identified in the Ottawa Charter. Developing personal skills is about providing information, education for health, and enhancing life skills (WHO,1986). It includes the development of health literacy, motor skills, and gaining an understanding of the relations between lifestyle diseases and risk behaviours. It promotes protective behaviours and provides the individual with the skills to be able to navigate the health system and critically analyse health information (PDHPE, 2022). It also encompasses a wider perspective and seeks to encourage lifelong learning that helps people to be active in all the dimensions of health in order to achieve better health (WHO, 1986). This means knowledge and skills in social settings, family contexts, spiritual matters, having a purpose to life, mental and emotional stability are all part of the development of personal skills (PDHPE, 2022). By doing so, it increases the options available to people to exercise more control over their own health and over their environments, and to make choices conducive to health (WHO, 1986).

Whitehead and Irvine (2011) already advanced that developing personal skills is not an easy task, resulting in this action not being developed as much as expected. This was described some years ago by Wise and Nutbeam (2007) who identified that much of this health promotion action remains to be done and that its influence on population health has not yet been realised.

The majority of 'health promotion' work often comes in the form of behaviourally oriented 'health education', focusing on the first part of the Ottawa definition of health promotion. Clinically located developing personal skills practice often takes place in hospital or clinic-based settings and, where it does, has been criticised for its limited outcomes. The institutional base has continued to focus on individual behaviour change (Whitehead and Irvine, 2011).

**Box 5.2**

### Definition of 'Developing personal skills' action of the Ottawa Charter for Health Promotion

Supporting personal and social development through providing information, education for health, and enhancing life skills. It increases the options available to people to exercise more control over their own health and over their environments, and to make choices conducive to health. Action is required through educational, professional, commercial, and voluntary bodies, and within institutions.

McQueen and Salazar (2011) stated that this could be explained because of the words 'information, education and enhancing', embedded in the statement of the Ottawa Charter, that are critical concepts and principles. Information is a rather passive concept, education is about learning, and skills are tools that an individual takes on. Their developments were, to some extent, responses to unduly simplistic, individual behavioural health interventions, which supports Whitehead and Irvine's (2011) perspective on this. The Ottawa Charter makes clear that efforts to develop personal skills through traditional health education methods are only a part of a more complex and sophisticated set of tools to promote good health. It is not just about skills and knowledge specific to behaviours and lifestyles.

Despite this discussion, and the myriad of behind-the-scenes debates on this, health education was already playing a strong role in the area of developing personal skills. The Ottawa Charter seemingly offered a broader vision for health promotion, but in doing so seemed to imply that health education was a limited approach. The Ottawa Charter recognised that active participation by people to directly affect their health and the broader determinants of it was paramount (McQueen and Salazar, 2011).

---

## Point to Ponder 5.2

We are increasingly aware of the importance of promoting the active participation of the population in order to ensure sustainable health care. However, its implementation from the nurses' point of view continues to be a challenge. One of the main barriers found was the nurses' controlling approach, influenced by organisational issues, where nurses exerted control over patient care, which impacted the patient participation (Tobiano et al., 2016). Other difficulties encountered were the lack of teamwork and patients' taking on passive roles.

This reality should not be discouraging since nurses have a crucial role in promoting patient participation (Oxelmark et al., 2018). One first and essential step could be to make an effort to respect the patients' view and accept patient as a part of the care team.

---

The development of personal skills requires again a multi-sectoral approach for achieving its full potential. Wise and Nutbeam (2007) also stress that the active engagement of clinical health professionals (such as nurses) is 'critical', as such it is necessary to reorient nurse education and training to changing attitudes and behaviours. Finally, another solution to appropriate strategic responses lies in health promotion practitioners being empowered to be realistic about what they can do and to determine within their own unique context the strategic approach that will help them to reach their desired goals (Whitehead and Irvine, 2011). This stands for nurses as much as any other healthcare professional with health promotion as part of their remit.

## Nurses as Central to Lead the Change

The Ottawa Charter retains its importance and all policy makers and professionals working to promote positive health should revisit and take heed of its principles (Thompson et al., 2018). It is a reality that the majority of agents tend to think health is still mostly about health care, hospitals and professionals. We need a fundamental change of direction and a new way of thinking. Health and well-being are about so much more than the absence of disease. They are about life and freedom, being all that we can be, and living life to the full; about our relationships, how we live, and what happens to us at work and at school. And they are about confidence and control, and the quality of our lives. Because of this, our health as individuals is intimately connected to the health of our communities and our society and, ultimately, our environment and our planet. Crisp (2020) also stresses in his book the importance of 'home', and it also suggests the even more powerful idea that we can 'create health'. Creating health practices is directly related to health promotion, and with the mentioned radical change needed to realise Ottawa Charter actions and principles. In this regard, for several decades nursing has been touted as the health profession most likely to initiate and lead health-promotion movements. Nurses are in a unique position to serve as leaders and role models to activate communities for health promotion, and especially in driving and developing the strategic lines addressed in this chapter (Whitehead, 2011).

Nurses with their values-driven, holistic view of health, and their frequent and continuing contact with individuals, are well equipped to walk alongside the individuals, guiding and supporting them, as they take control of their health and their communities (Crisp, 2020). Further they are the single largest group of healthcare providers, playing a vital role in making health-promotion and illness-prevention services available to all population groups (Whitehead, 2011).

---

### Tutorial Trigger 5.2

Nurses are in a unique position to drive and develop strategic lines for increasing health-promotion practices.

How do you think you could contribute to this in your daily practice?

---

## How can nurses integrate this health-promoting vision in this daily routine?

'Creating health' practices is partly about attitudes and behaviours, but it is also about putting as many tools as possible into the hands of individuals and communities so they can understand what is happening, ask the right questions and make decisions (Crisp, 2020). As health is influenced by a variety of factors, there is a greater need than ever to implement health-generating practices for people having a greater control and awareness of these determinants that affect and increase their health and well-being. To achieve this, it is necessary for nurses to work together with the client, looking for the meeting point between nurses' scientific-technical expertise, and the expertise of the person's experience in their context. A context in which each person develops (or not) personal skills, in which an adequate support network is present (or not), and in which a support network is present (or not), and in which socio-economic characteristics have a privileged influence on the individual and his or her health.

For creating health, nurses must work under an equal 'co-production' approach, listening to clients to understand their circumstances, lives and preferences, all of which will influence the success of treatment and whether they follow their advice or not (Crisp, 2020).

──────── Time to Reflect 5.2 ────────────────────────────────

It is known that the nurse-patient relationship is one of the aspects that affects the client's quality of care. In this relationship it is increasingly essential to acquire an equal 'co-production' approach. However, how do you think this approach translates into your professional work? What aspects of daily practice would change if nursing professionals worked under this approach?

────────────────────────────────────────────────────────────

Health-promoting practices implies helping the person to grow, and this includes accompanying the person/family/group to rediscover themselves, to increase their awareness of all the potential they have to achieve their health goals and to live a full life. Each individual has the capacities and potential to achieve their own goals. All have resources, individual and environmental, although they are not always aware of them and do not always mobilise them. Nurses must accompany in this self-discovery, to be able to give back to this person, to this family, the leadership of the care of their own health. Adopting health-creating practices by promoting alliances with other sectors, listening to the person and their family, focusing on their strengths and virtues, on the strengths of their communities, and inspiring them to contribute in some way to this health-creating 'movement' could help to advance in reorienting services and in developing personal skills. Doing so, we could respond to the prevalent urgency towards the empowerment of individuals to truly take control over a hospital environment. Other examples are collected by Whitehead and Irvine (2011), such as the development of a new generation of 'nurse health champions' as integral health improvement facilitators of health promotion in acute healthcare services – sitting within the notion of a wider 'health education' role, and within the framework of where a health-promoting health services strategy can be located in both acute and community-based clinical practice.

Finally, it is important to take into account that the nursing workforce remains very much a sleeping giant. Its huge size means that nurses have enormous potential as agents of social control and change in promoting health and well-being. It does not take too much imagination to understand what the impact might be if over half a million people became empowered, assertive and articulate agents of change for better health promotion (Whitehead and Irvine, 2011). Thus, more concerted and well-planned attempts to engage with and mobilise large numbers of health professionals are necessary, nursing in particular (Catford, 2014).

---

### Research in Brief 5.1

Actions are necessary to increase the number of nurses committed to health promotion; however, the first step to this is to ensure that nurses themselves promote their own health. Moreover, nurses act as role models for patients; hence, their health promotion is significant as it affects both their own and their patients' lifestyles. Nurses' health promotion varies depending on the environment and circumstances surrounding their professional practice. A recent study aimed to investigate the factors affecting nurses' health promotion behaviours (Zeng et al., 2021). In their study they included 19,422 nurses and they analysed general and lifestyle characteristics of the participants and the effect on health promotion behaviour. The results showed that hospital levels, working years, nightshift status and monthly income were predictors of health-promoting lifestyle behaviours. Therefore, hospitals should develop health-promotion programmes to promote healthy lifestyles among nurses who are negatively affected by the variables mentioned above. In addition, as nurses, we must promote health in the first place with our co-workers, other nursing professionals. When we experience the effects of health promotion in our own lives, we will be more empowered to do it with our clients.

---

## Summary

This chapter has explored nuanced elements of two of the five health-promotion actions covered in the Ottawa Charter. It provides an important foundation for understanding how both strategies have been developed across the years, as well as the difficulties and challenges that still exist for its full implementation. This chapter also has outlined different proposals to achieve it and specialise with a focus on the nursing profession. Being aware of these aspects is essential so that all health agents could promote health across all the social framework, including both health services and other sectors.

—— Key Points ————————————————————————

- Reorienting health services and developing personal skills are still both influenced mainly by the prevalence of the biomedical approach in the whole social framework, including professionals' education and research, and a limited vision of the role of healthcare services and health professionals for introducing health-promotion practices, beyond health education, and its role building alliances with other sectors.
- For its enhancement it is necessary to promote an attitudinal and behavioural change at professional and organisational level, starting with the realisation that health and well-being cannot be extended only from healthcare services, but instead by individuals and communities themselves. In this regard, nurses are well positioned to empower people to be aware of all their strengths and possibilities, as well as how they can sum and contribute to their environment.
- Our patterns of health service are becoming unsustainable calling for an action which requires moving towards more efficient and positive models of care. Therefore, there is a need to reorient the system itself by involving health-promotion leaders more actively in system development.
- Active engagement of health professionals, such as nurses, is essential. Consequently, it is necessary to reorient their education and training to changing attitudes and behaviours towards a 'creating health' practice. Nurses must work together with the client under a framework of equal 'co-production' and with the conviction that each person has all the necessary resources to achieve their goals.

## References

Alami, H., Gagnon, M.P., Ghandour, E.K. and Fortin, J.P. (2017). La réorientation des services de santé et la promotion de la santé: une lecture de la situation. *Santé Publique 29*(2), 179–84.

Catford, J. (2014). Turn, turn, turn: time to reorient health services. *Health Promotion International 29*(1), 1–4.

Crisp, N. (2020). *Health is Made at Home; Hospitals are for repairs*. SALUS Global Knowledge Exchange.

Haugan, G. and Eriksson, M. (2021). *Health Promotion in Health Care – Vital Theories and Research*. Springer. doi:10.1007/978-3-030-63135

International Council of Nurses. (2021). Nurses: a voice to lead a vision for future healthcare. International Council of Nurses. Available at: www.icn.ch/system/files/documents/202105/ICN%20Toolkit_2021_ENG_Final.pdf

López-Dicastillo, O., Canga-Armayor, N., Mujika, A., et al., (2017). Cinco paradojas de la promoción de la salud. *Gaceta Sanitaria 31*(3), 269–72. Available at: https://dx.doi.org/10.1016/j.gaceta.2016.10.011

McQueen, D.V. and Salazar, L. (2011). Health promotion, the Ottawa Charter and 'developing personal skills': a compact history of 25 years. *Health Promotion International 26*(2), 194–201. doi:10.1093/heapro/dar063

Oxelmark, L., Ulin, K., Chaboyer, W., Bucknall, T. and Ringdal, M. (2018). Registered Nurses' experiences of patient participation in hospital care: supporting and hindering factors patient participation in care. *Scandinavian Journal of Caring Sciences 32*(2), 612–21. doi.org/10.1111/scs.12486

PDHPE. (2022). The Ottawa Charter as an effective health promotion framework. Developing personal skills. Available at: https://pdhpe.net/better-health-for-individuals/what-strategies-help-to-promote-the-health-of-individuals/the-ottawa-charter-as-an-effective-health-promotion-framework/developing-personal-skills/

Thompson, S., Watson, M. and Tilford, S. (2018). The Ottawa charter 30 years on: still an important standard for health promotion. *International Journal of Health Promotion and Education 56*(2), 73–84.

Tobiano, G., Marshall, A., Bucknall, T. and Chaboyer, W. (2016). Activities patients and nurses undertake to promote patient participation. *Journal of Nursing Scholarship 48*(4), 362–70. doi.org/10.1111/jnu.12219

Whitehead, D. (2011). Health promotion in nursing: a Derridean discourse analysis. *Health Promotion International 26*(1), 117–27. https://doi.org/10.1093/heapro/daq073

Whitehead, D. and Irvine, F. (2011). Ottawa 251—'All aboard the Dazzling Bandwagon'—developing personal skills: what remains for the future? *Health Promotion International 26*(2), 245–52. doi:10.1093/heapro/dar072

Wise, M. and Nutbeam, D. (2007). Enabling health systems transformation: what progress has been made in re-orienting health services? *Promotion & Education 2*, 23–27.

World Health Organization. (2018). Multisectoral and intersectoral action for improved health and well-being for all: mapping of the WHO European Region. Available at: www.euro.who.int/__data/assets/pdf_file/0005/371435/multisectoral-report-h1720-eng.pdf

World Health Organization. (1986). The Ottawa Charter for health promotion. *Health Promotion, 1*(1), iii–v.

Zeng, W., Shang, S., Fang, Q., He, S., Li, J. and Yao, Y. (2021). Health promoting lifestyle behaviors and associated predictors among clinical nurses in China: A cross-sectional study. *BMC Nursing 20*(1), 230. https://doi.org/10.1186/s12912-021-00752-7

Zeydani, A., Atashzadeh-Shoorideh, F., Abdi, F., et al., (2021). Effect of community-based education on undergraduate nursing students' skills: a systematic review. *BMC Nursing 20*(1), 233. https://doi.org/10.1186/s12912-021-00755-4

Ziglio, E., Simpson, S. and Tsouros, A. (2011). Health promotion and health systems: some unfinished business. *Health Promotion International 26*, ii, 216.

# Introduction to Section 2

# Theoretical Underpinnings, Global Health and the Future of Health Promotion and Health Education

Section 2 of this book identifies some of the core skills that are required for health education and health promotion and details some of the processes involved covering topics such as health needs assessment and evaluation. This second section of the book starts with Chapter 6 which presents a model that combines a lifespan- and a settings-based approach to health promotion whereby both are brought together to provide a framework for planning, implementing and evaluating health promotion and health education interventions. Chapter 7 then moves on to consider the key attributes and skills that are needed in order for nurses to be effective in the promotion of health and for health education. The discussion draws on recognised national and international standards and ways of working and also discusses the challenges that nurses might face in their health-promotion role. Focusing on population groups rather than individual patients, Chapter 8 presents guidance about how we might assess health needs beginning with the concept of need, considering how health might be measured, exploring what health needs assessment is about, and explaining different approaches to assessing health need. Chapter 9 is focused on evaluation for health promotion. It considers the nature of health promotion interventions and what evaluation is about, and outlines various approaches to evaluation including theory-based and participatory approaches. The chapter offers nurses practical strategies for undertaking evaluation for health-promotion interventions. The focus of this second section of the book broadens in Chapter 10 where we turn to global health. This chapter considers the importance of health education and health promotion in a contemporary global context. It forefronts the need to move beyond reactive responses to health crises towards using health promotion and health education as powerful approaches to addressing global health challenges, highlighting the nurse's role in this. Finally, in this section, we explore the future of health promotion and health education for health professionals in Chapter 11. The chapter considers the changing landscape of health promotion and health education, drawing together important lessons from recent disciplinary development, policy, technological advancements and changing evidence.

# 6

# A Lifespan-Settings-Based Framework for Health Promotion

## Dean Whitehead

## Introduction

In the mid-1980s, the World Health Organization (WHO, 1986) released the highly influential *Ottawa Charter for Health Promotion*. One of the milestones of the charter was that it paved the way toward the development of a series of 'settings-based' health-promotion strategies, where specific health-related settings were designated for special attention (WHO, 1986). The Ottawa Charter supported certain settings being nominated as unique social systems for enabling health-promotion activities and strategy. These initially included a raft of proposed settings; being hospitals, communities, schools, workplaces, cities, villages, islands, and the home and family. Other settings have since been added to that original list which now includes health-promoting universities (HPU), and health-promoting prisons (HPP) (Watson et al., 2004; Whitehead, 2006a) – as well as other nursing-specific unique settings such as health-promoting nursing homes and churches. More recently, we have witnessed the explosion of 'virtual' settings as a mainstay of health-promotion strategy, particularly through the emerging discipline of health communication (Jenkins et al., 2020).

The notion of *settings*, related to healthcare practice and health-promotion/health-education processes, has been championed for some time now. For instance, Hesman states that 'health promotion takes place in "settings" – environments where people learn, work, play and love' (Hesman, 2007: 175). Complementing this, Dooris (2004: 58) states that 'peoples' lives straddle settings'. Closely related to the context of settings is *lifespan*. In line with Hesman's sentiment people also learn, work, play and love across their lifespan – from birth to death. Therefore, it seems 'sensible' to bring lifespan and settings together when planning, implementing and evaluating our health-promotion and health-education interventions with our clients and families. While it seems sensible to promote such a framework – only Whitehead (2011) has proposed and developed such a framework/model. This chapter focuses on this framework and elaborates on it here in terms of its 'logical and structured' approach to health promotion and health-education practice.

By the end of this chapter the reader will be able to:

1. Understand the context of health-promoting settings and their close relationship with lifespan.
2. Appreciate the main distinct types of settings and where they 'sit' within the continuum of lifespan.
3. Explain how Whitehead's (2011) Model/Framework brings settings and lifespan together to inform health promotion/health education process.

**Key terms**

Health promotion/promoting settings, lifespan, continuum, framework/model

## The Health Promotion Setting/lifespan Framework/Model

In nursing, we tend to think of health-promoting settings in terms of clinical health services i.e., health-promoting hospitals and, in terms of the Ottawa Charter (WHO, 1986), this often relates to the 'developing personal skills' key action strategy (Whitehead and Irvine, 2011). However, nurses potentially work in all settings (particularly those working in community/Primary Health Care settings) – although their practice may often be governed by medical models of health which have the potential to constrain and limit practice. The more that we can 'work out' which setting/s our practice sits in and where in the lifespan we are engaging with our clients, the more likely that our practice will be less constrained and limited.

Figure 6.1 is designed to visually illustrate and represent this chapter's focus on the health-promoting lifespan continuum and its stages, as they relate to various

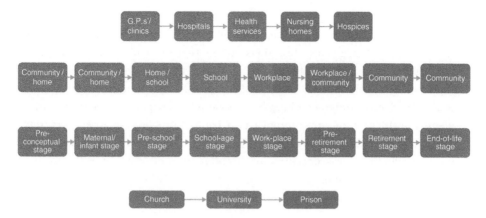

**Figure 6.1**   The Lifespan/Setting continuum

established settings. It is intended to draw the reader immediately to its central premise of 'whole' lifespan as a continuum and how it relates to specific settings at given times. The other main continuum associates related settings as an 'actual' sequence that is likely to be experienced by most people as a routine 'rites of passage' progression through the lifespan. The two more peripheral outer continuums acknowledge 'potential' health-related settings and settings that may not make up the 'normal' sequence of most individuals' life health journey. In line with the presented model, this chapter outlines common settings as they relate, directly or indirectly, to how nurses at the same time interact with their clients across their lifespan.

---

### Tutorial Trigger 6.1

Think about any recent health-promotion/health-education encounters you have been involved in. Identify what type/s of health promotion setting these encounters have occurred in (refer to Figure 6.1 to assist) – and what stage/s of the lifespan are the clients that you have engaged with on?

---

## The health promotion lifespan continuum – related to settings

### Pre-conceptual stage

In the not-too-distant future it is foreseen that the influence of biomedical technology, such as gene sequencing, genome therapy and stem cell treatments, will heavily influence and pre-determine the lifelong health status of individuals. This will often occur at the time of in-vitro fertilisation or even before conception. Butler and colleagues (2008) have hinted at the possibility that one day soon, we may witness genetic alteration techniques that will postpone ageing-related diseases and extend lifespan. They believe, as others do too, that this will herald a new era of preventive medicine and health promotion related to extending a healthy lifespan (Butler et al., 2008; Kirkwood, 2008; Olshansky et al., 2006). Interestingly, Richard et al.'s (2010: 454) study, describing Public Health Nurses' practices, states that they identify health promotion as prompt action 'before a problem has arisen' occurring over a lifelong period and 'could begin even *in utero* for a better outcome later'. The most notable global pre-conception health promotion intervention is the advocation of folic acid in common food products, such as bread and supplements, to help prevent developmental disabilities in children (Argyridis, 2019).

## Maternal / infant stage

This is an important stage of any individual's health development and an indicator of future health status in individuals. Domian et al. (2010) highlights the active health promotion role of Public Health Nurses working with disadvantaged mothers in their *My Baby and Me* comprehensive parenting intervention programme. In these ways, it is anticipated that young women will meet midwives and nurses before the momentum of pre-conception care is lost and before attitudes to breast-feeding are established. This type of intervention is at the heart of current public health policy around childbirth and child-care services. Housten and Cowley (2002) suggest that health promotion and empowerment are central to health-visiting practice, where individual needs assessment complements the principles of partnership-working in a health-promoting way.

## Kindergarten / pre-school stage

The concept of health-promoting schools (HPS) is one of the more visible in the nursing and general health promotion literature. However, the notion of health-promoting pre-schools, day-care education or kindergartens is not well established (Dresler et al., 2009). McKey and Huntington (2004) discuss the implications for nursing in child health practice related to the highly topical and relevant issue of pre-school childhood obesity. They state that nurses working in this area need to develop an understanding of the complex and often emotive issues at hand and an awareness of the reality of people's lives when devising health promotion strategies for this target group. Perren (2006) provide novel findings that help to put in place lifelong anti-bullying strategies as they impact the mental health of individuals and peer groups. They investigated varying bullying behaviours of children at the level of pre-school kindergarten and later links to mental health states throughout the lifespan. The outcomes were especially linked to how children fared when they moved into the school setting.

## Point to Ponder 6.1

An on-going debate is the question 'when is the best age to start formally educating children related to health and lifestyle promotion?' Is it kindergarten age – or later? Even more controversial is when to introduce sexual health for instance. This varies from country to country, and within countries as well.

## School stage

The school setting is seen as one of the most important health-related growth and frontline defence areas for health-promotion and health-education intervention, where health-promotion policies are a vital and integrated part of national curricula and health services (Tossavainen et al., 2004; Dressler- and Whitehead, 2009). From this position, the general Health-Promoting School (HPS) movement has come of age with a notable body of nursing-related literature. Specific publications, such as the *Journal of School Nursing*, highlight important emerging health-promotion agendas in this setting.

It is vital that health professional disciplines and services intervene at the initial stages of the lifespan continuum to instil healthy practices that younger people will then take with them into their young and middle-adult lives and beyond. Specific groups, such as school nurses, health visitors and specialist community public health nurses will have more obvious involvement in this setting. Furthermore, the role of student nurses, on schools-based placements, is highlighted by Laughlin et al. (2010). They report their *Healthy Living Project* where students' practicum experiences involved active application of health promotion aligned to specific community-based school projects. They combined service learning with research as part of a growing partnership with local primary and secondary schools.

## Research in Brief 6.1

Lee et al. (2020) reported on the English Wessex Healthy School Award Scheme and the Hong Kong Healthy School Award Scheme as a detailed system to analyse whether each school had reached the standard of a model Health Promoting School reflecting a more holistic appreciation and understanding of all the effects of school-based health promotion with positive award-related changes. They found that not many schools are able to implement the Health Promoting School strategy in its entirety and recommend that core indicators are needed as a starting point for wider implementation. The Hong Kong Healthy School Award Scheme is still ongoing. Lee et al. identify that the framework for Health Promoting School should go beyond improvement of health literacy to enable a more efficient system for education as a good investment in children's overall health and well-being.

Lee, A., Lo, A., Li, Q. et al. Health Promoting Schools: An Update. *Appl Health Econ Health Policy*, 18, 605-23 (2020). https://doi.org/10.1007/s40258-020-00575-8

## University/higher education stage

Universities and other higher education settings are not always going to figure in the lives of all clients. Increasingly now, however, greater numbers of individuals are accessing this type of setting as a 'routine' follow-on to post-16 school education (Dooris, 2009). The university may not be seen as somewhere where clinical nurses directly work or influence the health of individuals. However, most nurses in the world train and are educated through university, college, or polytechnic-based diploma/degree awards. They then often go on to remain in such institutions as they prepare for post-graduate studies. Universities and the like, therefore, can be viewed as testing grounds where the theoretical and practical components of delivered health promotion serve as a valuable starting or continuity point for clinical practice. The university can be seen as not only a good breeding ground for nurses to learn broad health policy and health-promotion skills, but also a useful location for disseminating these skills to both a localised and wider audience (Whitehead, 2004a). There are, so far, only a few examples of nursing-based health promotion in the university setting. For instance, Huyhn et al. (2000), as part of a university-based teaching-learning community clinical practicum programme, report how nursing students helped to set up a health information internet site within an underserved inner-city high school. The programme allowed these students to experience, at first hand, the sustainable practices of community-oriented participation. Local solutions to community health problems were uncovered and credibly linked to the university sector.

---

### Tutorial Trigger 6.2

There is a high likelihood that you are reading this text as part of a higher education course/programme that you are enrolled in. If this is the case, reflect on how this setting around you influences your health promotion practice - and to what extent you see this setting as health promoting i.e., disability and inclusion, healthy lifestyle influence etc.

## Workplace stage

The health-promoting workplace is fast gaining pace as one of the more important health-promotion settings (Shain and Kramer, 2004; Whitehead, 2006c). It holds a unique place where the health and wellbeing of workers inevitably impacts on the health of individuals within the workplace setting, their families, the local community, and society at large (Noblet and LaMontagne, 2006; Mills et al., 2007). It would also be remiss not to consider the further health contribution that such environments make on those for which health services are primarily designed – the client. Kearsey (2003) has already highlighted that healthy workplaces also equate to healthier people. Subsequently, and in line with the public health commitments of health service organisations, the extension of a positive healthy culture in the workplace is the potential influence on the health of immediate and wider family groups of health employees. As such, Ennals (2002) reminds us that we are obliged to consider the world beyond the workplace; the one where nurses are also engaged as citizens. In this sense, it is wise to consider the image that health services project into the communities that they serve. This is not just through the health standards and status of its patient outcomes but also through the health status of its local workforces. Similarly, Lavoie-Tremblay et al. (2008) stress the role of current nurses in creating healthy workplace environments for the sake of the next generation of nurses to follow. This will help to temper the effects of projected nurse shortages and keep the momentum of health-promoting services going forward. It is at this point that a unique cycle is added to Figure 6.1. Particularly, with soon-to-be new mothers (majority of births occurring at age of early employment) and fathers, health behaviours at this point profoundly influence the previously discussed pre-conception stage of the lifespan continuum.

Runciman et al. (2006) report on their nursing-led health promotion study into work practices of community nurses with older people. Their survey revealed that, where effective and creative group work at the interdisciplinary, multidisciplinary, and multi-agency levels occurs, then effective health promotion activity is subsequently evidenced in the workplace. The barriers to effective health promotion in the workplace existed where there was a lack of planning (especially involving clients), audit and evaluation, and where there was a lack of resources and funds. Effective workplace health promotion may even serve to extend the productive working lives of individuals who might, otherwise, contemplate earlier retirement. Tourangeau and Cranley (2006) investigated the intention of 13,000 Canadian nurses to remain in employment as they progressed towards retirement. From measuring predictors to remain or leave employment, they concluded that strategies needed for nurses to remain employed included employment practices that reflected moral integrity, incorporated clear communication systems, maximised employee involvement in decision-making, promoted praise and recognition, and an established shared vision and goals.

## Unemployment/welfare/detention stage

The link between work and socio-demographic status and healthy ageing is well established (Maltby, 2004). It is not to suggest that people who are unemployed or receiving welfare will go to prison. However, there are established links between long-term unemployment, low income, geographical location, and race that correlate to a higher incidence of criminality and penal incarceration in these sections of society that nurses encounter (Hek et al., 2006). Establishing health-promotion strategies within the prison setting is notably difficult as forced detention works counter to the health-promoting principles of negotiation, autonomy and humanism (Whitehead, 2006a). However, regarding nursing roles, Hek (2006) et al. (2006) elaborates on the growing and significant primary healthcare role of penal nurses whose priorities are to address social and health needs of their clients – as well as to improve their individual health status and to prevent re-offending and protect the wider community. Whether dealing with prison-based or unemployed clients, much of the health-promotion work within this stage would involve nurses from various disciplines introducing or re-orienting affected individuals to programmes that rehabilitate them to become active and productive members of their local community workforce. Laverack and Labonte (2000) advocate the targeting of traditionally complex social groups, such as unemployed clients, into health-promoting community empowerment and advocacy schemes. For those affected long-term in this stage, part of the health-promotion strategy needed would be effective preparation, working alongside those who have always worked in what would constitute the following pre- and post-retirement stages. The potential role for nurses in formulating and implementing health promotion programmes in various settings with people who are unemployed has been highlighted (Harris et al., 2009). Martin et al. (2010) describe their nurse-developed *welfare-to-wellness-to-work* health promotion programme. Through skills and knowledge development, they report positive participant outcomes in terms of increased self-esteem, self-care and self-empowerment.

## Pre-retirement stage

This is a stage of the lifespan continuum that has not been well researched and was only recognised as an actual stage on the continuum a couple of decades ago (Lethbridge, 2001). This is even though the need to promote healthy active ageing, to offset the impact of an ageing population on national resources and ensure a high quality of life in older age, has been well established. Secker et al. (2004) refer to this stage as the 'midlife' part of the continuum. They report their evaluation of a national pre-retirement health initiative in England. Their findings indicated that health improvement services could be effectively targeted at people in midlife and that service settings and style played an important part in the engagement of this usually neglected client group. Against the known backdrop demographic of the 'baby boomer' generation of the early 1960s, this generation is in or nearing this stage which most commonly falls within the midlife/pre-retirement age of 55–65 years. From a settings-based point of view, most health promotion activity is likely to occur either in the workplace or, from a social point of view, within the local community. It may also include, as part of or separate to, settings such as health-promoting churches (Peterson et al., 2002).

###### —— Time to Reflect 6.1 ——

It is widely reported that the healthcare professions (especially nursing, for instance) have an ageing workforce - with many of the 'baby boomers' due for retirement or already past the traditional retirement age (60-65 years of age). What implications do you think this has for the healthcare professions? How can the professions ensure that its workforce is retirement-ready and supported for a healthy retirement?

## Retirement stage

Where pre-retirement ends, and actual retirement begins is an important stage in the health status of individuals and their closest ones. De Vaus et al. (2007) report on their prospective longitudinal Healthy Retirement Project study. They found that retiring gradually allows for clients to make preparatory changes to their current and future lifestyle. They suggest that healthcare policies and work practices that promote control of retirement decisions for clients will enhance overall well-being later in life. When actual retirement occurs, health promotion is of considerable importance for retirees for sustaining a productive and healthy societal role and function. It is a significant area for healthcare workers, responsible for drafting policies and programmes, to consider helping improve health and wellness in older adults. For nursing, such is the level of health-promotion interest and active engagement at this stage of the lifespan that a well-crafted nursing-specific systematic review has been conducted (Wilson and Palha, 2007). Although the age of retirement can vary significantly between individuals, professions and countries, the general rule is that this age group commences around the 65-year-old mark.

Kennedy (2006) identified that health-promoting environments found in some naturally occurring retirement communities may be a low-cost community-based means of sustaining both the health and well-being of older people. He reported on the efforts to link biomedical and psychosocial services within naturally occurring retirement communities which assist seniors in their own homes. The desired outcomes were optimal health and independence relevant to, and mutually desired by, both health and social service providers. Wilson and Palha (2007) conducted a qualitative content analysis systematic review of the literature related to health promotion of adults at the age of retirement. Four themes emerged from the analysis of this literature. These were: (a) the considerable effect of retirement on retiring individuals and thus the need for support for more positive retirements, (b) identifying and overcoming barriers to health promotion at retirement, (c) evaluating the methods by which health promotion is introduced for positive and long-term change, and (d) describing the short- and long-term benefits of health promotion at retirement. Hitt et al. (1999), in their study, identified that most centenarians enjoyed a healthy and independent lifespan usually right up to a rapid terminal decline. Their 'compression of mortality paradigm' reported the more positive view that 'the older an individual gets the healthier they have been' – rather than the more commonly held view of 'the older people get the sicker they become'.

### End-of-life/palliation stage

Rosenberg and Yates (2010: 201) suggest that health promotion and palliative care may appear as 'conceptually incongruent fields'. Similarly, Kellehear (2008: 139) stresses that health promotion and palliative care can appear as both contradictory and strange companions; with dying patients there is no room for preventive advice. However, he goes on to highlight that palliative care is closely related to health promotion as its premise is based on holistic and humanistic therapeutic care. In this sense, the role of the nurse is to develop personal skills for clients, develop participatory relationships, educate, and inform clients and families, offer health and death education, social support, and strengthen community action and community participation. Rosenberg and Yates (2010) propose then that end-of-life palliative care is very amenable to the application of health-promotion practice. Richardson (2002) mirrors much of the above sentiment aligned to the role of community-based palliative care nurses. In turn, they have been able to offer a previously absent definition for health promotion in nursing-based palliation. Both Berg and Sarvimäki (2003) and Whitehead (2003) have also highlighted the importance and place of wider existential components of health promotion that can be linked to this stage. In this context, clients draw on existential forces to either help overcome adversity or give strength in facing a peaceful death. For dying patients, existential strength can offer hope and, for some, fulfilment. Fulfilment, in this case, may relate to the previously mentioned notion of faith-related or transcendental beliefs around potential 'afterlife' considerations. From a settings-based perspective, this stage of the lifespan continuum could potentially involve health-promoting nursing homes (Wass, 2000) and health-promoting hospices (Richardson, 2002).

## The potential 'other' settings

It may not always be prudent to refer to all the recognised health promotion settings from the point of view of a health-promotion lifespan continuum. For instance, despite their prominent place in nursing, direct healthcare-related settings such as acute health-promoting hospitals, GPs, clinics, nursing and rest homes, and hospices are not really addressed in this chapter. They are, however, represented in Figure 6.1. These types of settings are already comprehensively addressed within the mostly nursing-based literature (i.e., Bensberg et al., 2003; Chan and Wong, 2000; Cullen, 2002; Johnson and Baum, 2001; McInlay et al., 2005; Pelikan, 2007; Richardson, 2002; Wass, 2000; Watson, 2008; Whitehead, 2004c; Whitehead, 2005). However, they are not always a natural part of a person's health journey, or it is often difficult to predict when such episodes will occur. When they do occur, they tend to be short-term and are not usually the most desirable situations for the implementation of health-promotion initiatives. It is more appropriate, instead, to consider chronic illness and disability events in the context of social models of community intervention that promote recovery, rehabilitation and self-management of clients. Such examples are the increasing number of strategies that promote initiatives such as the *Hospital in the Home* and *Home Healthcare* (Duke and Street, 2003; Thome et al., 2003). Similarly, other 'potential' non-healthcare service settings that individuals may or may not encounter have already been detailed in this chapter i.e., universities and prisons – or are more generalised or peripheral to detail separately i.e., churches (Gosline and Schank, 2003; Peterson et al., 2002; Watson et al., 2004; Whitehead, 2004a; Whitehead, 2006a). However, because they potentially still hold a major place in the health journey of many, these settings are still identified in Figure 6.1. For instance, in DeHaven et al.'s (2004) review of health promotion in faith and religious-based organisations, its role is seen as extensive. Furthermore, the role of nurses figures in the review.

---

### Point to Ponder 6.2

The health-promoting settings movement remains fluid. Different settings are being proposed/added quite frequently. The 'astute' health practitioner will keep an eye open for new and evolving settings in the context of health promotion.

---

## Summary

The concept and impact of health-promotion settings is well established in the healthcare literature (Dooris, 2005; Poland et al., 2000; Whitehead, 2010; Whitelaw et al., 2001). What is less established, however, is the linking up of all settings as they potentially impact individuals, groups and communities at various times in their lives. Thinking beyond the scope of the immediate practice or setting to consider the links between, and influences of, other settings has enormous positive health benefits for those that work in and access them. Poland and colleagues stress the importance and uniqueness of settings-related 'place' in the literature and its profound impact on health strategy (Poland et al., 2005: 171). This includes nursing-based research in this field. They go on to state that the more common views of settings-related 'space and place' (either a geometric entity that impacts directly on the health of health professionals and their clients or as a 'locus or container' for health and healthcare activities) are sensible and pragmatic, but they remain 'under-theorised and rarely explicit foci of attention'. Current evidence, in most settings and across the lifespan continuum, suggests that concerted and universal health promotion reform is still to be realised in nursing – but that it is being worked towards. It is hoped that the perspective in this chapter, in linking all these contexts so that nurses view and practise their health promotion across the whole gambit of both linked-up settings and a linked-up lifespan continuum, will help to broaden called for health promotion reform in nursing and extend the healthcare repertoire of nurses.

─── **Key Points** ───────────────────────

- When we plan for a health promotion strategy it is important that we acknowledge the 'context' of where our clients are situated. Different settings demand different types of approaches – so health practitioners need to be aware of at least the main types of health-promoting settings that influence practice.
- When we consider health-promoting settings it is prudent to also consider issues of lifespan. Different settings tend to affect people differently at different times on the lifespan continuum.

## References

Argyridis, S. (2019). Folic acid in pregnancy, *Obstetrics, Gynaecology & Reproductive Medicine 29*(4), 2019, 118–20.

Bensberg, M., Kennedy, M. and Bennetts, S. (2003). Identifying the opportunities for health promoting emergency departments. *Accident and Emergency Nursing 11*, 173–81.

Berg, G.V. and Sarvimäki, A. (2003). A holistic-existential approach to health promotion. *Scandanavian Journal of Caring Sciences 17*, 384–91.

Butler, R.N., Miller, R.A., Perry, D. et al. (2008). New model of health promotion and disease prevention for the 21st century. *BMJ 337*(a399), 149–50.

Chan, F.Y.S. and Wong, G.K.C. (2000). Health promotion in hospitals: the attitudes of health care professionals. *The Hong Kong Nursing Journal 36*(2), 7–15.

Cullen, A. (2002). Health promotion in the changing face of the hospital landscape. *Collegian 9*, 41–2.

DeHaven, M.J., Hunter, I.B., Wilder, L., Walton, J.W. and Berry, J. (2004). Health programs in faith-based organisations: are they effective? *American Journal of Public Health 94*, 1030–6.

De Vaus, D., Wells, Y., Kendig, H. and Quine, S. (2007). Does gradual retirement have better outcomes than abrupt retirement? Results from an Australian panel study. *Ageing & Society 27*, 667–82.

Domian, E.W., Baggett, K.M., Carta, J.J., Mitchell, S. and Larson, E. (2010). Factors influencing mothers' abilities to engage in a comprehensive parenting intervention program. *Public Health Nursing 27*, 399–407.

Dooris, M. (2004). Joining up settings for health: A valuable investment for strategic partnership? *Critical Public Health 14*(1), 49–61.

Dooris, M. (2005). Healthy settings: Challenges to generating evidence of effectiveness. *Health Promotion International 21*, 55–65.

Dooris, M. (2009). Holistic and sustainable health improvement: The contribution of the settings-based approach to health promotion. *Perspectives in Public Health 129*, 29–36.

Dresler, E., Whitehead, D. and Coad, J. (2009). What are New Zealand children eating at school? A content analyses of 'consumed versus unconsumed' food groups in a lunch-box survey. *Health Education Journal 68*, 3–13.

Dresler-Hawke, E. and Whitehead, D. (2009). The Behavioral Ecological Model as a framework for school-based anti-bullying health promotion interventions. *Journal of School Nursing 25*, 195–204.

Duke, M. and Street, M. (2003). Hospital in the home: constructions of the nursing role – a literature review. *Journal of Clinical Nursing 12*, 852–9.

Ennals, R. (2002). Partnerships for sustainable healthy workplaces. *The Annals of Occupational Hygiene 46*, 423–8.

Gosline, M.B. and Schank, M.J. (2003). A University-wise Health Fair: A Health Promotion Clinical Practicum. *Nurse Educator 28*(1), 23–5.

Harris, E., Rose, V., Ritchie, J. and Harris, N. (2009). Labour market initiatives: potential settings for improving the health of people who are unemployed. *Health Promotion Journal of Australia 20*, 214–20.

Hek, G., Condon, L. and Harris, F. (2006). An emerging role for nurses working in prisons. *Prison Service Journal 166*, 42–4.

Hesman, A. (2007). Creating Supportive Environments for Health. In J. Wills (Ed.), *Promoting Health: Vital Notes for Nurses* (pp. 175–93). Oxford: Blackwell Publishing.

Hitt, R., Young-Xu, Y., Silvr, M. and Peris, T. (1999). Centenarians: the older you get, the healthier you have been. *The Lancet 354*, 652.

Housten, A. and Cowley, S. (2002). An empowerment approach to needs assessment in health visiting practice. *Journal of Clinical Nursing 11*, 640–50.

Huyhn, K., Kosmyna, B., Lea, H., et al., (2000). Creating an adolescent health promotion. INTERNET.SITE: A community partnership between university nursing students and an inner-city High School. *Nursing and Healthcare Perspectives 21*, 122–6.

Jenkins, E.L., Ilicic, J., Barklamb, A.M. and McCaffrey, T.A. (2020). Assessing the credibility and authenticity of social media content for applications in health communication: Scoping Review. *Journal of Medical Internet Research 22*(7), e17296. doi: 10.2196/17296

Johnson, A. and Baum, F. (2001). Health promotion hospitals: a typology of different organizational approaches to health promotion. *Health Promotion International 16*, 281–7.

Kearsey, K. (2003). Your work your health: whether patient or health care provider, a healthy workplace is key to well-being. *Registered Nurse Journal 15*(1), 16–19.

Kellehear, A. (2008). Health promotion in palliative care. In G. Mitchell (Ed.), *Palliative Care: A Patient-centred Approach* (pp.139–56). Abingdon, Oxon, UK: Radcliffe Publishing.

Kennedy, G.J. (2006). Naturally occurring retirement communities: An expanding opportunity for health promotion and disease prevention. *Primary Psychiatry 13*, 33–5.

Kirkwood, T. (2008). A systematic look at an old problem. *Nature, 451*, 644–7.

Laughlin, A., Pothoff, M., Schwartz, M., Synowiecki, B. and Yager, A. (2010). Combining service learning and research: partnering with schools. *Nurse Educator 35*, 188–91.

Laverack, G. and Labonte, R. (2000). A planning framework for community empowerment goals within health promotion. *Health Policy and Planning 15*, 255–62.

Lavoie-Tremblay, M., Wright, D., Desforges, N., Gelinas, C., Marchionni, C. and Drevniok, U. (2008). Creating a healthy workplace for new-generation nurses. *Journal of Nursing Scholarship 40*, 290–7.

Lee, A., Lo, A., Li, Q. et al. (2020). Health promoting schools: An update. *Applied Health Economics and Health Policy 18*, 605–23. Available at: https://doi.org/10.1007/s40258-020-00575-8

Lethbridge, J. (2001). *Pre-retirement Health Checks and Plans: A literature review*. London: Health Development Agency.

Maltby, T. (2004). Ageing and the Transition to Retirement: a Comparative Analysis of European Welfare States. Aldershot: Ashgate.

Martin, C.T., Keswick, J.L. and LeVeck, P. (2010). A welfare-to-wellness-to-work program. *Journal of Community Health Nursing 27*(146), 1099–1106.

McKey, A. and Huntington, A. (2004). Obesity in pre-school children: Issues and challenges for community based child health nurses. *Contemporary Nurse 18*, 145–51.

McKinlay, E., Plumridge, L., McBain, L., McLeod, D. et al. (2005). 'What sort of health promotion are you talking about?' a discourse analysis of the talk of general practitioners. *Social Science & Medicine 60*, 1099–106.

Mills, P.R., Kessler, R.C., Cooper, J. and Sullivan, S. (2007). Impact of a health promotion program on employee health risks and work productivity. *American Journal of Health Promotion 22*(1), 45–53.

Noblet, A. and LaMontagne, A.D. (2006). The role of workplace health promotion in addressing job stress. *Health Promotion International 21*, 346–53.

Olshansky, S.J., Perry, D., Miller, R.A. and Butler, R.N. (2006). In pursuit of the longevity dividend. *The Scientist 20*, 28–36.

Pearce, C., Leask, J. and Ritchie, J. (2008). Tapping midwives' views about the neo-natal hepatitis B vaccine: how welcome is a move towards a health promoting orientation? *Health Promotion Journal of Australia 19*(2), 161–3.

Pelikan, J.M. (2007). Health Promoting Hospitals: assessing developments in the net-work. *Italian Journal of Public Health 5*, 261–70.

Perren, S. and Alasker, P.D. (2006). Social behaviour and peer relationships of victims, bully-victims, and bullies in Kindergarten. *Journal of Child Psychology and Psychia-try 47*, 45–57.

Peterson, J., Atwood, J.R. and Yates, B. (2002). Key elements for church-based health pro-motion programs: outcome-based literature review. *Public Health Nursing 19*, 401–11.

Poland, B., Green, L. and Rootman, I. (2000). *Settings for Health Promotion: Linking Theory and Practice*. London: Sage Publications.

Poland, B., Lehoux, P., Holmes, D. and Andrews, G. (2005). How place matters: unpacking technology and power in health and social care. *Health and Social Care in the Community 13*, 170–80.

Richard, L., Gendron, S., Beudet, N., Boisvert, N., Soleil Suave, M. and Garceau-Brodeur, M-H. (2010). Health promotion and disease prevention among nurses working in local Public Health Organisations in Montreal, Quebec. *Public Health Nursing 27*, 450–58.

Richardson, J. (2002). Health promotion in palliative care: the patients' perception of therapeutic interaction with the palliative nurse in the primary care setting. *Journal of Advanced Nursing 40*, 432–40.

Rosenberg, J.P. and Yates, P.M. (2010). Health promotion in palliative care: the case for conceptual congruence. *Critical Public Health 20*, 201–10.

Runciman, P., Watson, H., McIntosh, J. and Tolson, D. (2006). Community nurses: health promotion work with older people. *Journal of Advanced Nursing 55*, 46–57.

Secker, J., Bowers, H., Webb, D. and Llanes, M. (2004). Theories of change: what works in improving health in mid-life? *Health Education Research 20*, 392–401.

Shain, M. and Kramer, D.M. (2004). Health promotion in the workplace: framing the concept; reviewing the evidence. *Occupational and Environmental Medicine 61*, 643–8.

Thome, B., Dykes, A-K. and Hallberg, L.R. (2003). Home care with regard to defini-tion, care recipients, content and outcome: systematic literature review. *Journal of Clinical Nursing 12*, 860–72.

Tossavainen, K., Turunen, H., Jakonen, S., Tupala, M. and Vertio, H. (2004). School nurses as health counsellors in Finnish ENHPS schools. *Health Education 104*(1), 33–44.

Tourangeau, A.E. and Cranley, L.A. (2006). Nurse intention to remain employed: under-standing and strengthening determinants. *Journal of Advanced Nursing 55*, 497–509.

Wass, A. (2000). *Promoting Health: The Primary Health Care Approach*. 2nd edn. Sydney, Australia: Harcourt.

Watson, M. (2008). Going for gold: the health promoting general practice. *Quality in Primary Care 16*, 177–85.

Watson, R., Stimpson, A. and Hostick, T. (2004). Prison health care: a review of the literature. *International Journal of Nursing Studies 41*, 119–224.

Whitehead, D. (2003). Beyond the metaphysical: health-promoting existential mechanisms and their impact on the health status of clients. *Journal of Clinical Nursing 12*, 678–88.

Whitehead, D. (2004a). Health Promoting Universities (HPU): the role and function of nursing. *Nurse Education Today 24*, 466–72.

Whitehead, D. (2004b). Health promotion and health education: advancing the concepts. *Journal of Advanced Nursing 47*, 311–20.

Whitehead, D. (2004c). The European Health Promoting Hospitals (HPH) Project – how far on? *Health Promotion International 19*, 259–67.

Whitehead, D. (2005). Health Promoting Hospitals (HPH): the role and function of nursing. *Journal of Clinical Nursing 14*, 20–7.

Whitehead, D. (2006a). Health Promoting Prisons (HPP) and the imperative for nursing. *International Journal of Nursing Studies 43*, 123–31.

Whitehead, D. (2006b). The Health Promoting School (HPS): what role for nursing? *Journal of Clinical Nursing 15*, 264–71.

Whitehead, D. (2006c). Workplace health promotion: the role and responsibilities of health care managers. *Journal of Nursing Management 14*, 59–68.

Whitehead, D. (2010). Settings Based Health Promotion. In D. Whitehead and F. Irvine (Eds), *Health Promotion and Health Education in Nursing: A Framework for Practice* (pp. 95–120). Houndsmills, Basingstoke, UK: Palgrave Macmillan.

Whitehead, D. (2011). Before the cradle and beyond the grave: a lifespan/settings-based framework for health promotion. *Journal of Clinical Nursing 20*(15–16), 2183–94.

Whitelaw, S., Baxendale, A., Bryce, C., MacHardy, L., Young, I. and Witney, E. (2001). 'Settings' based health promotion: a review. *Health Promotion International 16*(4), 339–53.

Wilson, D.M. and Palha, P. (2007). A systematic review of published research articles on health promotion at retirement. *Journal of Nursing Scholarship 39*, 330–7.

WHO (1986) *Ottawa Charter for Health Promotion*. Geneva: World Health Organization.

# 7

# Core Health Promotion and Health Education Skills

Susan Thompson

## Introduction

Health promotion is a complicated business, any discipline which seeks to influence all people in all settings with the aim of improving the health status of the whole of the world's population is bound to be. Nurses therefore need a high level of knowledge, skills and experience to confidently engage with their patients on a one-to-one basis, but also to act as a patient advocate and lobby for change at a more strategic level. This chapter will outline the key attributes and skills required for effective nursing practice in health promotion and health education, drawing on recognised national and international standards, regulation and ways of working. The chapter will then go on to discuss the challenges and pitfalls nurses may face in their health promotion role.

By the end of this chapter the reader will be able to:

1. Outline the nurse's role in health promotion and education.
2. Gain knowledge of the skills and attributes needed to practise health promotion and education.
3. Explore behaviour change models and techniques.
4. Discuss the potential challenges for nurses undertaking health promotion and education roles within their practice.

## Key terms

Behaviour change, Ottawa Charter, health promotion role in nursing, transtheoretical model, motivational interviewing

## The role of nurses and midwives within health promotion and health education

To be effective and competent in their health-promotion and education role nurses need training in the skills and attributes required. They also need some guiding principles and ways of working which are evidence-based and can direct their work. As we have seen in the previous chapter the journey started with the World Health Organization's Ottawa Charter of 1986, (WHO, 1986) and has continued to this day, seeking to raise the profile of the profession, establish health promotion as a discipline and provide direction for governments and practitioners. In 2005, the 6th Global Conference in Health Promotion (WHO, 2005) resulted in the Bangkok Charter which outlined five key principles necessary to guide effective health promotion policy (please see Box 7.1 for details).

### Box 7.1

### The World Health Organization: Five key principles necessary to guide effective health promotion policy (WHO, 2005)

1  That health promotion is context driven and should take account of the social and economic determinants of health and health inequalities.
2  That health promotion should address the different dimensions of physical, social, mental and spiritual health.
3  That all governments and all levels of government have a duty to improve the health of their citizens.

4 That it should be acknowledged that good health is intrinsically beneficial to the social and economic status of nations.

5 That people at an individual or community level should be fully engaged and participate in improving health status for themselves and others.

---

When discussing nursing practice, numbers 1, 2 and 5 of the key principles seem to be most relevant. Treating people as individuals and taking account of the context in which they live their lives by being holistic (that is taking into account the entirety of their existence) is essential for compassionate working (Nursing and Midwifery Council, n.d.). There is much talk of health equality, ensuring non-discrimination, but rather than delivering the same care to everyone regardless, this actually means a careful assessment by the nurse of the specific needs of that individual or community and adapting care to suit. The aim is to work in true partnership with patients and facilitate true choice (Coulter and Collins, 2011; Dy and Purnell, 2012; Oakley, Johl and Holber, 2018). These are all cornerstones of modern practice, so nurses and midwives already have key principles of health promotion enshrined in their existing practice (Nursing and Midwifery Council, n.d.).

## Point to Ponder 7.1

Western medicine has been dominated by the medical model for centuries and has been seen as paternalistic and autocratic. In recent decades there has been a move to see patients as partners in care, however, this still exists within a medical model framework. The vast majority of decisions and policy making comes from government organisations and is very 'top down'. Often consultations with the general public are designed to do little more than make minor changes to policies already largely written. Continual failure to properly engage at the outset and involve the public in decision making works against the idea of partners in care and may continue to undermine health promotion practice.

---

Nurses already possess many of the skills needed for health-promotion practice. Essential components are excellent communication skills and a non-judgemental approach (Thompson, 2014). Assessment of individuals' circumstances, their knowledge, attitudes and motivation should be the first step in facilitating healthy behaviour. The ability to use a strength-based approach to supporting people through change coupled with a true commitment to working in partnership with patients and families are key for effective and successful health-promotion activities (Gottlieb, 2013).

Some nurses in senior roles will have the remit to influence policy at a strategic level and be able to achieve real change at either a local, national or even global level. In-depth knowledge of their patients and their needs will enable them to act as true advocates within their speciality (Nsiah, Siakwa and Ninnoni, 2019). Within the UK, senior nurses acting as Governing Body Nurses (GBN) can be appointed to Clinical Commissioning Groups. These are bodies established as a result of the Health & Social Care Act (2012) in England and are tasked with directly commissioning healthcare services at a local level. The aim of such appointments is to ensure nursing expertise is inputted into the decision-making process. Nurses therefore have the potential to influence the health status of their patients at multiple levels.

## Standards for Nurse Education

In the United Kingdom (UK), the responsibility for regulating nursing (and midwifery) falls to the Nursing and Midwifery Council (NMC). This body acts to fulfil the legislative Nursing and Midwifery order 2001 to produce and maintain sets of standards for pre-registration nurse education and registered nurses and midwives. Approved Educational Institutions (AEIs) and healthcare providers, commonly referred to as 'practice partners' have the day-to-day responsibility for delivering pre-registration courses which are approved as fit for purpose in accordance with standards set by the NMC (NMC, 2018a).

Registered nurses are required to work to a set of proficiencies or standards set by the NMC which demonstrate the knowledge and skills nurses must exhibit when caring for their patients in every setting (NMC, 2018b). These proficiencies have been grouped into seven platforms. Platform number 2 is entitled Promoting Health and Preventing Ill Health and specifies that: "Registered nurses play a key role in improving and maintaining the mental, physical and behavioural health and well-being of people, families, communities and populations" (NMC, 2018b, p. 10).

The document then goes on to state 12 outcomes or proficiencies that registered nurses must maintain in order for them to fulfil this specific role. These proficiencies include; understanding the principles of health promotion, having knowledge of epidemiology, understanding inequalities in health, providing health information and aiding health literacy, helping people through behaviour change, undertaking health screening and vaccination and promoting and protecting health. This is a comprehensive list and the fact that this is the second out of seven platforms perhaps gives a sense of the importance given to health promotion as a core nursing role.

Globally, standards for nurse education vary remarkably with some countries accepting secondary level education as an entry to the profession, whereas others require university degrees (WHO, 2009). The World Health Organization has sought to standardise nursing educational programmes to a limited degree. However, it has concentrated its efforts on structure and governance rather than dictating actual curricula content, which is left to the individual countries and education providers. Programme graduates are nevertheless required to demonstrate competence in their field of practice and, crucially, an understanding of the wider determinants of health, an important first step on the road to promoting health within the populations they serve (WHO, 2009). In low-income countries high rates of preventable disease provide much scope for nurses to practice health promotion although, unfortunately, this practice is often constrained by lack of resources.

## Key skills and attributes required for health promotion and education

### Health communication

Good communication can be instinctive but can also be learnt and therefore taught. Pre-registration nursing programmes generally place an emphasis on communication skills early on in their programmes of study. Nevertheless, it is worth revisiting key principles and techniques within this chapter as excellent communication skills are an essential prerequisite for effective health promotion and education practice.

In the twentieth century there was an emphasis on improving communication within the healthcare setting, a recognition perhaps of the paternalistic and hierarchical communication methods which had dominated prior to this. As a consequence, there emerged a series of researchers and practitioners who revolutionised health communication and whose influence is still dominant to this day. One of these giants and their relevance to nursing and midwifery practice will be considered here.

Carl Rogers (1957) believed in the following core principles for effective communication which he termed a person-centred approach:

- Clients' needs should be put at the centre of interactions.
- All of us have within ourselves a capacity for growth and change.
- The professional's role is to act as mere facilitators to bring out clients' inner strength and ability to change.
- The client remains firmly in control and does the bulk of the work.

Rogers also stated that those using communication in a therapeutic environment needed to possess three core conditions (please see Box 7.2).

---

**Box 7.2**

## Carl Rogers' Core Conditions (Rogers, 1957)

- *Acceptance or Unconditional Positive Regard* which is...
  - ○ being non-judgemental
  - ○ treating the individual with respect
  - ○ not criticising
  - ○ seeing the person not just the behaviour
- *Congruence (Genuineness/Honesty)* which is...
  - ○ being sincere
  - ○ being honest
  - ○ being open within professional boundaries
- *Empathy* which is...
  - ○ being able to imagine the other person's experience
  - ○ being able to understand the other person's view/position

---

### Tutorial Trigger 7.1

Think of a time in your nursing and midwifery career when you came across a patient whose behaviour you felt was unacceptable.

Did you struggle to be non-judgemental and did this affect the level of respect you gave to that patient?

Were you able to be honest and open with that patient?

Were you able to empathise and take the patient's past history and past and present specific circumstances into account?

---

Sometimes it is hard for us to uphold Rogers' principles, but in order for us to work effectively with patients they are a crucial starting point and without these core conditions being in place our interactions and the care patients receive will inevitably suffer. Building a relationship is key here and to do that there needs to be open, honest, respectful communication between both parties and for that to happen there needs to be trust. Trust takes time to build, although generally within most societies the caring professions are luckily afforded a basic level of trust which can be built upon (Dinc and Gastmans, 2013; Sheehan and Fealy, 2020).

Certain communication techniques are also very useful tools. Use of minimal prompts such as 'I understand', 'OK', 'right' etc. along with non-verbal encouragements like nodding, smiling and maintaining an open posture will all help to convince the patient that you are giving them your full attention. Techniques such as paraphrasing, reflecting, silence, clarifying and summarising will convey to the patient that they are being listened to and engender a feeling within the patient that they are respected and understood (Egan, 2002; Rogers, 1961).

## Health needs assessment and agenda setting

Health needs assessment happens at various levels. They may be conducted to explore the health needs of a particular geographical locality, a certain demographic such as children or older people, or those with a particular condition, diabetes for example (Kelly, Powell and Bartle, 2012; Thompson, 2014). These strategic needs assessments are generally conducted by public bodies such as health services or local government. Nurses may be involved at this strategic level as a representative on a board such as the Joint Strategic Needs Assessment ones in the UK (Department of Health and Social Care, 2013). Most of the time however nurses are involved in patient health needs assessment working on a one-to-one basis, usually around supporting people through behaviour change and self-care. Health-promotion interactions are no different from routine patient interactions in that they need to start with assessment. It cannot be stressed enough that this is probably the most important stage in the process of supporting people through behaviour change and cannot be rushed. Too often practitioners rush in with advice before any understanding of the person sitting before them or their circumstances. This often results in alienation, resentment and a stubborn unwillingness on the part of the patient to change (Thompson, 2014). The assessment process needs to establish both the patient's level of knowledge regarding health determinants and also their level of motivation for change. How much do they understand about their condition, its causes, the effects of various behaviour choices or how self-care actions may improve their condition? It is obviously important here to fill in any gaps in knowledge without falling into the trap of either preaching or being condescending.

Crucial to this is an understanding of the patient's individual circumstances. It is also essential that patients are allowed to set their own goals and go at their own pace rather than being dictated to by such things as service targets or policy agendas (Petersen and Alexander, 2001; Thompson, 2014). Both can limit freedom to completely pursue the patients' goals, especially if services are specifically set up for certain issues which do not coincide with the priorities of patients. Although health professionals have a responsibility to raise such issues and discuss ways to help patients improve their health status, forcing issues onto patients will just result in alienation and possibly a reluctance to seek out health services in the future. It is important not to impose the value systems and goals of others onto patients who do not share them (NMC, n.d.). A useful thought in keep to mind throughout, is that patients and their families are 'partners' in care, they are being worked *with*, not being done *to*. It is important not to allow any sense of judgement to creep into interactions or, at least, to be aware of this. After all, we are all guilty of failing to take appropriate actions to reach our optimum health potential.

## Helping people with behaviour change

When working on a one-to-one basis with patients, nurses are in an ideal situation to start conversations around behaviour change. In 2014 the UK Government's Department of Health launched its new framework called Every Contact Counts aimed at encouraging behaviour change. This encouraged staff to give opportunistic, appropriate and timely advice on health and well-being to patients/service users, their carers, staff and communities they come into contact with (Department of Health, 2014). Its aim being that: 'Every healthcare professional should "make every contact count": use every contact with an individual to maintain or improve their mental and physical health and wellbeing where possible' (NHS Future Forum, 2012: 11). This initiative was on the back of evidence that brief advice lasting no more than three minutes has been shown to increase a person's chance of quitting smoking by up to 3 per cent (Cochrane Collaboration, 2008) and also the 5As model of change (ask, advise, assess, assist, and arrange) (Glasgow, Emont and Miller, 2006; Haseler, Crooke and Haseler, 2019). Although 3 per cent seems like a small proportion, if this is scaled up to the number of consultations healthcare staff have with their patients on a daily basis it equates to a large number of people.

Despite this, there was resistance to the requirement to routinely raise the subject of change with patients at every consultation as the framework was advising. It was thought that this would create a barrier between health professionals and patients and might possibly cause them not to present to health care in the future, due to the emphasis now placed on their behaviour. This was also a time in the UK of sweeping public service funding cuts and the framework was viewed cynically as a cheap option to use existing staff rather than maintain specialist health promotion services. In the most recent National Institute of Clinical Excellence (NICE) guidelines (2018) this aspect has been dropped due to insufficient evidence that this policy was either being followed or was effective. Nevertheless, it is important not to completely disregard opportunistic advice by health professionals because, if done with due consideration, it may prompt patients to improve their health status and may be a crucial first step towards behaviour change (Public Health England, 2020). An important and useful technique that can be used to raise the issue of behaviour change is motivational interviewing.

## Motivational interviewing

Motivational interviewing (MI) emerged in the 1980s as a challenge to the predominant model of advising patients on behaviour change, which at the time consisted largely of coercive, confrontational interactions between practitioners and patients. This tactic sought to pressurise patients into behaviour change by laying out the stark facts and risks that patients were taking because of their 'irresponsible behaviour'. In contrast MI offers a way of eliciting from people *their own* thoughts, concerns, views and ideas about change, so motivation is *evoked* rather than installed. MI has proven especially effective when used with people who are ambivalent to behaviour change as 'it is designed to strengthen an individual's motivation for and movement toward a specific goal by eliciting and exploring the person's own reasons for change within an atmosphere of acceptance and compassion' (Miller and Rollnick, 2012: 5). The MI practitioner aims to identify discrepancy in their patient, the mismatch between the health goals that the patient holds and their current behaviour, which is working in opposition to these goals. Importantly however it is the patient who needs to voice this, thus indicating that they are no longer ambivalent but positively considering and desiring change (Rosengren, 2017). There are many publications and courses on MI available to nurses who wish to further explore and practise this technique as MI has been proven to be very effective in supporting people through behaviour change (Lindson-Hawley, Thompson, and Begh, 2015; Rubak et al., 2005).

## Stages of change (Transtheoretical model)

In addition to the above, another excellent tool for health promotion is the trans-theoretical model which enables the nurse to assess patient motivation, then supports the patient through the stages of the change process. The strength of this

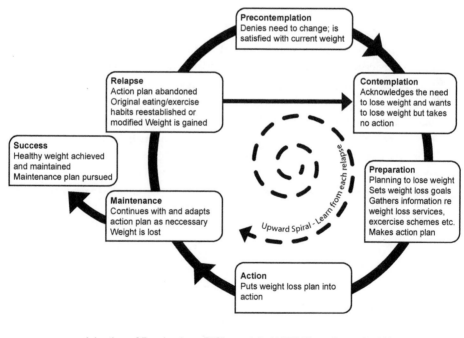

Adaption of Prochaska + DiClemente's (1983) Transtheoretical Model
to Show Stages of Change for Clients Undertaking Weight Loss

**Figure 7.1** The Stages of Change (Transtheoretical Model)

model is its straightforwardness and ease of use – it is easy to understand and apply (Prochaska and DiClemente, 1984; Thompson, 2014).

MI and the communication skills that have already been discussed should be used in conjunction with this model. First of all comes assessment. For example, questions asked such as 'do you feel that you would like to lose weight?' can open up the conversation and identify where the patient is in the cycle of change. Are they very negative, not at all interested in change? If so, they are in the pre-contemplative stage of the cycle. At this point a reiteration of the issues that their weight is causing them and an open-door approach to any future change of heart is all that is needed. As has been made clear, labouring the point just alienates the patient and destroys the caring relationship, so it should be left and maybe revisited at a future date. Mostly however you will find patients are in the contemplative phase when they acknowledge the need to change, would like to change but doubt their capacity to change or are putting it off. At this point information should be provided regarding support services available, discussions regarding their own individual circumstances, what have they tried before? what problems do they foresee? and an in-depth conversation which will move the patient onto the next stage – planning to change. Once goals, a timescale, support and resources to help have been identified this plan can be put into action. During the action phase contact should be maintained with the patient to ensure the plan is working and potentially adapt the plan as necessary to promote success. Hopefully, the patient will move into the maintenance phase, in which they maintain their changed behaviour. Often, of course, patients relapse and either revert to their previous behaviour or a version of it. It needs to be stressed to the patient that this is very common and should not indicate that they are incapable of change. At this point they re-enter the cycle at contemplation again and either work with the practitioner to adapt their plan, or maybe take a break and try again later. Behaviour change is hard, and the patient should not be made to feel guilty or incapable (Norcross, Krebs and Prochaska, 2011).

---

## Tutorial Trigger 7.2

If you were working with a patient who is a regular smoker and wanted to discuss lifestyle change:

- How would you identify at what stage your patient was at in the cycle of change?
- What questions would you ask for each stage?
- What might the client reply?

How would you move them on to the next stage - if appropriate?

## Research skills

All nurses and midwives need research skills to search for quality information, analyse, critique this and implement findings in their work. The nursing and midwifery professions regard research skills as an essential professional skill and a driver for change (NMC, n.d.; NHS England, 2021). New approaches to care are crucial if the profession is to continue to move forward and utilise research findings to enhance patient experience and improve outcomes. With regard to health promotion this means keeping up to date with new research within your area of expertise, new policy decisions and new evidence-based initiatives and services that may be available to your patients. This signposting function is crucial as nurses, especially those working in hospitals, often see patients for relatively short periods of time. Behaviour change is a long-term process so knowledge of effective interventions and where patients can go to access ongoing support is crucial. In addition, new techniques emerge because of ongoing research. Such new developments seek to improve the effectiveness of professionals working with patients, so it is important to keep up to date with new ways of working which have been proven to be both evidence-based and effective.

### Research in Brief 7.1

This review sought to bring together and interrogate a range of research regarding nurses' health promotion practice. Multiple databases were searched and 40 research papers which included quantitative, qualitative and empirical studies were analysed in depth. Research covered nurses' perceptions of their health promotion role, the theoretical basis they used for their practice, an assessment of their skills and expertise and their ability to perform the role. The review found that nurses either work from an individual, holistic, patient-oriented theoretical base, or a chronic disease, medically oriented stance. Health promotion concepts such as empowerment and working within the personal circumstances of the patient on ill-health prevention was important for nurses, however there was little knowledge or application of health and social care policy. Nurses exhibited a range of health-promotion knowledge and skills including knowledge of the wider determinants of health and advocacy, communication and partnership working skills. Nevertheless, organisational restraints compromised nurses' health-promotion work including lack of time and health education material. The culture of the individual organisation and managerial attitudes and commitment was also cited as being a factor in the importance given to nurses' health-promotion roles.

Kemppainen, V., Tossavainen, K. and Turunen, H. (2013). Nurses' roles in health promotion practice: an integrative review. *Health Promotion International*, 28(4), 490-501. doi: 10.1093/heapro/das034

## Challenges for Nurses in Practising Health Promotion

Globally, nurses and midwives make up almost 50 per cent of the world's healthcare workers. However, they also make up more than 50 per cent of the current shortfall in health workers, with South-East Asia and Africa being especially affected. It is estimated that for the United Nations Sustainable Development Goals for health and well-being to be met by the year 2030 the world will need an additional nine million nurses and midwives in employment (WHO, n.d.) (a). In 2020 The World Health Organisation produced its report: The State of the World's Nursing (WHO, 2020). This report called for a much greater investment in nursing education, jobs and leadership throughout the world. A WHO dataset examining the global work-force found that despite nurses forming the bedrock of healthcare services only 6% of nurses working in community care were actively involved in health promotion, disease prevention and rehabilitation (WHO, n.d.) (b).

In 1986 the Ottawa Charter sought to elevate the status of health promotion, tasking healthcare systems worldwide to reorient themselves away from diagnosis and treatment of disease and to invest more resources in health promotion and prevention (WHO, 1986). However, more than 30 years on, the dominance of the biomedical model remains entrenched within healthcare systems, with resources for health promotion seemingly to decrease year on year in some countries (Thompson, Watson and Tilford, 2018). This has severe ramifications for nurses' involvement in health promotion as most nurses work within the biomedical model in secondary and primary care institutions which are focused on the diagnosis and treatment of existing disease (Iriarte-Rotata et al., 2020; Watson and Thompson, 2019).

Much of the global burden of disease is non-communicable (NCD), such as cardiovascular diseases, cancer, diabetes, chronic respiratory diseases and mental health disorders. The United Nations has a Sustainable Development Goal (3.4) of reducing global deaths from non-communicable disease by one third by 2030 (United Nations, 2015). Nurses are ideally placed to influence the success of this target. In the UK, Governing Body Nurses (GBNs) have the potential to bring their unique, patient-focused experience and knowledge of holistic care to influence commissioning decisions (RCN, 2012). However, research has shown that clinical expertise is often sidelined in the face of cost effectiveness, budgetary constraints and performance management (Berg, Barry and Chandler, 2008). This added to suggestions of gender bias has left many GBNs dissatisfied with the role and what they are able to achieve within it (Allan et al., 2017). Nevertheless, as time has passed, more and more GBNs appear satisfied that they are contributing positively to the commissioning process and that their voice is being heard. Possibly, it has taken some time to recognise the contributions that nurses can make in what was initially proposed as a wholly medical body (Demsey and Minogue, 2017; O'Driscoll et al., 2018). Professional organisations aim to support their registered members to fulfil their health promotion role. Within the UK the Royal College of Nursing has produced resource frameworks which detail evidence-based practice and provide advice and information for practitioners to utilise when working with their patients (RCN, 2016). Chapter 10, Global health and Chapter 11, The future of health promotion and health education for health professionals pick up the discussion in this section in more detail.

───── Time to Reflect 7.1 ──────────────────────────────

Think of your day-to-day practice. How much of this time is devoted to health promotion and education? Would you like to spend more time with your patients on this aspect of your role? What is stopping you doing this? Is it:

Time restraints? Lack of knowledge of services available? Lack of confidence? Lack of training in certain techniques? Something else?

Think of ways that you can fulfil your health-promotion role within the constraints you are working with.

## Summary

This chapter has outlined the attitudes and skills that nurses need to regularly promote health as a core aspect of their practice. However, it has acknowledged that the dominance of the medical model and restraints associated with clinical care often get in the way of providing health promotion and education. Issues such as short-term patient contact and lack of influencing power especially at junior levels can seem insurmountable. Nevertheless, as practitioners we all need to do what we can within our own sphere. Some roles have more scope and time for health promotion than others, but everyone can act as a role model and influencer, be a teacher to junior staff and students and change the victim-blaming, simplistic culture, to a more nuanced dialogue and so improve the physical and mental well-being of the patients we serve.

───── Key Points ───────────────────────────────────

- Nurses have a duty to undertake health promotion and education as part of their day-to-day practice.
- Generally, they already possess many of the skills required to be successful in this role.
- More specific training in using certain models and techniques is available.
- Nurses need to challenge time and organisational constraints which often see health promotion squeezed out in favour of clinical care delivery.

# References

Allan, H., Dixon, R., Lee, G., Savage, J. and Tapson, C. (2017). Governing body nurses' experiences of clinical commissioning groups: An observational study of two clinical commissioning groups (CCGs) in England. *Journal of Research in Nursing 22*(3), 197–211.

Berg, E., Barry, J. and Chandler, J. (2008). New public management and social work in Sweden and England. Challenges and opportunities for staff in predominantly female organisations. *International Journal of Sociology and Social Policy, 28*(3–4), 114–28.

Cochrane Collaboration. (2008). *Physician Advice for Smoking Cessation (Review).* London. Wiley and Sons.

Coulter, A. and Collins, A. (2011). Making Shared Decision Making a Reality: No decision about me, without me. London: King's Fund.

Demsey, A. and Minogue, V. (2017). The governing body nurse as a clinical commissioning group nurse leader. *Nursing Standard. Royal College of Nursing (Great Britain) 31*(26). Retrieved from https://pubmed.ncbi.nlm.nih.gov/28224866/

Department of Health. (2014). *A Framework for Personalised Care and Population Health for Nurses, Midwives, Health Visitors and Allied Health Professionals.* London: Department of Health.

Department of Health and Social Care. (2013). *Joint Strategic Needs Assessments and Joint Health and Wellbeing Strategies, Statutory Guidance.* London: Department of Health and Social Care.

Dinc, L. and Gastmans, C. (2013). *Trust in nurse-patient relationships: A Literature Review.* Retrieved from https://www.researchgate.net/publication/235681860_Trust_in_Nurse-Patient_Relationships_A_Literature_Review

Dy, S. and Purnell, T. (2012). Key concepts relevant to quality of complex and shared decision making in healthcare: A literature review. *Social Science and Medicine 74,* 582–7.

Egan, G. (2002). *The Skilled Helper.* Pacific Grove, CA: Brooks/Cole.

Gottlieb, L.N. (2013). *Strength-based Nursing Care: Health and healing for person and family.* New York: Springer.

Glasgow, R.E., Emont, S. and Miller, D. (2006). Assessing delivery of the five 'As' for patient-centered counseling. *Health Promotion International 21*(3), 245–55. doi: 10.1093/heapro/dal017

Haseler, C., Crooke, R. and Haseler, T. (2019). Promoting physical activity to patients. *British Medical Journal* l5230. doi: 10.1136/bmj.l5230

Iriarte-Roteta, A., Lopez-Dicastillo, O., Mujika, A., Ruiz-Zaldibar, C. and Hernantes, N. (2020). Nurses' role in health promotion and prevention: A critical interpretive synthesis. *Journal of Clinical Nursing 29*(21–2), 3937–49.

Kelly, M.P., Powell, J.E. and Bartle, N. (2012). Health Needs Assessment. In Detels, R., Karim, Q.A., Baum, F., Li, L. and Leyland, A.H. (Eds). Oxford Textbook of Global Public Health. 7th ed. Oxford, Oxford University Press.

Kemppainen, V., Tossavainen, K. and Turunen, H. (2013). Nurses' roles in health promotion practice: An integrative review. *Health Promotion International 28*(4), 490–501. doi: 10.1093/heapro/das034

Lindson-Hawley, N., Thompson, T. and Begh, R. (2015). *Motivational Interviewing for Smoking Cessation.* Cochrane Database of Systematic Reviews. doi: 10.1002/14651858.cd006936.pub3

Miller, W.R. and Rollnick, S. (2012). *Motivational Interviewing – Helping People Change,* 3rd ed. New York: Guilford Press.

NHS England. (2021). Making research matter: Chief Nursing Officer for England's strategic plan for research. Available at: https://www.england.nhs.uk/publication/making-research-matter-chief-nursing-officer-for-englands-strategic-plan-for-research/

NHS Future Forum (2012). The NHS's role in the public's health. London, NHS Future Forum.

National Institute of Care Excellence (NICE). (2006). *Rapid Review of brief interventions and referral for smoking cessation.* Retrieved from https://www.nice.org.uk/guidance/ng92/evidence/brief-interventions-and-referral-for-smoking-cessation-pdf-4788922142

National Institute of Care Excellence (NICE). (2018). Guidance NG92 *Stop smoking interventions and services.* Retrieved from https://www.nice.org.uk/guidance/ng92

Norcross, J.C., Krebs, P.M. and Prochaska, J.O. (2011). Stages of change. *Journal of Clinical Psychology 67*(2), 143–54.

Nsiah, C., Siakwa, M. and Ninnoni, J. (2019). Registered Nurses' description of patient advocacy in the clinical setting. *Nursing Open 6*(3), 1124–32. doi: 10.1002/nop2.307

Nursing and Midwifery Council (NMC). (n.d.) *The Code.* Retrieved from www.nmc.org.uk/standards/code/

Nursing and Midwifery Council (2018a) *Programme Standards: Standards for pre-registration nursing programmes.* Retrieved from www.nmc.org.uk/globalassets/sitedocuments/standards-of-proficiency/standards-for-pre-registration-nursing-programmes/programme-standards-nursing.pdf

Nursing and Midwifery Council (NMC). (2018b). *Future Nurse: Standards of proficiency for registered nurses.* Retrieved from www.nmc.org.uk/globalassets/sitedocuments/standards-of-proficiency/nurses/future-nurse-proficiencies.pdf.

Nursing and Midwifery Council (NMC). (2019). *Standards of Proficiency for Midwives.* Retrieved from www.nmc.org.uk/globalassets/sitedocuments/standards/standards-of-proficiency-for-midwives.pdf

Oakley, C., Johl, R. and Holber, N. (2018). Holistic patient centred care. *British Journal of Nursing, 27*(4). doi: 10.12968/bjon.2018.27.4.S3

O'Driscoll, M., Allan, H., Lee, G., Savage, J., Tapson, C. and Dixon, R. (2018). Do governing body and CSU nurses on clinical commissioning groups really lead a nursing agenda? Findings from a 2015 Survey of the Commissioning Nurse Leaders' Network Membership. *Journal of Nursing Management 26*(3), 245–55. doi: 10.1111/jonm.12485

Petersen, D.J. and Alexander, G.R. (2001). *Needs Assessment in Public Health: A Practical Guide for Students and Professionals.* New York: Kluwer Academic.

Prochaska, J. and DiClemente, C. (1984). *The Transtheoretical Approach: Crossing traditional boundaries of change.* Homewood, IL: Dow Jones/Irwin.

Public Health England. (2020). Behaviour change: guides for national and local government. Available at: https://www.gov.uk/government/publications/behaviour-change-guide-for-local-government

Rogers, C. (1957). The necessary and sufficient conditions of therapeutic personality change. *Journal of Consulting Psychology 21*(2), 95–103.

Rogers, C.R. (1961). *On Becoming a Person: A therapist's view of psychotherapy.* Boston: Houghton Mifflin,

Royal College of Midwives (RCM). (2017). *Stepping up to Public Health: A new maternity model for women and families, midwives and maternity support workers.* London. Royal College of Midwives. Retrieved from https://www.rcm.org.uk/media/3165/stepping-up-to-public-health.pdf

Royal College of Nursing (RCN). (2012). *Nurse membership on Clinical Commissioning Group governing bodies.* Retrieved from https://www.rcn.org.uk/__data/assets/pdf_file/0007/467611/ccgs_2.pdf

Royal College of Nursing (RCN). (2016). *Nurses 4 public health–. The Value and Contribution of Nursing to Public Health in the UK: Final report.* London: RCN. Retrieved from https://www.rcn.org.uk/clinical-topics/public-health/the-role-of-nursing-staff-in-public-health

Rosengren, D.B. (2017). *Building Motivational Interviewing Skills: A practitioner workbook (Applications of Motivational Interviewing).* 2nd ed. New York: Guilford Press.

Royal Society of Public Health. (2020). *Impact pathways for everyday interactions.* Retrieved from https://www.rsph.org.uk/our-work/policy/wider-public-health-workforce/measuring-public-health-impact.html

Rubak, S., Sandbaek, A., Lauritzen, T. and Christensen, B. (2005). Motivational interviewing: a systematic review and meta-analysis. *British Journal of General Practice 55*(513), 305–12.

Sheehan, R. and Fealy, G. (2020). Trust in the nurse: Findings from a survey of hospitalised children. *Journal of Clinical Nursing 29*(21–2), 4289–99. doi: 10.1111/jocn.15466

Thompson, S.R. (2014). *The Essential Guide to Public Health and Health Promotion.* Abingdon: Routledge.

Thompson, S.R., Watson, M.C. and Tilford, S. (2018). The Ottawa Charter 30 years on: still an important standard for health promotion, *International Journal of Health Promotion and Education 56*(2), 73–84. Retrieved from https://www.tandfonline.com/doi/abs/10.1080/14635240.2017.1415765?journalCode=rhpe20

United Nations General Assembly. (2015). *Transforming our World: the 2030 Agenda for Sustainable Development.* Retrieved from https://sdgs.un.org/goals

Watson, M.C. and Thompson, S. (2019). Nursing crisis: Missed opportunities in promoting the health of the country. *British Medical Journal,* Rapid Response December 2019.

World Health Organization. (1986). *First International Conference on Health Promotion, Ottawa, 21 November 1986.* Retrieved from www.who.int/teams/health-promotion/enhanced-wellbeing/first-global-conference

World Health Organization. (2005). *Summary overview and background to Health Promotion: Globalization, health challenges and the Bangkok Charter 6th Global Conference on Health Promotion in Bangkok, Thailand 7–11 August 2005.* Retrieved from www. who.int/healthpromotion/conferences/6gchp/mediacentre/hpr_backgrounddoc_ summary.pdf

World Health Organization. (2009). *Global standards for the initial education of professional nurses and midwives.* Retrieved from www.who.int/hrh/resources/standards/en/

World Health Organization. (2020). *State of the World's Nursing Report – 2020.* Retrieved from www.who.int/publications/i/item/

World Health Organization. (n.d.) (a). *Nursing and Midwifery.* Retrieved from www. who.int/news-room/fact-sheets/detail/nursing-and-midwifery

World Health Organization. (n.d.) (b). *Improving Health Workforce Data and Evidence.* Retrieved from www.who.int/activities/improving-health-workforce-data-and- evidence

# 8

# Assessing Health Needs

Ivy O'Neil

## Introduction

Assessing a population's health needs is the first step in any healthcare planning activity and fundamental in promoting health, particularly given scarce resources worldwide. According to the WHO's 2020 report, the top global causes of death are associated with cardiovascular, respiratory and neonatal conditions. They can be grouped into communicable, non-communicable and injuries. In 2019, the top ten causes of death were ischaemic heart diseases; stroke; chronic obstructive pulmonary disease; lower respiratory infection; neonatal conditions; trachea, bronchus and lung cancers; Alzheimer's disease and dementias; diarrhoea disease; diabetes and kidney diseases. Seven out of ten leading causes of death were non-communicable. However, in low income countries, the top ten causes of death are neonatal conditions, followed by lower respiratory infections; ischaemic heart disease; stroke; then diarrhoeal diseases; malaria; road injuries; tuberculosis; HIV/AIDS and cirrhosis of liver. Although it's falling significantly, people in these countries are still more likely to die from communicable diseases than non-communicable diseases. In addition, with Covid-19 infection in recent years, it is crucial to assess the current disease burden in order to plan healthcare interventions. But, as we see later in this chapter, disease is only part of the picture of health needs.

Health Need Assessment (HNA) became a common term in the 1990s. In the UK, the 1990 Community Care Act gave local authorities lead responsibility to assess people's needs in their community and plan health care accordingly. It also contributed to ongoing debates on the 'concept of needs'. Worldwide, the growth of consumerism in the 1980s, economic concerns and the need to tackle health inequalities meant that HNA was important for planning services to help allocate resources, to shape and prioritise services. It is a tool aimed at steering health services strategies, identifying unmet needs and giving direction for service development.

In this chapter, we focus on population groups, not individual patients. Population groups can be geographical, community or people with specific health conditions. This chapter is about understanding HNA and how we determine health needs, based on our understanding of 'health' and 'needs', looking at different perspectives and its role in planning healthcare interventions.

By the end of this chapter the reader will:

- Understand what HNA is and how health needs are determined based on our understanding of 'health' and 'needs'.
- Explore the concepts of 'needs'.
- Explore different approaches to HNA – epidemiological, economic or sociological.
- Understand the different HNA models, frameworks or processes.

## Key terms

Epidemiology, community development, Community-Based Participatory Research (CBPR), needs, health needs, Health Needs Assessment (HNA), Joint Strategic Needs Assessment (JSNA), Precede-Proceed Model (PPM), Rapid Participatory Appraisal (RPA)

## Health Needs Assessment (HNA)

HNA is a systematic method for reviewing health issues facing a population, leading to agreed priorities and resources to improve health and reduce health inequalities (Cavanagh and Chadwick, 2005). It is a systematic approach to ensure health services use resources most efficiently to improve the health of the population (Wright, Williams and Wilkinson, 1998), a systematic method of identifying unmet health and healthcare needs of a population and making changes to meet these needs. It provides an excellent opportunity to listen to local voices and involve stakeholders in service planning, promote interagency collaboration and increase ownership and sustainability of service provision (Currie, 2016). Acknowledging limitations of the data used, results are analysed and services planned from the outset, and subsequently, health outcomes can be reviewed and needs assessment developed (Higginson, Hart, Koffman, Selman and Harding, 2007).

For nursing professions, hospital or community, HNA forms part of holistic and integrated care. In the busy practice setting however, there is a danger of failing to see the strategic wood for the immediate trees. The busy-ness of the workplace can work against strategic planning. Professionals often focus on immediate care rather than wider population health and social care needs. Assessing individual needs is a skill of all healthcare professionals. It forms the basis for planning care and has its own narrative in 'person-centred' care. However, planning care for the whole community involves overviewing population health, whether they are your patients or not, so that unmet needs within that community can be identified and health service provision can be determined accordingly.

'Meeting need' is a founding principle of health care. There is a misconception that Public Health and HNA apply only in primary care. The social context of your patients is important. Community nurses, with a good understanding of local community within a multi-professional team, are indeed best placed to assess population needs. However, HNA is also important in secondary services. The health needs of the community where the hospital is situated (the geographic area) or the health needs of groups of patients in hospital setting (diabetes, coronary heart disease .... etc.) are important. Indeed, rehabilitation programmes and discharge preparation start before the patient is discharged, forming part of care planning. Treatment isn't simply about mechanistic and immediate interventions. It's about addressing the underlying causes of illnesses. A community-centred or place-based approach (settings approach to health promotion as discussed in Chapters 4 and 6) offers opportunities to improve health and well-being, reduce health inequalities and develop local solutions (Public Health England (PHE), Association of Directors of Public Health and Local Government Association, 2019). By integrating services and building resilience in communities, individuals can take control of their own health and factors influencing it.

──── Time to Reflect 8.1 ──────────────────────────────────────────

Think about the community around you, what do you think their health needs are?
    What makes you think that there is a need in these areas? Write down your thoughts.

────────────────────────────────────────────────────────────────────

## Defining Health

As we are looking at 'health' 'need' 'assessment', it will be useful to remind ourselves here what we mean by 'health' and look deeper at the concept of 'needs'. As discussed in Chapter 1: *Health and its determinants*, 'health' is a complex concept. The traditional 'medical model of health' measures health in terms of illness whereas the 'social model of health' recognises the many factors that influence health, as seen in the rainbow model of health by Dahlgren and Whitehead (1991). Antonovosky's salutogenic approach to health (1984) provides another perspective. Health is located somewhere along the health-ease-dis-ease continuum. The Sense of Coherence (SOC) in Salutogenesis is about comprehensibility, manageability and meaningfulness; similar to the concept of 'positive health'. However, this positive concept of health can seem vague and difficult to measure (Bowling, 2005).

Using Covid-19 as an example, daily newspaper bulletins are often about confirmed cases, hospitalisations, numbers dying, numbers vaccinated. However, important issues surrounding Covid-19 might include the lack of social support for people with mental health problems, isolation among older people, unreachable family and community support networks, or the fear and stress of contracting illness when meeting friends and family. Indeed, Mana (2021) felt that a salutogenic approach with a strong SOC is an important personal resource during this global crisis. It helps people cope with stress, helping to manage their mental health. For many older people, health can be less about 'the bits of their bodies that aren't working' and more about 'having a laugh', 'having something to do', 'seeing families and friends' (Reed, Cook, Childs and Hall, 2003).

There are also important cultural differences in perceiving health, including age, gender, socio-economic background and ethnicity. Meeting health needs is about improving the quality of life for all. In HNA, it is important to understand the purposes of HNA. What are we assessing? What are the stressors on health? What are we trying to achieve? Do we have the resources to achieve health gain?

## Defining Needs

The concept of needs is central to healthcare provision. Services have to be responsive and proactive to people's needs. Maslow's hierarchy of needs (1954) was one of the earlier motivation theories in psychology. With basic needs met, people would become better workers, constantly striving to move upward, from physical needs to safety and security, love and belongingness, dignity and self-esteem. For Maslow, only when basic needs are met can self-actualisation be achieved, a state of well-being. However, this can sometimes appear overly simplistic and linear. It implies that all higher needs, such as appreciation of relationships, only matter when lower-level needs are met (Higginson et al., 2007).

Bradshaw (1972) viewed needs based on individual's perception. His 'taxonomy of needs' sees 'normative needs' as defined by experts. 'Felt needs' are described as want and 'expressed needs' as demand. 'Comparative needs' are explained as equity. Doyal and Gough (1991) however, define needs in terms of physical survival and personal autonomy, for example, economic and physical security, accommodation, food, clothing, social relationships. 'Needs' is a relative term and based on value judgements. It changes over time, historically, over life courses and in different cultures. It starts with people's own lives, not filtered by what services can afford. Needs are defined by users in the context of their experience (Asadi-Lari, Packham and Gray, 2003; Currie, 2016).

In health practice, needs are largely defined by practitioners, how needs are managed; the accessibility of services and operating criteria. It is defined as demand for services, links to priority setting and resource availability. Practitioners often have a different perspective from their clients. Practitioner views are shaped by ideology, culture, policy and organisational factors. Service users' definitions of need, however, depend on their life experience and expectations. Based on Stevens and Raftery (1994), Wright, Williams and Wilkinson (1998) discussed the relationship between needs, demand and supply. The ideal would be providing services (supply) that meet the identified needs and demands (patient's expressed and felt needs as described by Bradshaw (1972)). When services fail to match needs, inequity arises. Services become inadequate, ineffective, irrelevant and fragmented.

Importantly, people have 'rights' as well as 'needs', their entitlement to receive care. Doyal and Gough (1991) considered health needs and autonomy not only the two universal human needs, but basic human rights. Legislation such as the European Convention on Human Rights; Human Rights Act 1998; United Nations Convention on the Rights of the Child, emphasise the public's 'right' to health care.

---

────── Time to Reflect 8.2 ──────────────────────────────

Think of the last time you assessed the health needs of a group of clients –

- How did you make your assessment?
- Who did you involve in information gathering and developing services?
- How did you prioritise the issues?
- What services have you developed, if any?

---

## Measuring Health

The HNA process is similar to any health research. The difficulties lie with our understanding of health; what being healthy means; medical or social model of health; positive or negative approaches to health; whose needs we are trying to meet, normative needs as seen by professionals or expressed needs as seen by the people themselves; how we reach population groups whom we find hard to reach. Robust data collection can be time-consuming and problematic. Professionals may also have different priorities and commitments. Resources might be limited. Action planning, implementation and evaluation can also be challenging (Tobi, 2016). Stevens, Raftery, Mant and Simpson (2004) and Tobi (2016) look at three different types of HNA – epidemiological (pattern of illness), comparative (services comparison) and corporate (views of stakeholders) assessment. In this chapter, we divide the approaches into epidemiological, economical and sociological.

## Epidemiology and epidemiological approach to measuring health

Epidemiology is the cornerstone of public health and is primarily disease-centred. It is the study of the distribution and determinants of health and disease frequency in populations to promote wellness and prevent diseases (Regmi and Gee, 2016). The basic principle of epidemiology is that diseases occur in patterns. Patterns are predictable and can be analysed systematically, allowing prediction and generalisation. The role of epidemiology is asking questions, such as what is the magnitude of a health problem – what, to whom, when, where, why and how diseases happen.

One of the main purposes of epidemiology is to break the link between cause and effect, ultimately improving health, both in communicable and non-communicable diseases. Understanding the characteristics of disease patterns provides scientific and measurable evidence leading to the control and prevention of ill-health. The core function is evaluating health and healthcare needs; establishing strategies and policies to meet the needs of the people; monitoring and evaluating any changes for health improvement (Williams and Wright, 1998).

Epidemiology is a population science. It compares groups of people with and without a disease, and groups exposed and not exposed to a possible risk factor. Understanding demography is important to the understanding and interpretation of epidemiological data as its findings are drawn from and applied to people. Population data such as population size, age distribution, socio-economic status … etc. are important in helping practitioners understand health patterns while deciding approaches to good health.

Decreases in mortality and fertility rates in recent decades with the improvement of medical technology and socio-economic environment have led to a change in population age distributions – both epidemiologic and demographic transitions (Gerstman, 2013). There is an increased number of older people as well as an increase in people's life expectancy. Patterns of illnesses have also changed from the domination of communicable towards non-communicable diseases, from genes and germ theory in the nineteenth century, to behavioural and lifestyle choices in the twentieth and twenty-first centuries, coupled with social, economic and environmental influences in health (Krieger, 2011). In this section, we discuss traditional epidemiology and not 'lay epidemiology' which is a term to describe how lay people understand and interpret health risks (Allmark and Tod, 2006) or other alternative theories such as social or ecological epidemiologic perspectives as discussed by Krieger (2011). Two main types of traditional epidemiology are considered here – descriptive and analytical epidemiology.

Health and diseases are influenced by multiple factors as discussed in Chapter 1: *Health and its determinants*. Disease patterns grow from the interactions between groups of individuals and environment over time – the susceptibility of the host such as genetics, age, gender; the capacity of the microbiological agent to cause disease and the influence of the environment such as air, water, food, overcrowding, showing a multifactorial causation theory. Descriptive epidemiology provides information on the frequency and distribution of diseases – what, who, where and when. It is about disease in terms of person, place and time. It can be studied via records and surveillance data, cross-sectional or longitudinal surveys, looking at quantifiable data such as mortality and morbidity, incidence and prevalence of illnesses, admission episodes, birth data such as premature, stillbirth and low birth weight. Analytical epidemiology identifies associations between disease and possible causes, risk factors, and modes of transmission contributing to the development of diseases – why and how, and can be studied using experimental designs such as randomised control trials or observational studies such as cohort studies or case-control studies, comparing groups of people (Gerstman, 2013; Krieger, 2011; Green, Cross, Woodall and Tones, 2019).

Epidemiology deals with the increase of cases and possibility of outbreak, why and how diseases happened, linking clusters of cases, so that risk of developing the disease can be measured and predicted, and prevention strategies can be planned. Epidemiological studies attempt to find the links between environment and health, to support evidence-based practice. Descriptive epidemiology looks for patterns, generates hypotheses. Analytical epidemiology tests hypotheses, studies the causes, effects and risk factors of diseases. A descriptive study of Covid-19 might be a case series describing person, place, and time of the people with Covid-19 whereas an analytical study is about studying the causes and risks of people getting Covid-19.

However, there are limitations in research studies such as chance, bias, confounding as well as practical and ethical considerations. Causal relationships or associations can be difficult to determine. Even with the well-known Bradford Hill criteria used in epidemiological studies, we need to be cautious with research findings (Lucas and McMichael, 2005). With our rapidly changing complex environment in the twenty-first century with a slow change in population genetics over time, risk factors are not constant and may become ubiquitous and an invisible cause of diseases (Pearce, 2011). Pearce viewed epidemiological research as a process of study rather than specific methods.

Using obesity as an example, there are numerous debates and studies about the causes of obesity ranging from genetic, high energy intake, inactivity, cultural and behavioural factors or other environmental variants that make up our obesogenic environment such as transport, energy resources and availability, education, indoor vs outdoor entertainment. Traditional epidemiological studies may not be sufficient to identify actual causes of illnesses. Different types of study designs including ecological studies or other methods within the non-randomised controlled trial paradigm could play a role both in finding the cause of illnesses and variations between different populations, environments and time periods.

There are many challenges in using epidemiological approaches to assess health needs. Research data can be influenced by many factors. Health statistics may be incomplete or misleading; data may be inaccurate or misinterpreted. Data collection processes may not be robust. Over-reliance on epidemiology may distract us from other investigations of ill-health. There are also critics who view epidemiology as a second-rate science. Causal relationships are inferred rather than observed, for example, smoking causes lung cancer (Parascandola, 1998).

Public health data can be obtained locally from census information, public health and research reports, population and community surveys, views of the people and stakeholders in the community; nationally from government reports such as those published in Public Health England in the UK, Centre for Disease Control and Prevention in the US, or internationally from Public Health Observatory or the World Health Organization.

The epidemiological approach to HNA can seem to measure the ill-health of a population – the higher the incidence of a particular illness, the higher its needs. Indicators such as mortality rates inform practitioners or policy makers how unhealthy the population is rather than what their needs are. Epidemiological approaches are based on the assumption that experts know best. They measure negative health, attempt to quantify illnesses, measure symptoms rather than causes of illnesses. The causes of ill-health and the interactions of social, economic and environmental factors are complex. A decrease in mortality rates does not necessarily mean a nation is healthier. It could mean additional morbidities in long-term conditions while also failing to address other, more positive, indicators of health. It reflects a 'medical model' of health, viewing needs as diseases and illnesses rather than people's experience (Williams and Wright, 1998).

Using a non-systematic literature review of descriptive epidemiological evidence, Bundle, O'Connell, O'Connor and Bone (2018) carried out a HNA to assess the risk of indoor overheating as part of the 2017 UK Climate Change Risk Assessment. It showed potentially fatal health hazards that require actions from service providers and policy makers at both individual and population level. In another example by Clarke, Beenstock, Lukacs, Turner and Limmer (2018), a quantitative cross-sectional survey for a school-based HNA on the importance of sexual orientation as a key factor contributing to the children and young people's mental and physical health, the team acknowledged that a qualitative component would have produced more in-depth data enabling a wider and deeper understanding of the issues. Research funded by the Joseph Rowntree Foundation showed that focusing on older people's infirmities (a 'deficit' model) was too limiting and pathological. Likewise a 'heroic model' (successful ageing only with heroics like 'bunjee jumping') did not reflect older people's own experiences and hopes of healthy ageing (Reed, Cook, Childs and Hall, 2003).

---

### Tutorial Trigger 8.1

Look into the public health department responsible for the health of the people where you work or live, e.g., the most recent report from your regional public health observatory, and locate the health issues mentioned in the report. What does it tell you? Does it reflect the health needs of the people around you? Based on your knowledge of these people, think about what being healthy means and different types of needs: is there anything you can add to the report about the health of them?

---

## Economic approach

From the policy maker's point of view, HNA often means 'Health Care Need' Assessment (HCNA). The terms HNA and HCNA are often used interchangeably (Tobi, 2016). Healthcare needs are defined as the capacity to benefit from health care – the greater ability to benefit, the greater the need (Stevens and Gillam, 1998; Tobi, 2016). It is about cost-effectiveness, a way to manage resources and justify the need for services. It's a common approach for health service managers, gaining evidence for service development. It attempts to show evidence-based decision-making – the rationing of costs, demand and supply. Words like 'impact', 'priority', 'effectiveness' and 'need' become interchangeable – an outcome-focused service, looking at the effectiveness of treatment to deliver significant health gain.

HNA using economic approaches is based on the assessment of needs on health service provision, focusing on 'health care' rather than 'health'. Indeed, needs assessment has been advocated as a means of containing the growth of health costs (Bradshaw, 1994; Currie, 2016; Stevens and Raftery, 1994, 1997). It can be highly political. The purpose of HNA becomes a justification for funding. The emphasis is also on achieving equity (Powell, 2006; Tobi, 2016). It also minimises the input of lay people in the decision of service provision (Asadi-Lari, Packham and Gray, 2003). In countries with few economic resources, the term 'ability' to benefit can also be problematic (Higginson, Hart, Koffman, Selman and Harding, 2007).

## Sociological approach

It has long been acknowledged that poverty and deprivation link to health and health inequalities (Marmot, Allen, Goldblatt, Boyce and Morrison, 2020;

Marmot, Allen, Goldblatt, Herd and Morrison, 2020; Williams, Buck and Babalola, 2020). Successive governments globally have used sociological tools to measure poverty and deprivation since the 1970s, such as the Index of Multiple Deprivations (IMD) used in England (Ministry of Housing, Communities and Local Government, 2019); Official Poverty and Supplemental Poverty Measure (Institute for Research on Poverty, 2021) and the Social Vulnerability Index (SVI) used by the Centre for Disease Control (CDC) in the US (Agency for Toxic Substances and Disease Registry (ATSDR), 2021). These are useful social and economic indicators measuring deprivation. It can also provide useful supportive information on community resources and assets, helping plan strategies for health improvement.

One of the aims of HNA, other than improving health, is to reduce health inequalities. Improving health and tackling health inequalities require actions on all factors that influence health. Sociological approaches are less pathological in measuring health. They encompass the essence of holistic health, the social model of health. According to Hooper and Longworth (2002), the three underpinning principles in HNA are:

- improving health and inequalities
- integrating the improvement in health into the planning processes
- involving people who know about the health issues in a community.

## Community development approach and participatory methods

A community HNA is a participatory and collaborative process examining population needs using community health information via consulting with local people and those working in the community. It includes lay perspectives for health. People in the community know their own situation best. A partnership project between hospital, public health and the nursing school is an example of a community HNA of a rural community in the US by Van Gelderen, Krumwiede, Krumwiede, and Fenske (2018) using a Community Based Collaborative Action Research framework. The process encouraged community engagement, ensuring local voices were heard, recognising strengths and assets within the community. It also supported people's abilities to make decisions to improve health. Such processes can be time-consuming, but can be fluid, dynamic and empowering.

Another study by Chhabra (2018) in a community-based hospital in Kenya used focus groups of community gatekeepers and affected community members (teachers, caregivers, community health workers and youth), followed by a quantitative survey with adolescents themselves to identify perceived community needs of orphans and vulnerable children with HIV. The study highlighted the broader impoverished social context and structure shaping their development and behaviour, showing they are at increased risk of poor physical, social and mental health.

The use of Community Based Participatory Research (CBPR) approaches is quite common in community HNA. The process involves community members, practitioners and researchers to provide insights and knowledge of a community, and identify barriers (Harmon et al., 2021). A Congregational HNA tool developed by Harmon et al. for faith organisations allowing a comprehensive assessment of individual, social and environmental health needs using CBPR approaches found that interdisciplinary work can be challenging. Academic partners tend to be more involved in the developmental stage with healthcare partners only at implementation onwards. This led to some hesitancy for healthcare partners to take ownership of the developed service. They also felt that trust among stakeholders and finding a common language between academics and the community challenging. It is therefore important to emphasise shared and equal power among partners.

CBPR promotes capacity building, empowering, educating and is context relevant. It enhances members' agency and capacity for achieving social change (Dugan et al., 2021). Involving people early in the process can provide insights into social, cultural and environmental contexts that determine health. However, community members are often only involved in interventions after the HNA has been conducted, with interventions decided by academic researchers and public health officials. A workforce HNA by Dugan et al. (2021) found that a tailored participatory survey including community members as equitable collaborators in every phase of the research process could identify health issues undetectable by conventional top-down methods and provided interventions that address root causes of poor health. A similar study by Jaegers et al. (2020) on workplace mental health interventions in rural and urban jails agreed CBPR was useful in identifying health needs to inform tailored and evidence-based health promotion and protection interventions.

Interventions based on CBPR can be more relevant, acceptable, appropriate, credible and compatible with the organisational culture. However, involving the community can be time-intensive and demanding on resources. There are other challenges including issues of informed consent, discrimination based on socio-demographic characteristics and misuse of power and privilege (Dugan et al., 2021).

## Rapid Participatory Appraisal (RPA)

RPA is a useful tool in assessing health needs from a community and sociological perspective, emphasising the WHO's primary healthcare principles of equity, participation and multi-sectorial cooperation (Annett and Rifkin, 1995). It is a profile of a community built from information on different aspects of the community including: (1) national, regional and local policies, (2) existing current services, and (3) socio-ecological factors influencing the health and composition of communities. Information is usually collected from interviews with key informants and stakeholders (Annett and Rifkin, 1995; Murray, 1999; Palmer, 1999). It can enhance decision-making, gaining insight into communities, identifying needs, setting priorities and developing services, offering a relatively quick and cost-effective means for service users to determine their own health needs, influence policy change and resource allocation, a first step in assessing needs and planning service provision (Palmer, 1999).

A key role in global nursing is the promotion of health and well-being, promoting the United Nations' Sustainable Development Goals (2016). Cho et al. (2018) used RPA to assess the health needs of a rural community in Vietnam. It is an effective way to collect comprehensive community data quickly within a cultural context. Paradoxically, it can be time consuming rather than rapid, as it requires commitment from team members. Bergeron (1999) found that relying primarily on qualitative methods can also be limiting. He suggested adding quantitative methods to enhance the findings.

RPA is useful in Community Diagnosis in the assessment of the health and healthcare needs of a local community, providing insights into the social and environmental factors that influence health in the community (Davison et al., 1999). Green, Cross, Woodall and Tones (2019) prefer the term 'community analysis' in profiling a community. It gives a broader remit for the process, emphasising the positive aspects of a community. Similarly, environmental scanning is another tool that healthcare organisations can use as part of strategic planning to examine a specific health issue, assessing community needs as well as for programme and policy development. It is a process of gathering and analysing information of an organisation's external and internal environments to inform change (Charlton et al., 2021). However, definitions and methodology lack clarity. Rowel (2005) felt this could weaken efficacy for public health practice as it can easily be confused with other HNA tools.

## Precede-Proceed Planning Model (PPM)

Precede-Proceed planning model (PPM) is a valuable health promotion model for planning health promotion interventions. It consists of two clear phases – assessment and implementation. It is population-centred with a social-ecological and educational emphasis. It is also context and quality of life focused, through active participation of stakeholders (Handyside, Warren, Devine, Drovandi, 2021a, 2021b; Porter, 2016). The model can provide practical guidance in the HNA process. In a narrative study on HNA by community pharmacy, Handyside, Warren, Devine, Drovandi (2021b) found that PPM is useful to gain insight into the health need of a local community and in the development and evaluation of community pharmacy interventions. However, application of the model as a tool for HNA was limited. None of their reviewed studies prioritised community health needs, actively engaged all stakeholders or used all elements of the model. Applications could have been further developed by applying public health principles advocated in the model more fully.

## Joint Strategic Needs Assessment (JSNA)

As can be seen in the social model of health, all local government functions link to and have impacts on our health. The public health reforms in 2013 in England were generally welcomed, to improve health outcomes. Since the reforms, there has been better integration between public health and the wider public service functions, but with some fragmentation of service provisions. The main concerns are about the ever-shrinking public health budget (Buck, 2020). Local authorities need to focus more on 'place' based population health systems, such as developments in transport, education and economic development rather than focusing on 'people' functions only, such as children's services, adult health and social care, culture and leisure (Buck, 2020).

JSNA is a process that helps analyse health needs to inform and guide commissioning of health and social care services within a local authority. UK NHS Commissioners and local authorities have a statutory obligation to carry out JSNA and agree joint health and well-being strategies, through the Health and Wellbeing Board (DH, 2011, 2013; Local Government Improvement and Development, 2011; Tobi, 2016). People from different parts of the community must be included in the process to ensure a genuine voice, including people with particular communication needs. Their views and experience of local services, their needs and assets should be included as part of qualitative evidence in the planning of services. The core function of a JSNA is to identify inequalities and involves the community in service planning, improving their health outcomes (Tobi, 2016).

A good JSNA should include an assessment of the assets, strengths and capacities of local communities. Health and well-being are shaped by social, economic and environmental determinants. The challenge of persistent health inequalities cannot be satisfactorily addressed by one agency. Partnership is part of the solution (Tobi, 2016). An example of this in assessing the hearing needs of local populations was co-produced by NHS England, the Local Government Association and the Association of Directors of Public Health and PHE (NHS England, 2019). It showed that evidence can be brought together to meet the health needs of people with hearing impairment.

With the already-mentioned concepts of positive health and Salutogenesis, assets are about the strengths (capabilities and skills) of people as against needs which can be framed as deficits. It asks questions such as what have we already got, in ourselves and in our community; what makes us strong and healthy?

Assets-based approaches such as JSNA promote well-being by building social capital. They mobilise the community to use its own assets to solve its own problems (Macdowall, Bonell and Davies, 2006). They aspire to more than deficit models such as the medical model of health and negative health, promoting the population as co-producers of health, not just consumers of health services; strengthen the capacity of individuals and communities, realising potential and contributing to equitable and sustainable health, social and economic development (Macdowall, Bonell and Davies, 2006). Some variants of asset-based approaches are asset mapping, asset-based community development, appreciative inquiry, participatory appraisal (Improvement and Development Agency (IDeA), 2010).

## HNA on Covid-19

Covid-19 since early 2020 has affected lives on an unimaginable scale, not only in deaths, long Covid, but also mental health and isolation. In addition, there have been long delays, suspension and inaccessibility of both urgent, routine treatment and preventive services, particularly for those already in at-risk groups. With the lack of opportunity for face-to-face community participatory work because of lockdown, qualitative information is restricted to individual telephone or smaller scale group internet interviews, for example, Skype, Zoom.

With the present Covid-19 crisis, there is an urgent need for a comprehensive HNA for health-promotion services both in primary and secondary care services.

Wilson et al. (2021) demonstrated how digital information can be used to support services. They fuse multiple data sources into health intelligence through a Health Intelligence Atlas (HI-Atlas) that provides visualisations to identify high-risk locations and ensure an equitable vaccination programme for all residents. HI-Atlas uses existing traditional surveillance data to generate appropriate health intelligence to support proactive, effective and efficient planning and monitoring of Covid-19 vaccine preparedness and distribution in counties and states in the US.

Epidemiological approaches using existing public health surveillance data can be valuable for HNA. Crowdsourcing of internet data in participatory public health research can assist in JSNA in our Big Data environment (O'Neil, 2019). Our current internet capability can provide opportunities for data collection within 'social distancing' regulations. In our digitally enhanced environment, many have become digitally skilled, although, one needs to be aware that there is a danger of widening the health inequality gap even further between those digitally skilled and those whose digital access, skills or aspirations are poor (O'Neil, 2019).

---

**Point to Ponder 8.1**

Think of your experience, when you planned your health promotion intervention, did you go through a systematic health need assessment process?

What are the challenges you have come across when assessing your client's or your community's health need?

---

## HNA Process

Quantitative measurement of health using epidemiological approaches is valuable in identifying population health issues. However, involving people in assessing their own health needs adds a more comprehensive dimension. HNA is an important activity for public health practitioners and many healthcare professionals. In the past 20 years, other than the above mentioned Rapid Appraisal, JSNA and CBPR, various frameworks and guidance have been published to help practitioners assess community health and compile HNAs. For example, the Community-as-Partner model as discussed by Anderson and McFarlarne (2008) is well-known in public health nursing for the development of community-based interventions. An example of community participation in teenage pregnancy prevention using this model with the community assessment wheel and the nursing process was demonstrated by Oyedele, Wright and Maja (2014). PHE also provided simple guidance for health visitors and school nurses to assess the health needs of children aged 0–19 (PHE, 2021). This guidance follows three stages in the process – identifying need, identifying assets and determining priorities for actions. Cavanagh and Chadwick (2005) also provided a detailed useful HNA guide based on Hooper and Longworth's HNA workbook (2002).

Assessing health needs and improving health outcomes is a cycle. The diagram below (Figure 8.1 – A Health Need Assessment Cycle) provides a simple guide for practitioners to complete an evidence-based HNA for their target population, showing the cyclical process. The data could be collected from:

- Existing quantitative data
  - demographic data (census, IMD index ... )
  - epidemiological data (mortality, morbidity, prevalence, incidence ... )
  - hospital data (admission, discharge, waiting list ... )
  - GP Practice data (patient records ... )
  - public health report / national statistics
  - service audits

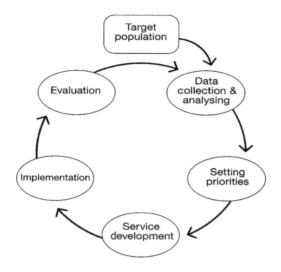

**Figure 8.1**  A Health Needs Assessment Cycle

- Existing qualitative data such as people's knowledge can be obtained via interviews or focus group discussions:
  - ○ practitioners and stakeholders knowledge
  - ○ community and service users knowledge
- Information gaps:
  - ○ Any gaps identified can also be added through quantitative or qualitative methods

## Summary

Health promotion is a social movement for justice in health. It is not just about improving health outcomes, but also about reducing health inequalities and promoting health equity. The principles of health promotion are clearly stated in the Ottawa Charter. The three broad activities are working with communities, influencing policies and communicating about health (Cross et al., 2021). Health promotion services need to be appropriate and accessible, meeting the unmet health needs of the people, tackling the root causes of ill-health. HNA is an important and necessary first step to service planning. To improve population health, we need to know what being healthy means and whose needs we are assessing as well as how to achieve health gain, looking into the factors influencing our health.

Epidemiological approaches in HNA are very useful to show people's health status. Making strategic and policy decisions about health matters also needs to involve the people themselves, listening to everyone's voices, including the multidisciplinary team as well as balancing available resources, making use of community assets and strengths. The sociological approach is empowering and enabling, provide a fuller insight of the health of the population. It is a cyclical and co-production health-promoting activity that needs to involve everyone throughout the different stages to achieve health gain (Dugan et al., 2021; Harmon et al., 2021).

There are other forms of assessment in health that students may come across which are not included in this chapter, for example, Health Impact Assessment, Integrated Impact Assessment, Health Equity Audit ... etc. Specifically, HNA is about the health of the population, the starting point is the people, whereas others are about measuring the impact of a programme or a policy, where the starting point is the service (Tobi, 2016).

This chapter has examined a range of approaches to HNA. It is important to be aware of the different implications depending upon the approach adopted. It is also important to be aware of different definitions of health and concepts of needs to understand how these different paradigms can influence our assessment of health. There is a wealth (but also a lack) of suitable evidence. In this chapter we have outlined some of the available sources. It is crucial to keep in mind the questions for which we are seeking answers, and not simply be driven by the available evidence.

---

### Point to Ponder 8.2

Consider Covid-19 (or any health issue or population group that you are interested in), use one of the systematic frameworks mentioned above, make a plan on how you would carry out a HNA in the community where you are based.

---

### ——— Key Points ———

- HNA is a systematic method of identifying unmet health and healthcare needs of a population.
- 'Needs' is a relative term and based on value judgements. Different people, different professionals view needs differently.
- Epidemiological, economical and sociological are three broad approaches to assess the health needs of a population.
- Health promotion services need to be appropriate and accessible, meeting the unmet health needs of the people, tackling the root causes of ill health.

# References

Agency for Toxic Substances and Disease Registry (ATSDR). (2021). *The Social Vulnerability Index (SVI) used by the Centre for Disease Control (CDC) in the US*. Available at: www.atsdr.cdc.gov/

Allmark, P.J. and Tod, A. (2006). How should public health professionals engage with lay epidemiology? *Journal of Medical Ethics 32*(8), 460–3.

Anderson, E.T. and Mcfarlarne, J. (2008). *Community as Partner: Theory and Practice in Nursing*. 5th Ed. Crawfordsville: Lippincott.

Annett, H. and Rifkin, S.B. (1995). *Guidelines for Rapid Participatory Appraisals to Assess Community Health Needs: A focus on health improvements for low income urban and rural areas*. Division of Strengthening of Health Services. Geneva: WHO.

Antonovosky, A. (1984). The Sense of Coherence as a determinant of health. In J.D. Matarazzo, S.M. Weiss, J.A. Herd and N.E. Miller (Eds)., *Behavioural Health: A handbook of Health Enhancement and Disease Prevention*. New York: John Wiley.

Asadi-Lari, M., Packham, C. and Gray, D. (2003). Need for redefining needs. *Health and Quality of Life Outcomes 1*, 34. Available at: www.hqlo.com/content./1/1/34

Bergeron, G. (1999). *Rapid Appraisal Methods for the Assessment, Design, and Evaluation of Food Security Programs*. Washington, D.C.: International Food Policy Research Institute. Available at: http://www.rmportal.net/framelib/rapid-appraisal-methods.pdf

Bowling, A. (2005). *Measuring Health: A Review of Quality of Life Measurement Scale*. 3rd Ed. United Kingdom: Open University Press.

Bradshaw, J. (1972). A Taxonomy of social need. In G. Maclachlan (Ed.), *Problems and Progress in Medical Care*. 6th Ed. Oxford: Oxford University Press.

Bradshaw, J. (1994). The conceptualisation and measurement of need: A social policy perspective. In J. Popay and G. Williams (Eds), *Research the People's Health*. London: Routledge.

Buck, D. (2020). *The English Local Government Public Health Reforms: An independent assessment*. London: The King's Fund.

Bundle, N., O'Connell, E., O'Connor, N. and Bone A. (2018). A public health needs assessment for domestic indoor overheating. *Public Health 161*, 147–53.

Cavanagh, S. and Chadwick, K. (2005). *Health Needs Assessment – a Practical Guide*. London: Health Development Agency.

Charlton, P., Kean, T., Liu, R.H., et al. (2021). Use of environmental scans in health services delivery research: A scoping review. *BMJ Open* 2021; 11:e050284. doi:10.1136/bmjopen-2021-050284

Chhabra, R., Teitelman, N., Silver, E.J., Raufman, J. and Bauman, L.J. (2018). Vulnerability multiplied: Health needs assessment of 13–18-year-old female orphan and vulnerable children in Kenya. *World Medical and Health Policy 1*(2), 129–45.

Cho, S., Lee, H., Yoon, S., Kim, Y., Levin, P.F. and Kim, E. (2018). Community health needs assessment: a nurses' global health project in Vietnam. *International Nursing Review 65*, 505–14.

Clarke, A., Beenstock, J., Lukacs, J.N., Turner, L. and Limmer, M. (2018). Major risk factors for sexual minority young people's mental and physical health: findings from a county-wide school-based health needs assessment. *Journal of Public Health* 41(3), e274–e282.

Cross, R., Warwick-Booth, L., Rowlands, S., Woodall, J., O'Neil, I. and Foster, S. (2021). *Health Promotion: Global Principles and Practice*, 2nd Ed. Oxfordshire: CABI.

Currie, C. (2016). *Approaches to the assessment of health care needs, utilisation and outcomes and the evaluation of health and health care by* Blackwood R. and Bindra, R. (2009). Available at: www.healthknowledge.org.uk/public-health-textbook/research-methods/1c-health-care-evaluation-health-care-assessment

Dahlgren, G. and Whitehead, M. (1991). *Policies and Strategies to Promote Social Equity in Health*. Stockholm: Institute of Future Studies.

Davison, H., Capewell, S., McNaughton, J., Murray, S.A., Hanlon, P. and McEwen, J. (1999). Community-oriented medical education in Glasgow: developing a community diagnosis exercise. *Medical Education 33*, 55–62.

Department of Health. (2011). *Joint Strategic Needs Assessment and Joint Health and Wellbeing Strategies Explained Commissioning for Populations*. London: HMSO.

Department of Health. (2013). *Statutory Guidance on Joint Strategic Needs Assessments and Joint Health and Wellbeing Strategies*. London: HMSO. Available at: www.gov.uk/government/uploads/system/uploads/attachment_data/file/223842/Statutory-Guidance-on-Joint-Strategic-Needs-Assessments-and-Joint-Health-and-Wellbeing-Strategies-March-2013.pdf

Doyal, L. and Gough, I. (1991). *A Theory of Human Need*. Basingstoke and London: Macmillan.

Dugan, A.G., Namazi, S., Cavallari, J.M., et al. (2021). Participatory survey design of a workforce health needs assessment for correctional supervisors. *American Journal of Industrial Medicine 64*, 414–30. Available at: https://doi.org/10.1002/ajim.23225

Gerstman, B.B. (2013). *Epidemiology Kept Simple*. 3rd Ed. Chichester, West Sussex: John Wiley & Sons.

Green, J., Cross, R., Woodall, J. and Tones, K. (2019). *Health Promotion, Planning and Strategies*. 4th Ed. London: Sage Publications.

Handyside, L., Warren, R., Devine, S. and Drovandi, A. (2021a). Health needs assessment in a regional community pharmacy using the PRECEDE-PROCEED model. *Research in Social and Administrative Pharmacy 17*, 1151–8.

Handyside, L., Warren, R., Devine, S. and Drovandi, A. (2021b). Utilisation of the PRECEDE-PROCEED model in community pharmacy for health needs assessment: A narrative review. *Research in Social and Administrative Pharmacy 17*, 292–9.

Harmon, B.E., Rose, N.E., Pichon, L.C., et al., (2021). Developing a Congregational Health Needs Assessment: Lessons learned from using a participatory research approach. *Progress in Community Health Partnerships: Research, Education, and Action 15*(1), 47–58.

Higginson, I.J., Hart, S., Koffman, J., Selman, L. and Harding, R. (2007). Needs assessments in palliative care: An appraisal of definitions and approaches used. *Journal of Pain and Symptom Management 33*(5), 500–5.

Hooper, J. and Longworth, P. (2002). *Health Needs Assessment Workbook*. London: Health Development Agency. Available at: www.hda.nhs.uk/publications

Improvement and Development Agency (IDeA). (2010). *A Glass Half-full: How an asset approach can improve community health and well-being*. The Local Government Association.

Institute for Research on Poverty. (2021). *How is Poverty Measured?* Available at: www.irp.wisc.edu/resources/how-is-poverty-measured/

Jaegers, L.A., Ahmad, S.O., Scheetz, G., et al. (2020). Total worker health needs assessment to identify workplace mental health interventions in rural and urban jails. *American Journal of Occupational Therapy 74*(3), 1–12. Available at: https://doi.org/10.5014/ajot.2020.036400

Krieger, N. (2011). *Epidemiology and the People's Health: Theory and Context*. New York: Oxford University Press.

Local Government Improvement and Development. (2011). *Joint Strategic Needs Assessment: A springboard for action*. Local Government Improvement and Development.

Lucas, R.M. and McMichael, A.J. (2005). Association or causation: evaluating links between environment and disease. *Bulletin of the World Health Organisation*, Oct., 83(10), 792–5.

Macdowall, W., Bonell, C. and Davies, M. (2006). *Health Promotion Practice*. Open University Press.

Mana, A., Grossi-Milani, R., Dolphine Fuentes Penachiotti, F., et al. (2021). Salutogenesis in the time of COVID-19: What coping resources enable people to face the crisis and stay well? International and longitudinal study. *Academia Letters*, Article 4322. Available at: https://doi.o2rg/10.20935/AL4322

Marmot, M., Allen, J., Goldblatt, P., Herd, E. and Morrison, J. (2020). *Build Back Fairer: The COVID-19 Marmot Review. The Pandemic, Socioeconomic and Health Inequalities in England*. London: Institute of Health Equity.

Marmot, M., Allen, J., Goldblatt, P., Boyce, T. and Morrison, J. (2020). *Health Equity in England: The Marmot Review 10 years on*. London: Institute of Health Equity. Available at: https://www.kingsfund.org.uk/publications/what-are-health-inequalities

Maslow, A.H. (1954). *Motivation and Personality*. New York: Harper.

Ministry of Housing, Communities and Local Government. (2019). *The English Indices of Deprivation* 2019 (IoD2019). *National Statistic release*. Available at: www.gov.uk/MHCLG

Murray, S. (1999). Experiences with 'rapid appraisal' in primary care: Involving the public in assessing health needs, orientating staff, and educating medical students. *British Medical Journal* 318, 440–4. Available at: http://bmj.bmjjournals.com/cgi/content/full/318/7181/440

NHS (National Health Service) England. (2019). *Joint Strategic Needs Assessment Guidance*. Local Government Association, the Association of Directors of Public Health and Public Health England.

O'Neil, I. (2019). *Digital Health Promotion: A Critical Introduction*. Cambridge: Polity.

Oyedele, O.A., Wright, S.C.D. and Maja, T.M.M. (2014). Community participation in teenage pregnancy prevention using the community-as-partner model. *International Journal of Nursing and Midwifery 6*(6), 80–9. doi: 10.5897/IJNM2014.0137

Palmer, C. (1999). Rapid appraisal of needs in reproductive health care in Southern Sudan: Qualitative studies. *British Medical Journal* 319, 743–8. Available at: http://bmj.bmjjournals.com/cgi/content/full/319/7212/743

Parascandola, M. (1998). Epidemiology: Second-rate science? *Public Health Reports* 113(4), 312–20.

Pearce, N. (2011). Epidemiology in a changing world: Variation, causation and ubiquitous risk factors. *International Journal of Epidemiology* 40, 503–12. doi:10.1093/ije/dyq257

Porter, C.M. (2016). Revisiting Precede–Proceed: A leading model for ecological and ethical health promotion. *Health Education Journal* 75(6), 753–64.

Powell, J. (2006). *Health Needs Assessment: A systematic approach*. London: National Library for Health.

Public Health England (PHE). (2021). *Population Health Needs Assessment: A guide for 0 to 19 health visiting and school nursing services*. Available at: www.gov.uk/government/publications/commissioning-of-public-health-services-for-children/population-health-needs-assessment-a-guide-for-0-to-19-health-visiting-and-school-nursing-services#what-is-health-needs-assessment

Public Health England, Association of Directors of Public Health, Local Government Association. (2019). *Health Inequalities: Place-based approaches to reduce inequalities*. GOV.UK website. Available at: www.gov.uk/government/publications/health-inequalities-place-based-approaches-to-reduce-inequalities

Reed, J., Cook, G., Childs, S. and Hall, A. (2003). *Getting Old is Not for Cowards. Comfortable, healthy ageing*. York: Joseph Rowntree Foundation, York Publishing Services.

Regmi, K. and Gee, I. (2016). *Public Health Intelligence*. Switzerland: Springer International Publishing.

Rowel, R., Moore, N.D. and Nowrojee, S. (2005). The utility of the environmental scan for public health practice: Lessons from an urban program to increase cancer screening. *Journal of National Medical Association* 97, 527–34.

Stevens, A. and Gillam, S. (1998). Needs assessment: From theory to practice. *British Medical Journal 316*, 1448–52.

Stevens, A. and Raftery, J. (1994). *Health Care Needs Assessment: The Epidemiologically Based Needs Assessment Reviews*. Oxford: Radcliffe Medical Press.

Stevens, A. and Raftery, J. (1997). *Health Care Needs Assessment: The Epidemiologically Based Needs Reviews, 2nd series*. Oxford: Radcliffe Medical Press.

Stevens, A., Raftery, J., Mant, J. and Simpson, S. (2004). *Health Care Needs Assessment: The Epidemiologically Based Needs Assessment Reviews*. Oxford: Radcliffe Medical Press.

Tobi, P. (2016). Health Needs Assessment. In K. Regmi and I. Gee, (Eds) *Public Health Intelligence*. Switzerland: Springer International Publishing.

United Nations. (2016). The Sustainable Development Goals 2016. *Working Papers, eSocial Sciences*. Available at: https://econpapers.repec.org/paper/esswpaper/id_3a11456.htm

Van Gelderen, S.A., Krumwiede, K.A., Krumwiede, N.K. and Fenske, C. (2018). Frameworks for community-based health promotion; Trailing the community-based collaborative action research framework: Supporting rural health through a Community Health Needs Assessment. *Health Promotion Practice 19*(5), 673–83.

Williams, R. and Wright, J. (1998). Health needs assessment: Epidemiological issues in health needs assessment. *British Medical Journal 31*, 1379–82.

Williams, E., Buck, D. and Babalola, G. (2020). *What are Health Inequalities?* The King's Fund. Available at: www.kingsfund.org.uk/publications/what-are-health-inequalities

Wilson, G.M., Ball, M.J., Szczesny, P., et al. (2021). Health Intelligence Atlas: A core tool for public health intelligence. *State of the Art Best Practice Paper Applied Clinical Informatics 12*, 944–53.

World Health Organisation (WHO). (2020). The top 10 causes of death. Available at: https://www.who.int/news-room/fact-sheets/detail/the-top-10-causes-of-death

Wright, J., Williams, R. and Wilkinson, J. R. (1998). Health needs assessment – Development and importance of health needs assessment. *British Medical Journal 316*, 1310–13.

# 9

# Evaluation

## Ebenezer Owusu-Addo

## Introduction

Following on from the previous chapter, the value of evaluation to assess both the outcomes and processes of health promotion programmes is discussed. The ability to plan and evaluate health promotion programmes are important skills for contemporary health-promotion practice. The chapter briefly describes the nature of health-promotion interventions and what evaluation is, and outlines various approaches to evaluation, including the role of experimental, theory-based and participatory approaches. The chapter demonstrates the value of evaluating outcomes and processes from programme delivery and offers nurses practical strategies to undertake evaluation. The role of health-promotion values in programme evaluation is also highlighted.

By the end of this chapter the reader will be able to:

1. Define the concept of evaluation in relation to public health/health-promotion programmes.
2. Understand the role of evaluation in evidence-based health promotion.
3. Examine the different approaches for programme evaluation; and
4. Discuss the considerations for effective health promotion programme evaluation.

### Key terms

Evaluation, evidence-based health promotion, health promotion values, health promotion interventions, indicators, participatory evaluation

## Evidence-based Health Promotion Practice

Evidence-based health promotion is a process of planning, implementing and evaluating programmes adapted from tested models or interventions in order to address health issues. Kahan and Goodstadt (2001) note that best practices in health promotion are 'those sets of processes and activities that are consistent with health promotion values/goals/ethics, theories/ beliefs, evidence, and understanding of the environment, and that are most likely to achieve health promotion goals in a given situation' (p. 47). To this end, evaluation has been identified as a best practice in health promotion (Owusu-Addo, Edusah and Sarfo-Mensah, 2015). The development of evaluation evidence is key to building the evidence base of health promotion.

## The Nature of Health Promotion Interventions

Health promotion interventions range in scope, scale, target population and settings. That is, by their nature, health promotion interventions are complex. Three categories of interventions have been identified in the literature, namely: simple, complicated and complex interventions (Ling, 2012; Rogers, 2008). Simple interventions are discrete and standardised in nature and can be manipulated under ideal conditions to produce the desired outcomes (Ling, 2012). Simple interventions consist of just a single component. Complicated interventions are linear in nature with interrelated but non-interacting components that are expected to function in a predictable way with outputs leading to desired and anticipated outcomes (Rogers, 2011).

While complex interventions share some of the traits of complicated interventions such as multiple components, these are characterised by interdependency, the role of human agency, a non-linear interaction between intervention components, and adaptation to changing conditions (Bamberger, Vaessen and Raimondo, 2015; Campbell et al., 2007). Complexities in interventions are determined by a broad range of factors including: the context within which the programme is designed and implemented; the specific components of the intervention; the interplay of programme beneficiaries and institutions, structure and agency; the possibility of determining anticipated outcomes; and prior knowledge of factors affecting success or failure (Bamberger et al., 2015; Owusu-Addo, 2019; Pawson, 2013).

Complex interventions, comprising multiple components and different levels, are often required to tackle the broader determinants of health. As complex interventions, health-promotion interventions are heavily context-dependent because their impacts are influenced by factors such as the policy environment, socio-economic conditions, organisational readiness, and the behaviour of the target beneficiaries.

Furthermore, health-promotion interventions tend to include a broad mix of components and may therefore achieve varied outcomes both intended and unintended, in different contexts (Owusu-Addo et al., 2015). These complexities have implications for the methodologies and methods that may be used in their evaluation. The implications of complexity for programme evaluation have been well discussed in the literature including the use of appropriate evaluation designs and methods, outcome patterns assessment, and the role of contexts in shaping outcomes (Barnes, Matka and Sullivan, 2003; Byrne, 2013; Campbell et al., 2007). Because of the nature of health promotion interventions, several approaches to evaluation have emerged including experimental, theory-based and participatory approaches.

## Defining Evaluation and Its Object

Evaluation has long been recognised as a core competency for health promotion practitioners (Barry, Battel-Kirk and Dempsey, 2012; Shilton et al., 2008), reflecting the vital contribution that evaluation can make to the design, implementation, impact and sustainability of health promotion policies and strategies. However, just like the concept of health, which is keenly contested (as discussed in Chapter 1: *Health and its determinants*), there is a difficulty in communicating what evaluation is to non-evaluators (LaVelle, 2011; Mason and Hunt, 2019).

One notable definition of evaluation is provided by Scriven (1991) who writes that evaluation is the systematic process to determine merit, worth, value or significance. The World Health Organization's (WHO) European Working Group on Health Promotion Evaluation (World Health Organization, 1998) also defines evaluation as: the systematic examination and assessment of the features of an initiative and its effects, in order to produce information that can be used by those who have an interest in its improvement or effectiveness. In its simplest form, an evaluation is to assess the extent to which interventions have achieved their goals (Green, Cross, Woodall and Tones, 2019).

Fleming and Parker (2020) provide a concise summary of the reasons for evaluation as follows:

- to assess how resources were deployed (*effort*)
- to assess whether what has been achieved was an economically sound use of resources (*efficiency*)
- to measure impact and outcomes and whether the intervention was worthwhile (*effectiveness*)
- to judge the adequacy and relevance of the delivery of the intervention (*execution*)
- to assess the overall benefits of the intervention (*efficacy*)
- to inform future plans
- to justify decisions to others.

Keeping with health promotion values of equity, participation and empowerment, Rootman and Goodstadt (2001) identify four key features that health promotion evaluations share. The first is participation – i.e., at each stage, the evaluation should involve all those with interest in the evaluand. Second, the eclectic nature of health promotion requires that evaluation draws on a variety of disciplines, and a wide range of information-gathering procedures should be considered for use. Third, evaluation should build the capacity of individuals, communities, organisations and governments to address important health promotion concerns. Last, evaluation should be appropriate: designed to accommodate the complex nature of health-promotion interventions and their long-term impact.

---

## Tutorial Trigger 9.1

As outlined above, health promotion evaluation should advance health promotion values. In what ways can evaluation be designed to help advance health promotion values? How might evaluation undermine health promotion values and principles?

---

# The Value of Evaluation in Health Promotion

There are several reasons why evaluation is important to health promotion practice. The growing burden of chronic diseases and persistent health inequalities, for example, call for continued development of evidence to inform effective health promotion and disease prevention strategies (Edwards, Stickney, Milat, Campbell and Thackway, 2016; Pettman et al., 2012). As observed by Naidoo and Wills (2016), health promotion is an 'uncertain business' meaning there are no guarantees that the outcomes of health promotion interventions will deliver what is anticipated or required of them. The implication here is that health promotors need to produce convincing evidence that health promotion actually does work (Whitehead, 2003). Evidence of what works, for whom, and in which circumstances is essential to inform policies and programmes that can address population health priorities. Evaluation has been identified as a key source of evidence providing information to a variety of audiences – including government bodies, funding bodies, and professional and client groups – that will satisfy questions of accountability and advance health promotion practice (Owusu-Addo, 2019; Owusu-Addo et al., 2015).

Evaluation makes a critical contribution to the evidence base for health promotion policy and programmes. Evidence generated through programme evaluation can provide contextually relevant insights for policy making and programming, reduce uncertainty in decision-making, enable accountability to funders by justifying the use of resources, facilitate organisational and programme level learning, improve effectiveness, and identify unexpected/unintended outcomes (Bauman and Nutbeam, 2013; Schwarzman et al., 2018; van Koperen et al., 2016).

More so, evaluation of health promotion interventions hold the promise of allowing policy makers, programme designers and managers to design and implement new ones. That is, evaluations help to determine what works well and what could be improved in a programme or initiative. Similarly, evaluation of health-promotion interventions is imperative to deliver the benefits of research into improved health outcomes (Bauman and Nutbeam, 2013; Owusu-Addo, 2022; Potvin and McQueen, 2008). From an ethical perspective, Green and South (2006) note that evaluation helps to ensure that interventions do no harm either directly, by 'squandering limited resources' on ineffective interventions or alienating community groups from and making them 'more resistant to other attempts to bring about change' (p. 5).

Despite the benefits that evidence from evaluation can bring to health-promotion practice, the routine inclusion of evaluation in the programme planning process remains problematic (Owusu-Addo, Cross and Sarfo-Mensah, 2017). Evaluation should be considered from the outset of programme development and integrated at all stages.

---

### Tutorial Trigger 9.2

Why is evaluation not always included in health-promotion programme planning, and what are the challenges of evaluating health-promotion programmes?

---

## Types of Evaluation

The types of evaluation reflect the various aspects involved in conducting a public health/health-promotion programme, including measuring the *impacts* and *outcomes* of the programme along with the delivery of health-promotion programmes focused upon measuring *process* (Owusu-Addo et al., 2015). It is also important to test the suitability and appropriateness of a programme in its early stages before it is well established; the measurement of this is called formative evaluation. Evaluations must be tailored to suit the activity and circumstances of individual programmes: no single type, design or method will be 'right' for all programmes (Bauman and Nutbeam, 2013).

### Formative evaluation

Formative evaluation occurs as part of programme planning. It is conducted to inform programme development and implementation. It provides information on achieving programme goals or improving a programme. For instance, mass media campaigns often use formative evaluation to develop and test concepts and messages. Bauman and Nutbeam (2013) identify four types of formative evaluation including pre-testing intervention methods and materials, understanding the target population or community through needs assessment, reviewing the problem and assessing previous efforts to address it, and using formative evaluation for programme planning. Generally, formative evaluation is the first step towards testing the underlying need for a programme and ascertaining its relevance to the target population. Formative evaluation is useful for determining the likelihood of intervention success or failure, as well as building a sound basis for subsequent process and outcome evaluations.

## Process evaluation

A process evaluation is a type of evaluation that assesses the type, quantity, and quality of programme activities or services – i.e., how the programme is being implemented (Ismail, Seabrook and Gilliland, 2021). It is a systematic, focused plan for gathering data/evidence to determine whether the programme model is implemented as originally intended and, if not, how operations differ from the initial plan. Process evaluation can be conducted alongside impact evaluation to assess the short-term impact of an intervention: the *health-promotion outcomes* (Bauman and Nutbeam, 2013).

Process evaluation has several benefits including the ability to determine the extent to which a programme or service is implemented as intended – i.e., intervention fidelity. A process evaluation can also provide programme designers and managers with information on the implementation process (Parry-Langdon, Bloor, Audrey and Holliday, 2003). This information can then be used to refine the delivery of a programme and improve its quality. Further, data from process evaluation may be useful in the interpretation of outcome data. For instance, if the programme is not achieving the expected outcomes, it may be because there are problems with intervention fidelity. Last, a process evaluation can help identify discrepancies between programme design and delivery and ultimately help to measure outcomes that more accurately reflect the programme as designed (Gerritsen et al., 2021). Despite these benefits of process evaluation, it is worth noting that while this type of evaluation may provide insight into why a programme is or isn't working, its intended purpose is not to provide evidence on programme effectiveness.

## Impact evaluation

This type of evaluation investigates whether programme objectives (intermediate effects) have been achieved or not. Appropriate measures here include changes in awareness, knowledge, attitudes, behaviours, and/or skills. The Glossary for Evidence-based Public defines impact evaluation as the type of evaluation that examines the initial effect of a programme on proximal targets of change, such as policies, behaviours, or attitudes (Rychetnik, Hawe, Waters, Barratt and Frommer, 2004).

The terms 'impact' and 'outcome' are used differently in public health and international development literature. In public health/health promotion, an outcome generally refers to the long-term, more global changes, while impact refers to short-term or immediate effects of an intervention. This is directly the opposite case in international development where outcome refers to the immediate effect of an intervention and impact to the long-term change/effect of interventions (White, 2014).

## Outcome evaluation

Outcome evaluation determines whether the programme goal (longer-term effect) has been reached or not. Outcome evaluation is also called summative evaluation in the sense that it can be used to make recommendations for future programme improvements as well as making an overall statement about the worth of a programme (Green and South, 2006). Appropriate measures here include changes in health conditions, quality of life, and behaviours. With respect to measuring programme effects (outcomes), both qualitative and quantitative methods of investigation are available. Table 9.1 provides examples of the various types of evaluations.

**Table 9.1**  Examples of different types of evaluations

| Type of evaluation | Author | Title of Study |
|---|---|---|
| Formative | Dixon-Ibarra, Driver, Van Volkenburg and Humphries (2017) | Formative evaluation on a physical activity health promotion programme for the group home setting |
| Process | Nguyen et al. (2013) | Sexual health promotion on social networking sites: a process evaluation of the FaceSpace Project |
| Impact | Grim, Hortz and Petosa (2011) | Impact evaluation of a pilot web-based intervention to increase physical activity |
| Outcome | Wyman et al. (2010) | An outcome evaluation of the Sources of Strength suicide prevention programme delivered by adolescent peer leaders in high schools |

**Point to Ponder 9.1**

Current trends in health care emphasise health promotion, quality of care improvement, and performance standards. This means that beyond the provision of direct, clinical services, there is an increased focus on the healthcare delivery system. Nurses are involved in (or managing) activities related to improving healthcare systems. For instance, evaluation of service delivery is an important aspect of nursing practice. Formative evaluation may need to be conducted to gauge the acceptability of exclusive breastfeeding intervention in a linguistically diverse population. To make valued contributions to these activities, nurses need to know the different types of evaluation, and when it may be appropriate to conduct a particular type of evaluation.

## Evaluation Approaches in Health Promotion

Various evaluation approaches have been used in health promotion. They have been influenced by the multidisciplinary nature of health promotion, and various research paradigms. Guba and Lincoln (2005) identified three paradigms in the evaluation world: positivism/post-positivism, interpretivism and pragmatism. Mertens (2008) added a fourth paradigm, that is, transformative, which provides a framework for evaluations that have a social justice and human rights lens.

Positivism and post-positivism are based on empiricism, a way of knowing that depends on perception of information through our five senses. Positivists claim that an external reality exists and that we can measure it objectively. Post-positivists challenged this concept of reality, positing that an external reality does exist, but can only be known probabilistically due to the limitation of human consciousness (Mertens, 2016). Interpretivists hold a divergent view that there is one reality out in the world waiting to be measured objectively. Rather, they view reality as being socially constructed by different stakeholders. Interpretivists' epistemological assumption is that the evaluator needs to be interactive with the stakeholders, building relationships that allow for the construction of reality to develop, rather than being detached from the stakeholders to avoid bias, as held by post-positivists (Patton, 2014). Pragmatism sits between post-positivism and interpretivism and is inclined towards the use of mixed methods to provide information that will help make evaluative judgements (Hall, 2013). These philosophical assumptions continue to shape the choice of evaluation designs and approaches in health promotion.

## Experimental and quasi-experimental approaches

The experimental and quasi-experimental approaches to programme evaluation are intended to produce unbiased conclusions about a programme's effectiveness. They are based on the principle of counterfactual analysis. Within the positivist and post-positivist traditions, randomised controlled trials (RCTs) are identified to be feasible and appropriate for evaluating health-promotion interventions and advancing health-promotion research (Rosen, Manor, Engelhard and Zucker, 2006). RCTs analyse what difference an intervention makes through comparing those in the intervention to a control group who do not receive it. Indeed, RCT designs are deemed as the 'gold standard' for gaining an unbiased estimate of intervention effects (Rychetnik, Frommer, Hawe and Shiell, 2002). While some have proposed that RCTs can be used to evaluate complex interventions if the right measures are instituted (Craig et al., 2012; White, 2013), it has been widely argued that RCTs are largely suitable for evaluating simple or complicated (but not complex) interventions (Ling, 2012; Pawson, 2013; Zimmerman et al., 2012). A major limitation is that RCTs have difficulties accounting for how intervention components interact with each other and with complex open systems in unpredictable ways. In fact the World Health Organization (1998) has even concluded that 'the use of randomised control trials to evaluate health promotion initiatives is, in most cases, inappropriate, misleading and unnecessarily expensive' (p. 5). Despite the criticisms levelled against RCTs, a recent systematic review of the approaches used to evaluate complex interventions found that RCTs still dominate the health evaluation literature (Minary et al., 2019).

Quasi-experimental designs (QEDs) are used when RCT is not possible but when a comparison group can be identified (Handley, Lyles, McCulloch and Cattamanchi, 2018; Stufflebeam and Coryn, 2014). It has been argued that the QEDs are generally more suited to the nature of health-promotion programme evaluations, where the programmes are complex and influenced by many factors (Gasparrini and Lopez Bernal, 2015). That is, QEDs are legitimate, necessary and useful in their own right, and can fully assess a programme's merit and worth. There are a range of QEDs, all of which aim to include the use of a comparison group (Handley et al., 2018) (see Table 9.2), the feature used in experimental designs. The difference with the QEDs is that the allocation to the groups is not random. While QEDs are useful and often adopted instead of RCTs for impact evaluation (White, 2013), it has been observed that they are greatly limited in their ability to answer questions about how and why programmes work or fail to work within particular contexts (Pawson, 2013; Van Belle et al., 2016). That is, experimental designs in general are quite limited in unpacking the 'black box' of complex interventions to explain how programmes' outcomes are produced. The limited applicability of experimental designs in health promotion has resulted in the call for participatory designs and the use of qualitative methods and/or mixed methods in gathering evidence in the evaluation of health-promotion programmes (Owusu-Addo, 2022; Owusu-Addo et al., 2015).

**Table 9.2** Quasi-experimental designs (QEDs)

| Design | Description |
|---|---|
| Pre-Post with Non-equivalent control group | In this design, the intervention is introduced at a single point in time to one or more sites, for which there is also a pre-test and post-test evaluation period. The pre-post differences between these two sites are then compared. That is, analysis is usually based on estimating the difference in the amount of change over time in the outcome of interest between the two groups, beginning with the intervention and moving forward in time. |
| Stepped Wedge Design | Intervention is rolled out over time, usually at the site level. Participants who initially do not receive the intervention later cross over to receive the intervention. Those that wait, provide control data during the time others receive the intervention, reducing the risk of bias due to time and time-dependent covariates. Can either be based on serial cross-sectional data collected by sites for different time periods (sites cross over), or by following a cohort of same individuals over time (individuals cross over). |
| Interrupted Time Series | Multiple observations are assessed for a number of consecutive points in time before and after intervention within the same individual or group. |
| Regression Discontinuity Design | This design requires control over assignment of participants to one or more treatment and control conditions through pre-testing. Unlike experimental designs that require random assignment to conditions, regression discontinuity designs assign units to conditions on the basis of a cut score on an assignment variable, often based on treatment need or merit. |

*Source*: Handley et al. (2018). Stufflebeam and Coryn (2014)

## Tutorial Trigger 9.3

1 Identify and define the most basic methodological requirement for conducting an evaluation based on experimental and quasi-experimental designs; then list the more general requirements for conducting a sound experimental study.
2 Distinguish between studies that assess the effects of health-promotion interventions and ones that assess the causes of observed outcomes; then discuss the applicability of randomised controlled experimental design to both types of studies.

## Participatory approaches

Participatory evaluation approaches have been used frequently in health promotion (Allard, Bilodeau and Gendron, 2008). Participatory evaluation is an approach that involves the stakeholders of a programme or policy in the evaluation process. At the heart of participatory evaluation approach is a lens of social justice on the evaluation process to critically examine stakeholders' assumptions about the health-promotion intervention and how outcomes are to be produced (Owusu-Addo, 2022). One of these forms is empowerment evaluation developed by Fetterman and Wandersman (2005). Fetterman and Wandersman (2005) defined empowerment evaluation as 'an evaluation approach that aims to increase the likelihood that programs will achieve results by increasing the capacity of program stakeholders to plan, implement, and evaluate their own programs' (p. 27). Qualitative methods, and participatory action research, are commonly used in empowerment evaluation.

Participatory approaches sit within the interpretive and transformative paradigms and align with the health-promotion values of empowerment and social justice, which make them imperative to adopt in evaluating health-promotion interventions. Mertens (2016) notes that the transformative paradigm helps organise thinking about how evaluators 'can serve the interests of social justice through the production of credible evidence that is responsive to the needs of marginalized communities' (p. 103). Participatory approaches help to elevate community and indigenous voices in the evaluation and also elucidate the broad range of impacts that health promotion interventions may achieve (Drawson, Toombs and Mushquash, 2017). It has been argued that in less participatory evaluation (whereby the evaluator treats stakeholders as research 'subjects' and only focuses on finding the so called 'truth' in a manner of reliable and valid data from the stakeholders) the values of the researcher feature prominently (Owusu-Addo et al., 2015). In contrast, actively involving the stakeholders in a collaborative manner has the potential to ensure that stakeholders' values, particularly those of the community, drive the evaluation agenda (Springett, 2001). Box 9.1 summarises the advantages and challenges of participatory evaluation.

---

**Box 9.1**

## Advantages and challenges of participatory evaluation

*Advantages of doing participatory evaluation:*

   a. identify locally relevant evaluation questions
   b. improve accuracy and relevance of reports
   c. establish and explain causality

d. improve programme performance
e. empower participants
f. build capacity
g. develop leaders and build teams
h. sustain organisational learning and growth

*Challenges in implementing and using participatory evaluation:*

a. time and commitment
b. resources
c. conflicts between approaches
d. unclear purpose of participation, or a purpose that is not aligned with evaluation design
e. lack of facilitation skills
f. only focusing on participation in one aspect of the evaluation process, e.g., data collection
g. lack of cultural and contextual understanding, and the implications of these for the evaluation design

*Source*: https://www.betterevaluation.org/en/plan/approach/participatory_evaluation

## Theory-driven evaluation

Theory-driven evaluation approaches are increasingly being used in programme evaluation. Conceptually, theory-driven evaluation explicates a programme theory, and empirically, it investigates how programmes cause intended or observed outcomes (Coryn et al., 2011: 203). Further, theory-driven evaluation focuses on unpacking the 'black box' of programmes to understand their inner workings, thereby exposing the programme logic to scrutiny.

'Black box' evaluation (Astbury and Leeuw, 2010; H.T. Chen and Chen, 1990) is a sobriquet often given to evaluation approaches such as experimental and quasi-experimental designs that are positivist in nature. It refers to the practice of evaluating interventions by focusing on the outcomes produced by the intervention without paying attention to how and why the outcomes are produced (Funnell and Rogers, 2011). In this way, policy makers and practitioners get little knowledge about the programme's mechanisms of change which are important for replication. To overcome the challenges associated with black box evaluations, theory-driven approaches to evaluation focus on building an understanding of how and why programmes work or fail to work. One of such commonly used theory-driven evaluation approaches is realist evaluation (Pawson, 2013; Pawson and Tilley, 1997).

## Realist evaluation

Among the array of theory-driven evaluation approaches (e.g., theory of change, contribution analysis etc.), realist evaluation (Pawson, 2013; Pawson and Tilley, 1997) has been adjudged as providing a holistic approach to evaluating complex social programmes with different causal mechanisms operating in different contexts (Bamberger et al., 2015; Marchal, Van Belle, Van Olmen, Hoerée and Kegels, 2012).

Realist evaluation is underpinned by realist philosophy of science which holds that there is a real world that can be known through human senses, cognitions, language and culture (Pawson, 2013). Realist evaluation sees programmes as open social systems and structures with real causal powers, and that programme participants respond differently to programmes in different contexts. The key question that realist evaluation seeks to address is 'what works, for whom, under what circumstances, and how' (Pawson, 2013: 15). Realist evaluation thus seeks to unpack programmatic 'black boxes'. Typically, realist evaluation aims to explain programme effectiveness by way of exploring how different programme mechanisms are triggered in particular contexts. This implies that programmes work differently in different contexts, therefore, a health-promotion intervention that works in one setting may fail in another setting as the 'mechanisms' needed for success are 'fired' to different degrees in different contexts.

Realist evaluation places emphasis on understanding how programmes generate outcomes and how causal mechanisms are shaped by programme contexts. In realist evaluation, programmes are said to be 'theories incarnate' (Greenhalgh et al., 2015; Pawson and Tilley, 1997). This means that any time that a programme is designed and implemented, it is testing certain sets of assumptions of policy makers and programme designers regarding how change might occur, even though these theories might not be explicit. To unpack this programme theory, Pawson and Tilley (1997) coined the realist evaluation heuristic 'Context + Mechanism = Outcome', to explain how context influences mechanisms to produce programme outcomes. The work of the realist evaluator therefore, is to elicit, test and refine context (C), mechanism (M) and outcome configurations (CMOCs) (i.e., the programme theory) to explain what works, for whom, under what circumstances, and how (Pawson, 2013).

*Context* implies the circumstances in which the programme plays out. Pawson (2013: 37) identifies four key contextual layers of a programme: individuals (i.e., characteristics and capacities of programme stakeholders), interpersonal relations (i.e., stakeholder relationships), institutional settings (i.e., rules, norms and customs local to the programme), and infrastructure (i.e., broader social, economic, political and cultural setting of the programme). Realist evaluation posits that the success of a programme is contingent on its location in an appropriate context. While other evaluation approaches such as experimental and quasi-experimental designs treat contexts as extraneous variables that have to be controlled, in realist evaluation, context is treated as an integral part of the programme (Davidoff, 2011; Pawson, 2013). A realist approach thus acknowledges that programmes are implemented in multiple, open and interacting systems, and recognises that particular aspects of programme context will have implications for whether and how the programme mechanisms operate to produce programme outcomes.

*Mechanisms* refers to a combination of resources offered by a programme and stakeholders' reasoning in response to these (Pawson and Tilley, 1997). Put differently, 'mechanisms' are not the programme activities, services or variables, but the response they trigger from stakeholders and the resulting outcomes (Weiss, 1997). For Elster, J. (2007: 36), mechanisms are the 'cogs and wheels that have brought the relationship between policies/programmes and outcomes into existence'. It is through the operation of programme mechanisms that we come to understand 'why' a programme works (Pawson and Tilley, 1997).

In realist evaluation, *Outcomes* implies outcome patterns that result from the firing of programme mechanisms both intended and unintended. The examination of programme outcomes in realist evaluation is not to draw conclusions about whether or not the programme works, but to examine outcome patterns in a theory testing role to check if the conjectured context-mechanism theories are confirmed (Pawson and Tilley, 1997).

The realist notion is that there is always an interaction between context and mechanisms, and that it is this interaction that produces programme outcomes. This makes the realist evaluation approach appropriate for the evaluation of health-promotion interventions, with multiple components implemented in diverse contexts, dependent on the dynamics of relationships among programme stakeholders (Owusu-Addo, 2019; Owusu-Addo, Renzaho and Smith, 2020).

Notwithstanding the merits of realist evaluation in terms of providing a sound framework for evaluation of complex programmes, challenges still remain in its application. The first challenge relates to the question of what constitutes a mechanism as there exist different conceptualisations of mechanisms within evaluation (Astbury and Leeuw, 2010; Dalkin, Greenhalgh, Jones, Cunningham and Lhussier, 2015). Second, context is multifaceted and operates at various levels of a system (political, social, organisational, individual), making it challenging in accounting for these in an evaluation (Owusu-Addo et al., 2020). Third, by focusing on assessing both the programme's impacts and the circumstances under which these are produced, realist evaluation and theory-driven evaluations in general tend to be resource-and time-intensive (Marchal et al., 2012).

**Research in Brief 9.1**

Cash transfers (CTs) are healthy public policy initiatives that focus on addressing poverty and vulnerability. Even though burgeoning evidence points to CTs' impact on the social determinants of health (SDoH), there is little evidence about how and why CTs work to influence the SDoH (Owusu-Addo et al., 2020). This study reports on a realist evaluation aimed at developing a middle-range theory that explains how CTs influence the SDoH by exploring programme mechanisms of change and associated contextual factors. The study found that at the meso level, key mechanisms of collaboration and intersectoral working, formalisation of roles of service providers, and a shared vision across sectors were important to both the implementation and outcomes of CTs. Contextual factors that influenced programme mechanisms at the meso level include active involvement of sector ministries and their decentralised departments in programme policy formulation and design, availability of resources, and availability of a single registry containing information on programme beneficiaries. At the micro level, programme mechanisms of change identified include household empowerment, needs prioritisation and choice making, risk-taking behaviour, programme awareness, and beneficiaries' voice in programme decision-making and implementation. This realist evaluation provides evidence-based understandings regarding CTs' mechanism of change in the contexts within which they operate, and can inform CT policy, design, implementation, adaptation and future evaluation.

Owusu-Addo, E., Renzaho, A. M. and Smith, B. J. (2020). Developing a middle-range theory to explain how cash transfers work to tackle the social determinants of health: A realist case study. *World Development 130*, 104920.

**Time to Reflect 9.1**

There are several approaches to health-promotion evaluation. There is nothing like the best evaluation approach. The nature of the health-promotion intervention and evaluation questions play a key role in the kind of evaluation approach that may be appropriate for the evaluation. Think about a health-promotion intervention that you are familiar with. It might be located in your own practice. What evaluation approach will be more appropriate for evaluating the intervention, and why?

## Planning Health Promotion Evaluation

This section provides practical steps in conducting programme evaluation in practice. The flow diagram in Figure 9.1 provides a summary of the key steps in carrying out programme evaluation.

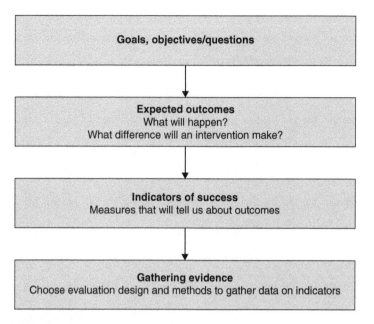

**Figure 9.1**  Steps in conducting evaluation

## Understanding the purpose of the evaluation – Goals, objectives and questions

An important step in planning health-promotion evaluation is to understand the purpose of the evaluation. Owen (2004) outlines key questions to reflect on in regard to the purpose of an evaluation: Is the evaluation for the purpose of determining the way a programme is to be implemented? synthesising information to aid programme development? clarifying a programme? improving the implementation of a programme? monitoring programme outcomes? or determining programme worth? It is also important to determine the audience for the evaluation prior to developing an evaluation plan. The evaluation questions need to reflect a comprehensive understanding of health-promotion programmes and what they are intended to address.

### Outcomes

Another important step in the evaluation plan is the identification of the outcomes to be measured. Bauman and Nutbeam (2013) note that health-promotion outcomes may range from the 'impact' of health-promotion interventions in the short term to health outcomes in the longer term (p. 7). As shown in Figure 9.2, health-promotion outcomes can be tracked at various stages of programme implementation. These include:

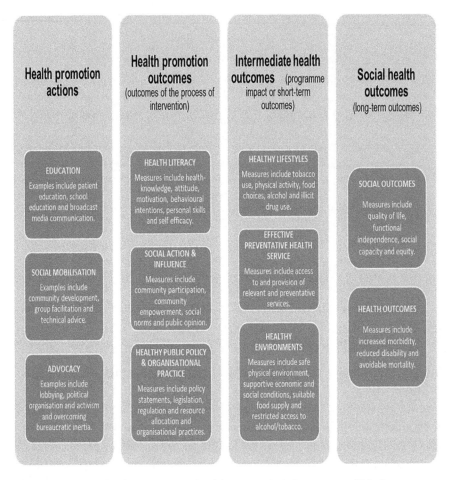

**Figure 9.2**   Levels of outcomes in health promotion. Bauman and Nutbeam (2013), p. 8

- long-term health and social outcomes – changes in health status (mortality and morbidity and well-being)
- health promotion outcomes – these represent immediate results of health-promotion activities. For example more women opt for skilled delivery (behaviour change)
- intermediate/short-term outcomes – for example women with increased knowledge and awareness of the benefits of skilled delivery

The Outcomes can be at *individual*, *organisational* or *community/population* level. They can be behavioural, educational, social, environmental and physiological.

## Choosing indicators

An indicator is a specific measure of programme performance that is tracked over time by the monitoring system. They are measures that allow us to assess change (i.e., capture key aspects of the programme and its effects) (Green and South, 2006), and are defined in terms of quantity, quality and time. They can be quantitative or qualitative. A review of a programme's logical framework (if any) and engagement with programme stakeholders are key sources of identifying programme indicators of success (Owusu-Addo et al., 2015). Table 9.3 provides the criteria for selecting indicators.

---

### Points to Ponder 9.2

Indicators are usually selected to capture key aspects of the programme and its effects. Consider what might be appropriate indicators for the following health promotion interventions:

- smoking cessation clinic
- healthy eating intervention in schools
- mass media campaign on safe sex practice among adolescents and young people

---

**Table 9.3**  Criteria for Indicator Selection

| Criteria | Description |
| --- | --- |
| Valid | Indicators should measure the condition or event they are intended to measure |
| Reliable | Indicators should produce the same results when used more than once to measure the same condition or event, all things being equal (e.g., using the same methods, tools or instruments) |
| Specific | Indicators should measure only the condition or event they are intended to measure |
| Sensitive | Indicators should reflect changes in the state of the condition or event under observation |
| Operational | Indicators should be measured with definitions that are developed and tested at the programme level and with reference standards |
| Affordable | The costs of measuring the indicators should be reasonable |
| Feasible | It should be possible to carry out the proposed data collection |
| Comparable | Indicators should be comparable (e.g., over time, across geographical lines) |

## Gathering evidence

This step entails making decisions regarding the choice of *evaluation design* approach and the methods of data collection. It is about linking outcomes, indicators and methods. Stern et al. (2012) note that the choice of evaluation design requires a reconciliation among three key elements: evaluation aims and questions, programme attributes (i.e., complex, complicated or simple programme), and appropriate designs and methods. This is to ensure that the evaluation approach chosen is able to effectively address the evaluation questions and the peculiarity of the evaluand. Similarly, Rogers et al. (2015) also note that the choice of evaluation design should be informed by the nature of the evaluand, the nature of the evaluation (i.e., purpose of evaluation and types of questions), and resources and constraints (i.e., expertise and time, and existing evidence from evaluation). Box 9.2 provides additional information on making decisions about the choice of evaluation design.

---

**Box 9.2**

### Choosing evaluation design

In choosing evaluation design don't ask, 'Which approach is best', ask:

- What is the purpose of the evaluation?
- What kinds of impact/outcome questions are being addressed?
- What are the main situational contingencies?
- How might you usefully combine or integrate multiple causal strategies, given the above?
- What is the most appropriate design, rather than the best design

---

The present era is predominantly and rightly characterised by methodological eclecticism. Mixed-methods (combining quantitative and qualitative data to answer particular evaluation question/s) are highly recommended in gathering evidence in evaluating health-promotion programmes (Bauman and Nutbeam, 2013; Green and South, 2006; Ridde and de Sardan, 2015). In recent times, mixed-method has come centre stage in scholarly work on research and evaluation with a specific field that for years now has had its own scientific journals (*International Journal of Multiple Research Approaches, Journal of Mixed Methods Research* and in 2013, its academic association, the Mixed Methods International Research Association (http://mmira. wildapricot.org).

As observed by the U.S. Department of Health and Human Services, Centers for Disease Control and Prevention (2011) sometimes a 'single method is not sufficient to accurately measure an outcome because the thing being measured is complex and/or the data method/source does not yield data reliable or accurate enough. Employing multiple methods helps increase the accuracy of the measurement and the certainty of your conclusions when the various methods yield similar results' (p. 63). The use of mixed-methods in evaluating programmes gives room for tri-angulation, stakeholder involvement, and validating quantitative findings via qualitative data which enriches the depth of analysis (Owusu-Addo et al., 2015). This is directly in line with calls for the use of 'judicial principle' where evidence is sought from different sources (Green et al., 2019).

## Summary

This chapter has examined evaluation and its value in providing credible evidence for evidence-based health promotion. It has brought to the fore the various types of evaluation and the approaches to health-promotion evaluation. Kok (1993) argues that inadequate planning and evaluation of programmes are the reasons why health promotion is not effective in some cases. It is therefore important that health-promotion professionals reflect critically on their practice and become skilled in programme planning and evaluation. In this chapter we have provided practical guidelines on how to conduct health-promotion evaluation that would advance health-promotion practice.

—— **Key Points** ——————————————————————————————

- Health-promotion evaluation should be informed by health-promotion values with clear strategies adopted in the evaluation, planning and implementation processes to advance these values in a way that would enable and empower individuals, institutions, organisa-tions and communities to gain control over their health and its determinants.
- Health-promotion evaluation should lay emphasis on working with people collabora-tively by adopting evaluation designs that value the dignity of all participants rather than adopting an approach that detaches the evaluator from the participants.
- Evaluation methods used in health-promotion evaluation should be flexible and diverse as a single method may give limited insight, but combination of methods may give a rich picture of intervention processes, impacts, outcomes and conditions for improvement.

# References

Allard, D., Bilodeau, A. and Gendron, S. (2008). Figurative thinking and models: tools for participatory evaluation. In *Health Promotion Evaluation Practices in the Americas* (pp. 123–47). Springer.

Astbury, B. and Leeuw, F. L. (2010). Unpacking black boxes: mechanisms and theory building in evaluation. *American Journal of Evaluation 31*(3), 363–81.

Bamberger, M., Vaessen, J. and Raimondo, E. (2015). *Dealing with Complexity in Development Evaluation: A practical approach.* Sage Publications.

Barnes, M., Matka, E. and Sullivan, H. (2003). Evidence, understanding and complexity: evaluation in non-linear systems. *Evaluation 9*(3), 265–84.

Barry, M.M., Battel-Kirk, B. and Dempsey, C. (2012). The CompHP core competencies framework for health promotion in Europe. *Health Education & Behavior 39*(6), 648–62.

Bauman, A. and Nutbeam, D. (2013). *Evaluation in a Nutshell: A practical guide to the evaluation of health promotion programs.* McGraw-Hill.

Bloom, B. (1986). Ralph Tyler's impact on evaluation theory and practice. *Journal of Thought*, 36–46.

Byrne, D. (2013). Evaluating complex social interventions in a complex world. *Evaluation 19*(3), 217–28.

Campbell, N.C., Murray, E., Darbyshire, J., Emery, J., Farmer, A., Griffiths, F., … Kinmonth, A.L. (2007). Designing and evaluating complex interventions to improve health care. *BMJ 334*(7591), 455–9.

Chen, H.-T. and Rossi, P.H. (1983). Evaluating with sense: The theory-driven approach. *Evaluation Review 7*(3), 283–302.

Chen, H.T. (1990). *Theory-driven Evaluations.* Sage.

Coryn, C.L., Noakes, L.A., Westine, C.D. and Schröter, D.C. (2011). A systematic review of theory-driven evaluation practice from 1990 to 2009. *American Journal of Evaluation 32*(2), 199–226.

Craig, P., Cooper, C., Gunnell, D., Haw, S., Lawson, K., Macintyre, S., … Sutton, M. (2012). Using natural experiments to evaluate population health interventions: New Medical Research Council guidance. *Journal of Epidemiology and Community Health 66*(12), 1182–6.

Cronbach, L.J. and Snow, R.E. (1977). *Aptitudes and Instructional Methods: A handbook for research on interactions.* New York: Irvington.

Dalkin, S.M., Greenhalgh, J., Jones, D., Cunningham, B. and Lhussier, M. (2015). What's in a mechanism? Development of a key concept in realist evaluation. *Implementation Science 10*(1), 1–7.

Davidoff, F. (2011). Heterogeneity: we can't live with it, and we can't live without it. *BMJ Quality and Safety, 20*(Suppl.1), i11–i12.

Dixon-Ibarra, A., Driver, S., Van Volkenburg, H. and Humphries, K. (2017). Formative evaluation on a physical activity health promotion program for the group home setting. *Evaluation and Program Planning, 60*, 81–90.

Donaldson, S.I. (2007). *Program Theory-driven Evaluation Science: Strategies and applications.* Routledge.

Drawson, A.S., Toombs, E. and Mushquash, C.J. (2017). Indigenous research methods: A systematic review. *International Indigenous Policy Journal 8*(2).

Edwards, B., Stickney, B., Milat, A., Campbell, D. and Thackway, S. (2016). Building research and evaluation capacity in population health: The NSW Health approach. *Health Promotion Journal of Australia 27*(3), 264–7.

Fetterman, D.M. and Wandersman, A. (2005). *Empowerment Evaluation Principles in Practice*. New York: Guilford Press.

Fleming, M.L. and Parker, E. (2020). *Health Promotion: Principles and practice in the Australian context*. Routledge.

Funnell, S.C. and Rogers, P.J. (2011). *Purposeful Program Theory: Effective use of theories of change and logic models* (Vol. 31). John Wiley & Sons.

Gasparrini, A. and Lopez Bernal, J. (2015). Commentary: On the use of quasi-experimental designs in public health evaluation. *International Journal of Epidemiology 44*(3), 966–8. doi:10.1093/ije/dyv065

Gerritsen, D.L., de Vries, E., Smalbrugge, M., Smeets, C.H., van der Spek, K., Zuidema, S.U. and Koopmans, R.T. (2021). Implementing a multidisciplinary psychotropic medication review among nursing home residents with dementia: a process evaluation. *International Psychogeriatrics 33*(9), 933–45.

Green, J., Cross, R., Woodall, J. and Tones, K. (2019). *Health Promotion: Planning and strategies*, 4th Ed. Sage.

Green, J. and South, J. (2006). *Key Concepts in Public Health Practice: Evaluation*. Maidenhead, Berkshire: Open University Press.

Greenhalgh, T., Wong, G., Jagosh, J., Greenhalgh, J., Manzano, A., Westhorp, G. and Pawson, R. (2015). Protocol—the RAMESES II study: developing guidance and reporting standards for realist evaluation. *BMJ Open 5*(8), e008567.

Grim, M., Hortz, B. and Petosa, R. (2011). Impact evaluation of a pilot web-based intervention to increase physical activity. *American Journal of Health Promotion 25*(4), 227–30.

Guba, E.G. and Lincoln, Y.S. (2005). Paradigmatic controversies, contradictions, and emerging confluences. In N. K. Denzin and Y. S. Lincoln (Eds), The Sage handbook of qualitative research (3rd ed., pp. 191–216). Thousand Oaks, CA: Sage.

Hall, J.N. (2013). Pragmatism, evidence, and mixed methods evaluation. *New Directions for Evaluation 2013*(138), 15–26.

Handley, M.A., Lyles, C.R., McCulloch, C. and Cattamanchi, A. (2018). Selecting and improving quasi-experimental designs in effectiveness and implementation research. *Annual Review of Public Health 39*, 5–25. doi:10.1146/annurev-publhealth-040617-014128

Ismail, M.R., Seabrook, J.A. and Gilliland, J.A. (2021). Process evaluation of fruit and vegetables distribution interventions in school-based settings: A systematic review. *Preventive Medicine Reports 21*, 101281.

Kahan, B. and Goodstadt, M. (2001). The interactive domain model of best practices in health promotion: Developing and implementing a best practices approach to health promotion. *Health Promotion Practice 2*(1), 43–67.

Kok, G. (1993). Why are so many health promotion programs ineffective? *Health Promotion Journal of Australia 3*(2), 12–17.

LaVelle, J.M. (2011). Planning for Evaluation's future: Undergraduate students' interest in program evaluation. *American Journal of Evaluation 32*(3), 362–75.

Ling, T. (2012). Evaluating complex and unfolding interventions in real time. *Evaluation 18*(1), 79–91.

Marchal, B., Van Belle, S., Van Olmen, J., Hoerée, T. and Kegels, G. (2012). Is realist evaluation keeping its promise? A review of published empirical studies in the field of health systems research. *Evaluation 18*(2), 192–212.

Mason, S. and Hunt, A. (2019). So what do you do? Exploring evaluator descriptions of their work. *American Journal of Evaluation 40*(3), 395–413.

Mertens, D.M. (2008). *Transformative Research and Evaluation*. New York: Guilford Press.

Mertens, D.M. (2016). Assumptions at the philosophical and programmatic levels in evaluation. *Evaluation and Program Planning 59*, 102–8.

Minary, L., Trompette, J., Kivits, J., Cambon, L., Tarquinio, C. and Alla, F. (2019). Which design to evaluate complex interventions? Toward a methodological framework through a systematic review. *BMC Medical Research Methodology* (1), 1–9.

Naidoo, J. and Wills, J. (2016). *Foundations for Health Promotion-E-Book*. Elsevier Health Sciences.

Nguyen, P., Gold, J., Pedrana, A., Chang, S., Howard, S., Ilic, O., … Stoove, M. (2013). Sexual health promotion on social networking sites: a process evaluation of the FaceSpace Project. *Journal of Adolescent Health 53*(1), 98–104.

Owen, J.M. (2004). Evaluation forms: toward an inclusive framework for evaluation practice. In M. C. Alkin (Ed.), *Evaluation Roots: Tracing theorists' views and influences*. Thousand Oaks: Sage Publication *356*, 370.

Owusu-Addo, E. (2019). *Cash Transfers as Social Policy for Tackling the Social Determinants of Health: A Realist Evaluation*. Monash University.

Owusu-Addo, E. (2022). Researching the practices of policymakers in implementing a social policy intervention in Ghana. In *Global Handbook of Health Promotion Research, Vol. 1* (pp. 469–8). Springer.

Owusu-Addo, E., Cross, R. and Sarfo-Mensah, P. (2017). Evidence-based practice in local public health service in Ghana. *Critical Public Health 27*(1), 125–38.

Owusu-Addo, E., Edusah, S.E. and Sarfo-Mensah, P. (2015). The utility of stakeholder involvement in the evaluation of community-based health promotion programmes. *International Journal of Health Promotion and Education 53*(6), 291–302.

Owusu-Addo, E., Renzaho, A.M. and Smith, B.J. (2020). Developing a middle-range theory to explain how cash transfers work to tackle the social determinants of health: A realist case study. *World Development 130*, 104920.

Parry-Langdon, N., Bloor, M., Audrey, S. and Holliday, J. (2003). Process evaluation of health promotion interventions. *Policy & Politics 31*(2), 207–16.

Patton, M.Q. (2014). *Qualitative Research & Evaluation Methods: Integrating theory and practice*: Sage Publications.

Pawson, R. (2013). *The Science of Evaluation: A realist manifesto*. Sage.

Pawson, R. and Tilley, N. (1997). *Realistic Evaluation*. Sage.

Pettman, T.L., Armstrong, R., Doyle, J., Burford, B., Anderson, L.M., Hillgrove, T., ... Waters, E. (2012). Strengthening evaluation to capture the breadth of public health practice: ideal vs. real. *J. Public Health (Oxf)* *34*(1), 151–5. doi:10.1093/pubmed/fds014

Potvin, L. and McQueen, D. (2008). *Health Promotion Evaluation Practices in the Americas*. Springer.

Ridde, V. and de Sardan, J.-P.O. (2015). A mixed methods contribution to the study of public health policies: complementarities and difficulties. *BMC Health Services Research 15*(3), 1–8.

Rogers, P., Hawkins, A., McDonald, B., Macfarlan, A. and Milne, C. (2015). Choosing appropriate designs and methods for impact evaluation. Canberra: Office of the Chief Economist, Australian Government.

Rogers, P.J. (2008). Using programme theory to evaluate complicated and complex aspects of interventions. *Evaluation 14*(1), 29–48.

Rogers, P.J., Forss, K, Marra, M. and Schwartz, R. (2011). Evaluating the Complex: Attribution, Contribution and Beyond: Comparative Policy Evaluation, Vol. 18. New Brunswick, NJ: Transaction Publishers. 33–52.

Rootman, I. and Goodstadt, M. (2001). *Evaluation in Health Promotion: Principles and perspectives*. WHO Regional Office Europe.

Rosen, L., Manor, O., Engelhard, D. and Zucker, D. (2006). In defense of the randomized controlled trial for health promotion research. *American Journal of Public Health 96*(7), 1181–6.

Rychetnik, L., Frommer, M., Hawe, P. and Shiell, A. (2002). Criteria for evaluating evidence on public health interventions. *Journal of Epidemiology & Community Health 56*(2), 119–27.

Rychetnik, L., Hawe, P., Waters, E., Barratt, A. and Frommer, M. (2004). A glossary for evidence-based public health. *Journal of Epidemiology & Community Health 58*(7), 538–45.

Schwarzman, J., Bauman, A., Gabbe, B., Rissel, C., Shilton, T. and Smith, B. (2018). Organizational determinants of evaluation practice in Australian prevention agencies. *Health Education Research 33*(3), 243–55.

Scriven, M. (1991). *Evaluation Thesaurus*. Sage.

Shilton, T., Howat, P., James, R., Burke, L., Hutchins, C. and Woodman, R. (2008). Health promotion competencies for Australia 2001–5: trends and their implications. *Promotion & Education 15*(2), 21–6.

Springett, J. (2001). Appropriate approaches to the evaluation of health promotion. *Critical Public Health 11*(2), 139–51.

Stern, E., Stame, N., Mayne, J., Forss, K., Davies, R. and Befani, B. (2012). DFID Working Paper 38. Broadening the range of designs and methods for impact evaluations. London: DFID.

Stufflebeam, D.L. and Coryn, C.L. (2014). *Evaluation Theory, Models, and Applications* (Vol. 50). John Wiley & Sons.

Van Belle, S., Wong, G., Westhorp, G., Pearson, M., Emmel, N., Manzano, A. and Marchal, B. (2016). Can 'realist' randomised controlled trials be genuinely realist? *Trials 17*(1), 1–6.

van Koperen, T.M., Renders, C.M., Spierings, E.J., Hendriks, A.-M., Westerman, M. J., Seidell, J.C. and Schuit, A.J. (2016). Recommendations and improvements for the evaluation of integrated community-wide interventions approaches. *Journal of Obesity, 2016*.

Weiss, C.H. (1995). Nothing as practical as good theory: Exploring theory-based evaluation for comprehensive community initiatives for children and families. *New Approaches to Evaluating Community Initiatives: Concepts, methods, and contexts 1*, 65–92.

White, H. (2013). An introduction to the use of randomised control trials to evaluate development interventions. *Journal of Development Effectiveness 5*(1), 30–49.

White, H. (2014). Current challenges in impact evaluation. *The European Journal of Development Research 26*(1), 18–30.

Whitehead, D. (2003). Evaluating health promotion: a model for nursing practice. *Journal of Advanced Nursing 41*(5), 490–8.

World Health Organization. (1998). *Health Promotion Evaluation: Recommendations to policy-makers: report of the WHO European Working Group on Health Promotion Evaluation*. Retrieved from https://apps.who.int/iris/bitstream/handle/10665/108116/E60706.pdf?sequence=1&isAllowed=y

Wyman, P.A., Brown, C.H., LoMurray, M., Schmeelk-Cone, K., Petrova, M., Yu, Q., ... Wang, W. (2010). An outcome evaluation of the Sources of Strength suicide prevention program delivered by adolescent peer leaders in high schools. *American Journal of Public Health 100*(9), 1653–61.

Zimmerman, B.J., Dubois, N., Houle, J., Lloyd, S., Mercier, C., Brousselle, A. and Rey, L. (2012). How does complexity impact evaluation? An introduction to the special issue. *The Canadian Journal of Program Evaluation = La Revue canadienne d'evaluation de programme 26*(3), v.

# 10

# Global Health

## Julian Pillay and Ruth Cross

## Introduction

This chapter highlights the importance of health promotion (HP) and health education (HE) in a contemporary global context. The chapter embeds the need to move
beyond reactive responses to health crises towards health-promotive and health
education approaches as powerful responses to current health challenges. Modern health challenges are outlined from a global perspective and include impactful
phenomena such as disease outbreaks, trends in disease patterns including the rise
in non-communicable diseases as well as climate change and political strife. Nurses
have a vital role to play in the promotion of global health and so, finally, the chapter considers the role of the nurse in disaster management and the specific part that
the International Council of Nurses has to play.

By the end of this chapter the reader will be able to:

1. Appreciate an overview of the history of global health and the global health
   agenda.
2. Outline some of the key global structures, systems and policies that support
   global health.
3. Define Sustainable Development Goal (SDG) 3 and provide a synopsis of key
   indicators that form part of the 2030 targets outlined, within the backdrop of
   contemporary global health.
4. State and outline some of the urgent health challenges as identified by the
   World Health Organization (WHO) and contextualise these challenges to
   possible health promotion efforts.

**Key terms**

Contemporary global health, Declaration of Alma-Ata; global health challenges, Millennium Declaration, Millennium Development Goals, Ottawa Charter Declaration, Sustainable Development Goals, World Health Organization

## Origins of Global Health

The concept of Global Health evolved from the study of public health, tropical medicine and international health and emerged as a distinct entity in the twenty-first century (Eliasz, 2018). Much of its basis has paralleled with public health in deeply entrenching the view that the health of a population is determined by the physical and social environment. Consequently, as the discipline of public health expanded, the importance of social and environmental factors on people's health was recognised and epidemiological tools were used to evaluate these factors. The trend of identifying disease patterns to determine causality has formed a strong basis for devising health-promotion interventions as part of a global health endeavour.

## The Foci of Global Health and the Emergence of the World Health Organization (WHO)

Much of the global health agenda recognises inequality as a driving force of illness and therefore advocates for social justice. This dates as far back as the industrial revolution where many physicians drew parallels between health and well-being and social justice (Palilonis, 2015). In 1851 the first international conference on public health took place in Paris in response to an ongoing cholera epidemic (Birn, 2009). The main intent of the event was to determine how the international community should respond to this public health emergency. As such, this marked a turning point in the history of global health as it was the first time that a critical health issue was addressed through international cooperation. This stimulated the onset of many such conferences held mainly on a needs basis over the next decades, until the World Health Organization (WHO) was initiated after which such gatherings became more regular.

The constitution of a newly envisioned WHO, signed by all members of the United Nations (UN) (61 countries) in July 1946 ushered in the first World Health Assembly in 1948 and a new chapter in global health (Eliasz, 2018). Since its inception, the WHO has been at the forefront of many key global health initiatives and ultimately the basis of the global health promotion agenda (please see Chapter 3: *A history of health promotion and health education* and Chapter 5: *The Ottawa Charter* for further details).

## Mandate of the World Health Organization (WHO) and the Culmination of the Declaration of Alma-Ata

From its onset, the WHO has held a broad mandate that encompasses research and data collection, health training (particularly emergency relief), epidemiological surveillance and setting international health standards. To this effect major successes have been achieved, for example, rolling out and expanding vaccination coverage, reducing the rates of childhood mortality and eradicating smallpox by 1980 (Markel, 2014). The inception of the WHO spearheaded a period of global and public health marked by centralisation within the WHO and the practice of direct aid from wealthier nations to poorer nations (Palilonis, 2015).

In 1978 the first-ever international conference on primary care, convened by the WHO and the United Nations Children's Emergency Fund (UNICEF), took place in the city of Almaty in Kazakhstan. The meeting culminated in the Declaration of Alma-Ata that has since been recognised as the watershed moment in the history of global health. This declaration endorsed the primary care approach to improving health, with a strong emphasis on the need to tackle the social, economic and political determinants of health (WHO, 1978). It also endorsed a vision of health for all by the year 2000 (Ibid.) and in so doing marked a turning point in the strategy of the WHO in moving beyond a focus of reducing infectious diseases towards the delivery of health care. During the subsequent years, many more non-governmental organisations (NGOs) formed to address specific regions, specific diseases or other determinants of health such as sanitation, clean water or food insecurity. At the same time, the WHO turned its attention to expanding primary care services over and above its traditional responsibilities, i.e., surveillance and prevention of infectious diseases.

## Global Health as a Shared Vision

The magnitude and intensity of the many global health challenges makes it difficult for any single country or agency to independently tackle them. Consequently, most organisations merge their ideas and resources for more impactful and sustainable health outcomes. International health organisations are generally divided into three groups: multilateral organisations, bilateral organisations, and non-governmental organisations (NGOs).

The prominent multilateral organisations are all part of the United Nations (UN). However, there are other non-UN organisations that are at the forefront of tackling global health challenges, such as the Global Fund to Fight AIDS, Tuberculosis and Malaria (International Medical Volunteers Association, 2022). Multilateral organisations that focus on global health involve multiple governmental as well as non-governmental support and include organisations such as the WHO – recognised as the premier international health organisation; the Pan American Health Organization – a regional field office for WHO in America; the World Bank – a leading institution in health and development that plays a critical role in global health by providing loans, credits and grants to poor countries for various developmental projects; the United Nations Children's Fund (UNICEF) – a key player in child health initiatives; and the Joint United Nations Programme of HIV/AIDS (UNAIDS) – a partnership towards achieving universal access to HIV prevention, treatment, care and support (Fogarty International Center, 2019).

Examples of bilateral organisations (i.e., a single government agency or a non-profit organisation that provides funding to developing countries) include the United States Agency for International Development (USAID) – the lead US Government agency that provides funding and support for global health initiatives; Centers for Disease Control (CDC) – part of the US Department of Health and Human Services responsible for implementing global public health initiatives; and non-governmental organisations (NGOs) – usually task-oriented, non-profit and voluntary organisations at local, national or international level – such as 'Doctors without borders', 'CARE International' and 'Population Services International' (University at Albany, 2022).

—— **Time to Reflect 10.1** ——————————————————————

Global health is characterised by the interaction between rich and poor societies/nations. Over the past decades, much of the global health agenda has been funded by wealthier nations as a mechanism of reducing the burden of disease in poorer societies. Yet, it is arguable that wealthy nations are the key drivers of poverty and are therefore accountable for the disparities in health. The support of poorer societies by wealthier nations is therefore a question of good will/generosity versus moral obligation through the principles of distributive justice.

## The Ottawa Charter Declaration

The first International Conference on Health Promotion (HP), meeting in Ottawa in November 1986 presented a 'Charter' for action to achieve Health for All by the year 2000 and beyond, thereafter referred to as the Ottawa Charter Declaration

(WHO, 1986). This conference was primarily a response to growing expectations for a new public health movement around the world. It built on the progress made through the Declaration on Primary Health Care at Alma-Ata as well as the WHO's targets towards meeting the 'Health for All' agenda.

The Ottawa Charter emphasises five aspects to comprehensively promote health. In (1) 'Building healthy public policy' governments should develop and implement policies that promote optimum health; (2) recognising that 'Creating a supportive environment' is necessary to facilitate healthy choices; (3) requiring 'Community participation' in order to promote healthy living and to encourage a shift from unhealthy practices to more healthy lifestyles in people/communities; (4) in 'Developing personal skills', interventions should be directed towards addressing group-specific needs as well as the determinants that influence behaviour; and (5) 'Re-orienting health service providers' towards more promotive and preventive practices than simply a focus on curative treatment – particularly through changing the attitudes of health providers (WHO, 1986). For further information please see Chapter 5: *The Ottawa Charter*.

Despite this clearly defined approach towards enabling health for all, the Ottawa Charter has, over the years received criticism for (1) largely having been developed by first-world countries that are typically more equipped to incorporate this agenda into a more efficient and effective healthcare sector than their third-world counterparts; and (2) being based on a multi-faceted approach to health care, that is largely determined by well-functioning sectors external to health and again, evidently less functioning/integrated in developing countries. For example, in countries such as South Africa, there were well developed policies on tobacco legislation and HIV prevention/treatment that were framed within the Ottawa Charter context (Taylor et al., 2009), but in requiring a multifaceted approach, South Africa did not have the resources, infrastructure and integrated approach for such policies to become doable. Without the necessary building blocks (i.e., all-inclusive inputs and well-integrated processes), the necessary outputs, outcomes and impact were less attainable.

A further matter that begs a question is around how relevant the Ottawa Charter is in current times amidst key modern challenges/changes such as globalisation and climate change to name a few. Consequently, a more contemporary approach towards unpacking the Ottawa Charter or potentially an expanded/modified charter may be more relevant, hence requiring deeper reflection and interrogation.

---

## Tutorial Trigger 10.1

The first International Conference on Health Promotion that took place in Ottawa in November 1986 presented a charter for action to achieve Health for All by the year 2000 and beyond. The charter incorporates FIVE key action areas in health promotion and THREE basic health promotion strategies.

Using the FIVE key action areas of the Ottawa Charter Declaration towards Health for All by 2000 and beyond, prepare a strategy map that provides a health-promotion plan to respond to the Covid-19 pandemic.

The strategy map should present key ideas/strategies in bullet point form for each of the five aspects identified and prepared as an A4 size flyer/pamphlet in landscape orientation.

---

## Research in Brief 10.1

The aim of this research was to describe and compare nursing health-promotion and prevention practice with the activities outlined in the Ottawa Charter in the light of the fact that nurses' potential for health promotion is often hindered by role confusion and a lack of understanding of what health promotion is. The research employed a critical interpretive synthesis examining data from 62 relevant papers determined by a range of inclusion and exclusion criteria. Thirty constructs were used to interrogate the papers, for example, 'evaluation', 'improving equity', and 'influencing policy'. The constructs were each aligned with one of the five action areas of the Ottawa Charter juxtaposed with activities in nursing practice as follows: (1) Addressing individuals' lifestyle factors vs. developing personal skills; (2) Focusing on environmental hazards vs. creating supportive environments; (3) Action on families vs. strengthening communities; (4) Promoting community participation vs. strengthening community action, and (5) Influencing policies vs. building healthy public policy. To guide this process the Ottawa Charter was used as a framework and an integrative grid was developed to categorise each activity under the five action areas and three strategies (advocacy, enabling, mediation) of the Charter. Research from a variety of work settings and countries was included. The paper concludes that there are significant mismatches between the Ottawa Charter's areas of action and strategies and nurses' practice in health promotion and prevention. Some of this was attributed to a misunderstanding about what health promotion entails, misunderstanding about different terms and role confusion. In addition, a lack of political will to support nurses beyond simply providing health education was highly impactful. Furthermore, the predominance of a biomedical model, lack of organisational prioritisation and research methodological flaws were also contributory factors. The implications for the wider global community included the highlighting of role confusion as one of the major barriers to developing nurses' capacity for health-promotion practice. In addition, conclusions included the observation that health promotion was often reduced to health education, a state that was reinforced by management strategies and organisational policies.

*Source:* Iriarte-Roteta, A., Lopez-Dicastillo, O., Mujika, A., Ruiz-Zaldibar, C., Hernantes, N., Bermejo-Martins, E. and Pumar-Méndez, M. (2020). Nurses' role in health promotion and prevention: A critical interpretive synthesis. *Journal of Clinical Nursing,* doi: 10.1111/jocn.15441

# The Millennium Declaration

In 2000, the Millennium Declaration was devised by heads of government within the framework of the WHO. This led to the emergence of the 'Eight Millennium Development Goals' which had a strong focus on health issues (UN, 2000) – see Box 10.1 Subsequently, discussions about global health, poverty alleviation and environmental sustainability became central issues at international political fora.

---

**Box 10.1**

## Eight Millennium Development Goals: United Nations, 2000

1   Eradicate extreme poverty and hunger
2   Provide universal primary education
3   Improve gender equality and empowerment of women
4   Reduce childhood mortality
5   Improve maternal health
6   Combat HIV/AIDS, malaria and other disease
7   Promote environmental sustainability
8   Develop global partnerships.

*Note*: Extracted from "United Nations Millennium Declaration" by UN, 2000, United Nations (Ed.)

---

# Contemporary Global Health

As is evident in the synopsis presented thus far of the evolution of global health, until the early twenty-first century, much of the efforts around global health focused on infectious diseases, nutrition and maternal/child health with less emphases on non-communicable diseases (NCDs) such as heart disease, diabetes and cancer that were regarded as diseases affecting the developed countries. It is now well recognised that many developing countries face a double burden of disease, i.e., both communicable and non-communicable diseases, which forms the basis of contemporary global health. However, over the last decades we have seen the further challenge in many developing countries, brought on by the confluence of HIV and tuberculosis with obesity and non-communicable diseases, poor outcomes for child and maternal health, and violence and injury constituting a quadruple burden of disease (Bradshaw et al., 2003). Schie et al. (2020: 466) define this quadruple burden of disease as 'conditions characterised as communicable, non-communicable, maternal and/or perinatal and trauma'. Nurses have a huge role to play in tackling this burden. However, the added burden placed on the healthcare system to deliver favourable outcomes within this climate creates an urgent need to expand health promotive efforts as a primary focus of health rather than reactive responses through curative approaches.

---

### Point to Ponder 10.1

'Global Health needs more health promotion than disease management; good work and income conditions for all; equal opportunities; the reduction of socio-economic and health inequalities; food sovereignty; responsible environmental policy; social security, peace, democracy and participation'. (Holst, 2020: 8)

The statement above neatly articulates the need for global health to embrace a multi-faceted, cross-cutting approach. It is therefore imperative that global health considers and emphasises the social, political and economic determinants of health to support the reduction of health inequalities within and among countries.

---

## The 2030 Agenda for Sustainable Development

'Leaving no one behind' is the hallmark of the Sustainable Development Goals (SDGs) adopted by the UN in September 2015 (United Nations Development Programme (UNDP), 2017). This 2030 Agenda for Sustainable Development, initiated by the UN and adopted by all UN member states, provides a shared blueprint for peace and prosperity for people and the planet, from a contemporary perspective (UN, 2015). The essence of this Agenda pivots around 17 SDGs, serving as an urgent call for action by all countries in a global partnership (UNDP, 2017). The Agenda recognises that striving towards global equity must be paralleled with strategies that improve health and education, reduce inequality and stimulate economic growth, amid the backdrop of environmental sustainability (UN, 2015).

The SDGs of the 2030 Agenda for Sustainable Development build on decades of effort by countries and the UN and provide a contemporary global context. Whilst the concept of health promotion, which forms a key component of public health, is embedded in many of the SDGs, SDG 3 is of particular relevance to health promotion. Defined as; Ensure healthy lives and promote well-being for all at all ages', this SDG proposes to, by 2030, achieve several measurable targets (UN, 2015) – see Box 10.2. Notwithstanding the 17 clearly defined SDGs, Mohammed and Ghebreyesus (2018) demonstrate the interconnectedness of the SDGs to each other. More importantly, the fact that even though SDG 3 focuses specifically on good health and well-being, good health and well-being contributes to almost all other SDGs/goals (Mohammed and Ghebreyesus, 2018).

**Box 10.2**

## Targets of SDG 3

- By 2030, reduce the global maternal mortality ratio to less than 70 per 100,000 live births;
- By 2030, end preventable deaths of new-borns and children under 5 years of age, with all countries aiming to reduce neonatal mortality to 12 per 1,000 live births or lower and under-5 mortality to 25 per 1,000 live births or lower;
- By 2030, end the epidemics of AIDS, tuberculosis, malaria and neglected tropical diseases and combat hepatitis, water-borne diseases and other communicable diseases;
- By 2030, reduce premature mortality from non-communicable diseases by one-third, through prevention and treatment and to promote mental health and well-being;
- Strengthen the prevention and treatment of substance abuse, including narcotic drug abuse and harmful use of alcohol;
- By 2030, reduce the number of global deaths and injuries from road traffic accidents by half;
- By 2030, ensure universal access to sexual and reproductive healthcare services, including family planning, information and education, and the integration of reproductive health into national strategies and programmes;
- Achieve universal health coverage, including financial risk protection, access to quality essential healthcare services and access to safe, effective, quality and affordable essential medicines and vaccines for all;
- By 2030, substantially reduce the number of deaths and illnesses from hazardous chemicals and air, water and soil pollution and contamination;
    a  Strengthen the implementation of the WHO Framework Convention on Tobacco Control in all countries, as appropriate;
    b  Support the research and development of vaccines and medicines for the communicable and non-communicable diseases that primarily affect developing countries, provide access to affordable essential medicines and vaccines, in accordance with the Doha Declaration on the Trade-Related Aspects of Intellectual Property Rights (TRIPS) Agreement and Public Health, which affirms the right of developing countries to use to the full the provisions in the TRIPS Agreement regarding flexibilities to protect public health, and, in particular, provide access to medicines for all;
    c  Substantially increase health financing and the recruitment, development, training and retention of the health workforce in developing countries, especially in least developed countries and small island developing States;
    d  Strengthen the capacity of all countries, in particular developing countries, for early warning, risk reduction and management of national and global health risks.

*Source*: 'Transforming our world: the 2030 Agenda for Sustainable Development', UN, Department of Economic and Social Affairs, 2015, United Nations.

## Contemporary Health Challenges

Against the backdrop of efforts towards the attainment of the SDGs, and in particular SDG 3, in the beginning of 2020 the WHO released a list of urgent, global health challenges. Box 10.3 presents each of the challenges identified by the WHO and summarises each, respectively. Evidently, much of the challenges centre around health issues in a far deeper manner than the simply operational and health coverage targets created through the SDGs.

---

**Box 10.3**

### World Health Organization's list of global health challenges, 2020

- *Elevating health in the climate debate*

  Air pollution kills an estimated 7 million people each year, while climate change causes more extreme weather events, exacerbates malnutrition and fuels the spread of infectious diseases

- *Delivering health in conflict and crisis*

  Conflict is forcing record numbers of people out of their own homes, leaving tens of millions of people with little access to health care

- *Making health care fairer*

  There is an 18-year difference in the life expectancy between rich and poor countries. Persistent and growing socio-economic gaps result in major discrepancies in the quality of people's health

- *Expanding access to medicines*

  About one-third of the world's population lack access to medicines, vaccines, diagnostic tools and other essential health products

- *Stopping infectious diseases*

  Infectious diseases continue to kill millions of people each year. Even vaccine-preventable diseases continue to kill hundreds of thousands each year

- *Preparing people for epidemics*

  Every year, the world spends far more responding to disease outbreaks, natural disasters and other health emergencies than it does preparing for and preventing them

- *Protecting people from dangerous products*

  Lack of food, unsafe food and unhealthy diets are responsible for almost one third of the current global burden of disease

- *Investing in the people who defend our health*

  Chronic under-investment in the education and employment of healthcare workers has led to health worker shortages globally

- *Keeping adolescents safe*

  More than 1 million adolescents aged 10–19 die each year. The leading causes of death include road injury, HIV, suicide, lower respiratory infections and interpersonal violence

- *Earning public trust*

  Public health is compromised by the uncontrolled dissemination of misinformation as well as the lack of trust in public institutions

- *Harnessing new technologies*

  Monitoring and regulating new technologies to circumvent ethical and social implications and to prevent the harm to people they are intended to help

- *Protecting the medicines that protect us*

  Anti-microbial resistance (AMR) threatens to reverse the gains made in medicine since the pre-antibiotic era

- *Keeping health care clean*

  Roughly one in four health facilities lack basic water services

  *Source*: 'Urgent health challenges for the next decade' by T.A. Ghebreyesus, 2020, WHO.

Any number of global challenges, that will impact health and health care, can be expected over the next decade, including infections such as Covid-19 as well as others related to global warming and climate change (Catton, 2020). It is estimated that the healthcare workforce comprises 50 per cent of nurses and midwives (WHO, 2016) who are therefore vital to achieving global health by acting as primary advocates towards shaping healthcare policy, practice and education (Klopper et al., 2019).

## Tutorial Trigger 10.2

'The world can't afford to do nothing' – this is the WHO's message in its 2020 report listing the most urgent health challenges for the decade ahead.

Choose any ONE of the 2020 Global challenges listed in Box 10.3. Develop a detailed Health Promotion plan, particularly identifying key strategies that can be implemented/supported by nurses.

## Global Threats to Public Health over the Last Three Decades

Over the last three decades, several infectious diseases have emerged as global threats.

In the 1990s HIV/AIDS and TB became a force that galvanised international cooperation between government and non-government organisations. Many emergency and relief funding agencies, as well as private philanthropists, came to the fore to address research and treatment of HIV/AIDS in the developing countries and expanded the field of global health (Brandt, 2013). In subsequent years, what began with the spread of the AIDS pandemic further developed into the emergence of several new infectious diseases. These include SARS (Severe Acute Respiratory Syndrome) which surfaced in Asia in 2002; H1N1 (Swine) flu in the northern hemisphere between 2009 and 2010; MERS (Middle-East Respiratory Syndrome) in 2012; Avian influenza from 2013 onwards; Ebola in Western Africa in 2014; Zika in the Democratic Republic of Congo in 2019 and its subsequent emergence in Brazil. Most recently, the coronavirus pandemic that originated in China and spread globally in catastrophic numbers has sparked global alarm. Despite widespread efforts to contain many of these pandemics globally, there are questions raised as to whether a reactive and curative approach to containment is/has been less effective than a more fervent health-promotion response. To further confound the challenge of containing rapidly emerging infectious diseases, is the epidemiological transition (i.e., the consequent exponential rise in non-communicable, chronic diseases coupled with re-emerging pandemics and infectious diseases) (Omran, 2005) for which a balance in global efforts is difficult to attain.

Compounded by the HIV and tuberculosis crisis in many developing countries as well as the emergence of trauma/violence as a threat to health care, the quadruple burden of diseases therefore beckons the need for an approach that moves beyond a focus on reactive and curative efforts. As stated previously, nurses have a huge part to play in addressing global health issues. From tackling maternal and infant mortality, to supporting people with chronic disease, to dealing with the effects of trauma and violence, such healthcare personnel are vital to the cause of maximising health gain at an individual, societal and global level. One area where nurses are specifically involved that is relevant to the discussion in this chapter is disaster management.

## Disaster Nursing

Worldwide we are seeing an increase in human-induced and natural disasters and the resulting devastating impact on people (Kalanlar, 2019). Such disasters include earthquakes, extreme weather events, flooding and contamination of water sources. Loke et al. (2021), among others, argue that nurses have a pivotal part to play in disaster management across the globe (Loke, Guo and Molassiotis, 2021). Nurses can contribute to disaster recovery in a number of ways including limiting morbidity and mortality and promoting positive health behaviours and they are 'one of the most important players in promoting health during disaster situations'

(Kalanlar, 2019). Nurses have been involved in disaster management and response since nursing was first established as a profession; however, disaster nursing as a distinct nursing speciality is still in its relative infancy in some parts of the world at least (Al Harthi, Al Thobaity, Al Ahmari and Almalki, 2020; Kalanlar, 2019). Disaster nursing is defined as 'the adaptation of professional nursing knowledge, skills, and attitudes in recognising and meeting the physical and emotional needs of disaster victims' (Rojas, 2020) and 'supporting the daily activities of communities as part of the disaster recovery process' (Harada, Zhuravsky, Marutani and Hickmott, 2021). The global coronavirus pandemic provides an excellent illustration of the role that nurses play in disaster management at a global level. Nurses were at the forefront of healthcare delivery as the pandemic took hold during the first half of 2020 and have also been at the helm in the subsequent vaccine rollouts in early 2021 in different countries.

Nurses have a key role to play in the four stages of disaster management outlined in Box 10.4. However, there are several challenges in preparing and supporting nurses working in disaster management. A scoping review identified several barriers faced by nurses responding to disasters (Al Harthi et al., 2020). These included '1) disaster nursing as a new speciality, 2) inadequate level of preparedness, 3) poor formal education, 4) lack of research, 5) ethical and legal issues and 6) issues related to nurses' roles in disasters' (Al Harthi et al., 2020). Loke et al. (2021) also argue that more disaster nursing research is needed in order to improve nurses' capacity to respond to global disasters.

---

**Box 10.4**

**Four Steps of Disaster Management**

*Before disaster occurs:*

*Step 1:* Identifying disaster risks
*Step 2:* Preparedness - including education and training, planning and policy

*After disaster begins:*

*Step 3:* Disaster response; implementing a disaster plan
*Step 4:* Disaster recovery; supporting a return to normality

> Note. Adapted from *'Challenges for nurses in disaster management*: a scoping review' by M. Al Harthi et al., 2020, *Risk Management and Healthcare Policy*, 13, 2627-2634.

---

It is vital for nurses (and other health professionals) to be prepared to respond appropriately and effectively to disasters (Kalanlar, 2019). However, Al Harthi et al. (2020) argue that disaster nursing, as a speciality, needs further development including improved disaster management education and training in order to enable nurses to respond effectively to disasters. Disaster nursing education is crucial in developing effective responses to disaster management (Kalanlar, 2019). As alluded to earlier in the chapter voluntary, or non-governmental, organisations are often part of a co-ordinated response to disasters. Nurses and midwives make up some of the core staff particularly of those organisations that have a medical or health focus. Many of these, such as the International Red Cross and Red Crescent Movement, are well recognised for their global efforts intervening to support people facing disaster.

## The Role of the International Council of Nurses

The International Council of Nurses (ICN) works closely with other global agencies such as the World Health Organization and the World Bank (see Box 10.5 for more information). The ICN has several functions including:

- ensuring quality nursing care for everyone
- ensuring the development of sound health policy
- advancing nursing knowledge
- ensuring a competent and satisfied nursing workforce.

Nursing is the largest healthcare profession in the world and the ICN is the largest network of health professions connecting millions of nurses. Any nurse who is a member of their country's national nursing association is automatically a member of the ICN. One of the primary purposes of the ICN is to influence policy at all levels, from the top down, and to ensure quality training and education for nurses (Kennedy, 2021). The ICN emphasises how one of the key roles of the nurse is to promote health.

### Box 10.5

**The International Council of Nurses**

The International Council of Nurses (ICN) was founded in 1899 and is a federation of over 130 national nurses' associations. The ICN represents more than 27 million nurses globally.

The *mission* of the ICN is 'to represent nursing worldwide, advance the nursing profession, promote the wellbeing of nurses, and advocate for health in all policies'. The *vision* of the ICN is 'the global community recognises, supports, and invests in nurses and nursing to lead and deliver health for all'.

The ICN seeks to align and integrate nursing with global health priorities (as identified earlier in this chapter). During the period 2017-2020 those priorities were as follows:

- universal health coverage
- non-communicable diseases
- primary health care
- human resources for health
- person centred care
- patient safety
- antimicrobial resistance
- mental health
- immunisation and,
- the Sustainable Development Goals.

During the global coronavirus pandemic, the ICN advocated for the nursing profession recognising the vital role that nurses were playing in caring for their communities and the increased demands on them. The President, Annette Kennedy, highlighted the mass trauma experienced by nurses in a context of nursing shortages and pressed governments to appropriately recompense, protect and support nurses (International Council of Nurses, 2021). As of 2021 the ICN endorsed the UK Nursing Times Covid-19: Are You OK campaign, which aimed to raise awareness of the impact of working through the global pandemic on nurses' mental health and well-being as well as ensuring that they had access to appropriate support. This was in recognition of the global shortage of nurses even before the pandemic took hold (Ford, 2021).

*Source*: International Council of Nurses website (www.icn.ch).

---

## Summary

The rapid succession of disease outbreaks has contributed to building international relations towards strengthened health. Consequently, global health has become more concrete and is currently ranked high on the international political agenda. However, global efforts often fall short of attaining a complete 'universal' approach as would be expected from a 'global' effort. Most experts would agree that the best way to improve health outcomes is simply to ensure that people have access to quality health care. Moreover, the transdisciplinary and interdisciplinary approach must become more explicit and most importantly, there is a dire need to move beyond the biomedical, clinical or genetic engineering approaches to carefully consider the complexity of health in all its dimensions and diversity. It is therefore imperative that public health, and within this the tenet of health promotion, remains the mainstay of all levels of care. Nurses remain vital to efforts to address and improve global health.

—— **Key Points** ————————————————————————

- Much of the global health agenda recognises inequality as a driving force of illness and therefore advocates for social justice.
- Global health must embrace a multifaceted, cross-cutting approach that moves beyond reactive and curative approaches.
- Nurses have an important part to play in the global health agenda bringing skill-sets and transferable skills that impact health outcomes at different levels.

# References

Al Harthi, M., Al Thobaity, A., Al Ahmari, W. and Almalki, M. (2020). Challenges for nurses in disaster management: a scoping review. *Risk Management and Healthcare Policy 13*, 2627–34.

Birn, A.-E. (2009). The stages of international (global) health: histories of success or successes of history? *Global Public Health 4*(1), 50–68.

Bradshaw, D., Groenevald, P., Laubscher, R., et al. (2003). Initial burden of diseases estimates for South Africa, 2000. *South African Medical Journal 93*(9), 682–8.

Brandt, A.M. (2013). How AIDS invented global health. *New England Journal of Medicine 368*(23), 2149–52. doi: 10.1056/NEJMp1305297

Catton, H. (2020). Global challenges in health and health care for nurses and midwives everywhere. *International Nursing Review 67*(1), 4–6.

Eliasz, M.K. (2018). A History of Global Health. In B. Sethia and P. Kumar (Eds), *Essentials of Global Health*. Elsevier Health Sciences.

Fogarty International Center. (2019). Nongovernmental Organizations (NGOs) working in Global Health Research. Retrieved 11 March 2022, from www.fic.nih.gov/Global/Pages/NGOs.aspx

Ford, S. (2021). International Council of Nurses. *Nursing Times*. Retrieved 14 June 2021, from www.nursingtimes.net/covid-19-are-you-ok/international-council-of-nurses-24-02-2021/

Ghebreyesus, T.A. (2020). Urgent health challenges for the next decade. *World Health Organization*. Retrieved 14 June 2021, from www.who.int/news-room/photo-story/photo-story-detail/urgent-health-challenges-for-the-next-decadeHarada, N., Zhuravsky, L., Marutani, M. and Hickmott, B. (2021). Cultural safety in disaster nursing. *Kai Tiaki Nursing New Zealand, 27*(2), 19–21.

Holst, J. (2020). Global Health – emergence, hegemonic trends and biomedical reductionism. *Global Health 16*(1), 42. doi: 10.1186/s12992-020-00573-4

International Council of Nurses. (2021). Gender inequalities exposed by COVID-19. Retrieved 14 June 2021, from www.icn.ch/news/gender-inequalities-exposed-covid-19-international-council-nurses-challenges-gender-bias

International Medical Volunteers Association. (2022). The Major International Health Organisations. Retrieved 11 March 2022, from www.imva.org/pages/orgfrm.htm

Kalanlar, B. (2019). The challenges and opportunities in disaster nursing education in Turkey. *Journal of Trauma Nursing JTN 26*(3), 164–70.

Kennedy, A. (2021). President's message. *International Council of Nurses*. Retrieved 14 June 2021, from www.icn.ch/who-we-are/presidents-message

Klopper, H.C., Madigan, R.N., Vlasich, C., Albien, A., Ricciardi, R., Catrambone, C. and Tigges, E. (2019). Advancement of global health: Recommendations from the global advisory panel on the future of nursing and midwifery (GAPFON). *Journal of Advanced Nursing 76*, 741–8.

Loke, A.Y., Guo, C. and Molassiotis, A. (2021). Development of disaster nursing education and training programs in the past 20 years (2000–2019): A systematic review. *Nurse Education Today 99*, 1–19.

Markel, H. (2014). Worldly approaches to global health: 1851 to the present. *Public Health 128*(2), 124–8.

Mohammed, A.J. and Ghebreyesus, T.A. (2018). Healthy living, well-being and the sustainable development goals. *Bulletin of the World Health Organization 96*, 590–90A. https://doi.org/10.2471/BLT.18.222042

Omran, A.R. (2005). The epidemiological transition: A theory of the epidemiology of population change. *The Milbank Quarterly 83*(4), 731–57.

Palilonis, M. (2015). An Introduction to Global Health and Global Health Ethics: A brief history of global health. Available on: ZSR Library at <wakespace.lib.wfu.edu/handle/10339/57141>

Rojas, K. (2020). What is Disaster Nursing? *Trusted Health*. Retrieved 14 June 2021, from www.trustedhealth.com/blog/what-is-disaster-nursing

Schie, K.E., Spies, E., Hyams, L.B., et al. (2020). Paediatric dysphagia within the context of South Africa's quadruple burden of disease, seen at a tertiary level hospital. *International Journal of Speech-Language Pathology 22*(4), 466–74.

Taylor, M., Meyer-Weitz, A., Jinabhai, C. and Sathiparsad, R. (2009). Meeting the challenges of the Ottawa Charter: comparing South African responses to AIDS and tobacco control. *Health Promotion International 24*(3), 203–10.

United Nations. (2000). *United Nations Millennium Declaration*. United Nations (Ed.).

United Nations. (2015). *Transforming our World: The 2030 agenda for sustainable development*. New York: United Nations, Department of Economic and Social Affairs.

United Nations Development Programme. (2017). Sustainable Development Goals. Retrieved 7 June 2021, from www.undp.org/sustainable-development-goals

University at Albany. (2022). Organizations working in Global Health. Retrieved 11 March 2022, from www.albany.edu/globalhealth/organizations-working-global-health

World Health Organization. (1978). Declaration of Alma-Ata. International Conference on Primary Health Care, Alma-Ata, USSR, 6–12 September 1978. Retrieved 7 June 2021, from www.who.int/hpr/NPH/docs/declaration_almaata.pdf

World Health Organization. (1986). Ottawa Charter for Health Promotion, 1986.

World Health Organization. (2016). Global strategic directions for strengthening nursing and midwifery 2016–2020. Geneva, Switzerland.

# 11

# The Future of Health Promotion and Health Education for Health Professionals

## Louise Warwick-Booth and Ruth Cross

## Introduction

While health education practice has remained relatively 'static' for several decades, health promotion is more fluid and ever-evolving – especially around the health policy space. Health promotion has 'struggled', for some time, against competing disciplines (especially medicine) to gain a strong evidence-based foothold when applying for government funding and as a discipline that sets and leads national health policy agendas. The overall health-promotion agenda is often at the behest of preventive medicine and public health. This chapter predicts the changing landscape and extent to which the current situation may change, evolve and adapt, reflecting upon the current policy and practice context within the UK and more globally. The chapter examines the changing health-promotion landscape, and draws together important lessons from recent disciplinary developments, policy, technological advancements, changing evidence and the impact of Covid-19.

By the end of this chapter the reader will be able to:

1. Understand the complexity of health promotion as a specific discipline.
2. Appreciate and describe the policy context in which health promotion and health education are situated within the UK, as well as more globally.
3. Understand how technological advancements and the changing evidence base underpinning practice enable health to be promoted.
4. Describe lessons from Covid-19 in relation to what they mean for the future of health promotion and health education for professionals.

## Key terms

Policy, global context, workforce education, technology, e-literacy, health promotion education

## Health Promotion as a Specific Discipline

Throughout this book we have argued that nurses play a central role in the promotion of health in a myriad of ways, these include health education and health promotion. As Hubley et al. (2021) state, health promotion is an essential component of most health and community workers' jobs, this includes nurses. The education of nurses in the fields of health education and health promotion is therefore crucial. Elsewhere in this book (please see Chapter 2: *Defining health promotion and health education*) we have discussed the definitional parameters of health education and health promotion. We established that health education was an important facet of health promotion and that health promotion is a distinct, specific discipline defined by a set of principles and values. We also differentiated between health promotion and public health as well as other related areas such as environmental health (please see the discussion in Chapter 3: *A history of health promotion and health education*).

---

### Point to Ponder 11.1

There is an ongoing discussion in the wider literature about the relationship between health promotion and public health. Some people view health promotion as an integral part of public health whilst other people view both as one and the same. However, some people argue, as we have here, that health promotion (whilst closely allied to public health) has a distinct identity that sets it apart from public health as defined by a specific set of values. Cross et al.'s (2021) view is that 'health promotion is a social movement with the central aim of tackling the social determinants of health [to] bring about social and health justice' (p. 1).

---

We have therefore determined that health promotion sets itself apart by a focus on empowerment, equity, tackling health inequalities, social justice and participation and that, more broadly, it is politically and ethically driven (Cross et al., 2021a; Watson et al., 2021). Simply put, health promotion is about 'improving the health status of individuals and communities' at all levels (Wills and Jackson, 2014: 19).

The Institute of Health Promotion and Education (Watson et al., 2021) published a position statement on health promotion in which it was stated that 'access to the educational programmes should be made available for all those involved in providing health promotion in whatever capacity and at whatever level' (p. 2). In many countries in the world nursing has now become a graduate profession and so universities have a huge role to play in educating these aspiring professionals about health education and health promotion during pre- and post-registration/ qualification programmes. Cross et al. (2021b, p. 187) point out that one of the key roles that universities play is 'to develop capacity in health promotion, thus developing the health promotion workforce and adding the human resources for health'. The education of nurses in health education and health promotion is vital to ensuring that they are able to carry out these parts of their role to the best effect; however, in practice there is often disparity in the ways in which nurses see themselves as health educators or health promoters and how much emphasis this is given in their day-to-day roles. In addition, as Iriarte-Roteta et al. (2020) argue, role confusion can impede nurses' potential to promote health. Many studies on the nurse's role in health promotion have found that their role is largely conceptualised as being a health educator rather than appreciating the wider range of activities that constitute health promotion (see for example Whitehead, 2011). In addition, health professionals often carry out what would be defined as health promotion activity but is not seen as such (Manning, 2017). This may be because, as Wild and McGrath (2019) point out, 'health promotion [can appear] to be related to anything and everything and this can make it feel less relevant to the day-to-day work of many nurses' (p. 29) yet health promotion is an integral part of the nurse's role (Evans et al., 2017) and is explicitly written into their codes of conduct. For example, the Nursing and Midwifery Council of the United Kingdom (2018) outlines seven standards of proficiency for nursing the second of which is 'promoting health and preventing ill health'. Wills and Jackson (2014) argue that health promotion is 'increasingly important' to nursing practice as it 'enhances the way in which health care and services are viewed, looking beyond the medical model to consider the broader influences on health' (p. 16). The nurse has a large role to play in this. All of this points to the importance of effective education for, and about, health promotion for workforce capacity and development in order for nurses to fulfil this essential component of their roles. As WHO (2015: 6) states, 'health workforce education, service delivery models, regulation, legislation and professional roles must continue to evolve and align with population needs'. This is necessary so that nurses are able to grasp the important difference between simply engaging in health education activities (such as giving advice and information) and working to empower people (Whitehead, 2018), both of which are influenced by the policy context underpinning practice.

## Policy Context

Policy is an ever-changing field, and the future work of healthcare professionals will always be affected by policy, as 'nursing needs policy, it provides the context to nurses' practice, roles, and knowledge and frames patients' day-to-day lives' (Annesley, 2019: 496). Health policy means several different things such as trying to improve population health, educate the workforce and ensure that government decisions are implemented and enacted through processes (Walt, 1995). Nurses working in the UK will all experience policy impacts as a result of reorganisations, restructures, target driven cultures and in most recent times constantly shifting guidance linked to government decisions about the management of Covid-19 (Warwick-Booth et al., 2021). Whilst healthcare policy is focused upon the provision of services to treat patients, health policy more generally now notes the need for prevention within health system models (NHS England, 2014, Kings Fund, 2021). Health policy also directly informs educational provision linked to workforce training requirements.

---

### Tutorial Trigger 11.1

Recognition of the complexities of contemporary nursing led to policy changes around educational requirements in the UK. Nurses now need to be qualified to degree level (from 2013) as this is an entry requirement for the role.

How do you think all degree level education for nurses enhances their practice? In your view is degree level education what is needed in terms of workforce training?

---

Degree level health education for future health professionals involves research training, and research evidence is important in practice, as Box 11.1 illustrates.

**— Research in Brief 11.1 —**

Research has shown that nurse education is important for patient survival and positive outcomes post-surgically in the USA (Kutney-Lee et al., 2013). Using nurse survey and patient discharge data from Pennsylvania in 1999 and 2006, this study illustrated that 'a ten-point increase in the percentage of nurses holding a baccalaureate degree in nursing within a hospital was associated with an average reduction of 2.12 deaths for every 1,000 patients - and for a subset of patients with complications, an average reduction of 7.47 deaths per 1,000 patients' (Kutney-Lee et al., 2013: 579).

Researchers estimated that if all of the hospitals in their study (134) had increased the percentage of nurses employed who had baccalaureate qualifications by ten points during the time period of the study, approximately 500 deaths among general, orthopaedic, and vascular surgery patients could also have been prevented. This study provides a strong level of evidence for improving the standards to which nurses are educated to, as a mechanism to promote health.

Kutney-Lee, A., Sloane, D.M. and Aiken, L.H. (2013). 'An increase in the number of nurses with baccalaureate degrees is linked to lower rates of post-surgery mortality.' *Health Affairs* (Millwood) *32*, 3, 579-86.

Nurse-led research can also influence the policy process in several ways, for example by informing agenda setting on workforce issues, providing evidence of effective interventions to inform policy discussions, and contributing to understandings of what works, as well as what does not for policy implementation (Ellenbecker and Edward, 2016). Policy implementation is executed through a complex system, with health professionals working as 'street level bureaucrats' (Lipsky, 2010) to put into practice the decisions made by those in power, such as government ministers and managers (Annesley, 2019; Blakemore and Warwick-Booth, 2013). Contemporary policy tends to focus upon:

1. The prevention of ill-health
2. The promotion of personal responsibility
3. Supporting people to take control of their own health (Public Health England, 2018).

## Point to Ponder 11.2

As a healthcare practitioner, to what extent are you able to tackle health improvement in your daily role? How does policy direct your work? Think about health advice linked to alcohol intake, smoking cessation and lifestyle changes here as starting points.

Health promotion as a discipline has been critical about the over-emphasis on curative medicine within policy approaches for many years (Kickbusch et al., 1990; Warwick-Booth and Rowlands, 2020). Despite the broad array of evidence to illustrate the ways in which the wider policy environment determines health outcomes (Bambra, 2019), policy makers remain focused upon healthcare services rather than wider determinants. Policy makers blame unwell citizens for their irresponsible behaviours without recognising that these are determined by wider environmental factors as well as a limited menu of healthy choices, arising from policy decisions (Bambra, 2019; Dowding, 2020). Policy which negatively impacts upon health outcomes also leads to increased pressure on the health services (Annesley, 2019). Consequently, it remains important for health professionals to understand policy processes, and to potentially influence them as agents of change (Hajizadeh et al., 2021). In summary, health policy underpins both nursing practice and health promotion education in the UK as well as further afield, and so now the chapter turns to examining the global policy context.

## Global Context

The policy context of health promotion education at a global level varies considerably from region to region and country to country. Global policy underpinning health-promotion efforts are largely driven by the World Health Organization's agenda as detailed in Chapter 3: *A history of health promotion and health education.* The global Covid-19 pandemic brought health education and health promotion to the fore. This will be discussed in more detail as a case study later in the chapter. It is sufficient to note here that the interconnectedness of modern life presents complex challenges for the promotion of health and requires multifaceted responses. The United Nations Millennium Development Goals (global targets for a 2015 deadline), and subsequent Sustainable Development Goals detail the scope of future challenges. These wide-ranging targets (17 in total) illustrate that the world's current global challenges, such as poverty, must be tackled by using strategies to improve both health and education (UN, 2022).

The state of education about health education and health promotion for healthcare professionals varies enormously across different contexts. Much of this variation is to do with how prominent health education and health promotion are within different countries; however, other factors such as resources, expertise and infrastructure also come into play. By way of examining the global context we will focus first on the global south and then turn to Canada for an example from the global north outside of the United Kingdom.

In relation to the global south, Anugwom (2020) maintains that health promotion is crucial to the achievement of health goals in Africa – for more information about how this might be realised please see Box 11.1. Whilst Anugwom (2020) recognises that the individual countries of the African continent are different, diverse and face specific structural challenges, he argues that there is a need to develop a culture of sharing evidence of what works for the promotion of health and, in relation to workforce development, training in health promotion needs to be tailored to different cadres of healthcare workers rooted in evidence of best practice. This applies to nursing as much as any other part of the healthcare workforce.

---

**Box 11.1**

## Health promotion's potential in Africa

Anugwom (2020) argues that several things need to happen in synergy for health promotion to achieve its full potential in the African context as follows:

- Legislation: political will is necessary to support policy that will improve healthcare delivery including public health governance and leadership.
- Finance: the health delivery system needs to be underpinned by appropriate funding.
- Organisational change: the health system needs to be robustly organised in order to cope with change and challenges.
- Gender inclusiveness: men and women need to be equal partners and collaborators.
- Mapping of priorities: health promotion should be pursued through capacity building, action planning, advocacy and multi-sectoral action.

*Adapted from Anugwom (2020)*

---

Liyanagunawardena and Aboshady (2017) point out that health education in the global south has been experiencing several challenges including insufficient infrastructure, outdated curricula and teaching methods, a lack of well-trained healthcare personnel, and cultural barriers that prevent open discussion about 'sensitive' topics such as sexuality.

As Keshavarz Mohammadi (2019) argues, health promotion has to be adaptable in order to be sustainable and that requires developing a critical mass of scholarship. In addition, the global political context of health is characterised by an increasing demand for services and support alongside decreasing resources (Palfrey, 2018). Against this backdrop the role of the nurse in promoting health is even more crucial. However, there is a global shortage of nurses. There is an estimated shortage of between 6 million (WHO, 2020) and 9 million nurses worldwide (Drennan and Ross, 2019). Nurses make up approximately half of the world's healthcare workforce so this is significant. At a global level nursing is consistently under-resourced however, adequately funding nurse-delivered care will save millions of lives a year (WHO, 2021).

──── Tutorial Trigger 11.2 ────────────────────────────────

Globally, education for nurses varies from country to country and region to region. Similarly, the focus on health education and health promotion within training also varies. How do you think training and education for nurses could incorporate greater emphasis on health education and health promotion? What would need to change?

## Technology and Health Promotion – How Has This Changed the Landscape?

──── Time to Reflect 11.1 ───────────────────────────────

Before you read the next section of this chapter on 'Technology and health promotion' take some time to reflect on the following:

Advances in technology have had a significant impact on the ways that nurses have worked over the past several decades. Their roles will continue to change as new developments take place. Reflect on how your role as a nurse (or trainee) has been impacted on by technology since you first started in it. Specifically consider your role as a health educator or health promoter. How might you have to adapt in future to use technology to support these aspects of your role? How might technology assist you to promote health?

Technology has advanced very quickly over the past few decades and is likely to continue to do so. This has considerably influenced the ways in which health is promoted and increased the potential for health communication in multiple ways. Many things that are commonplace now would have been unimaginable two or three decades ago. These include wearable technology to monitor different aspects of health and fitness status (for example, blood sugar levels, heart rate and energy expenditure), gamification (for example, active video games designed to encourage the user to move), telehealth (for example, monitoring or exchanging information about a person's health remotely) and web-based/enabled platforms (Naslund and Aschbrenner, 2019; O'Neil, 2019). Technology has not just changed how health promotion takes place, it has also changed (and is changing) how health professionals are trained in health education and health promotion.

Liyanagunawardena and Aboshady (2017) argue that e-learning (distance learning) has huge potential to address some of the development needs experienced by healthcare professionals in countries in the global south in relation to health education (and health promotion). They point out how this mode of delivery can decrease costs, increase access and provide a more consistent, efficient form of training in health education for healthcare professionals. Given how a massive amount of education had to transition to on-line delivery during the global Covid-19 pandemic it is likely that a lot will continue to take place via this medium in future. Educational courses and modules developed and delivered on-line through different mobile means are readily available and accessible to anyone with the hardware (i.e., a laptop or a smartphone) and it is likely that this type of provision will continue to burgeon (Morales et al., 2019). However, inequalities in access to technology create barriers to access for many, and there are differences in digital literacy which prevent several communities from participating in these new health-promoting activities (Koh et al., 2021).

Over the past two decades we have also seen the increasing use of social media which has huge potential for health promotion alongside the use of mHealth (mobile health) technology such as apps and IMS (instant messaging systems). Fox et al. (2020) point out that, whilst some see mHealth as a 'silver bullet' solution to many of the health delivery issues in the global south there are several challenges to be overcome such as 'the design, development, piloting, implementation and maintenance associated with mHealth' (p. 50). The use of social media in the promotion of health is crucial and Anugwom (2020) argues that platforms such as WhatsApp and blogs have huge potential for reaching young Africans particularly. As such, the use of mobile technology for health applications has increased enormously elsewhere as well, for example, in North America (Morales et al., 2019).

Liyanagunawardena and Aboshady (2017) argue for collaborations between the World Health Organization, educational institutions, e-learning providers and country health authorities in the global south to 'create customized health education courses to meet the needs of their populations' (p. 76). In addition, they point to how on-line learning could be used for continuing professional development for health professionals in resource-poor settings to address gaps in health education provision. Morales et al. (2019) point to the potential of mHealth as a vehicle for providing information and education about health promotion as well making the collection and monitoring of health data much more straightforward and enabling immediate feedback.

All of this points to the need for nurses to develop a set of e-skills and to possess an increasingly high level of e-literacy which also has implications for health-promotion education. E-literacy refers to technological proficiency (Van Winkle et al., 2017). As technology advances, the requirement for healthcare professionals to adapt and keep up with fast-paced change is very real and the same is true for health-promotion educators. In addition, the healthcare professional's role in supporting the development of eHealth literacy (electronic health literacy) in their patients and clients is increasingly important – this being about the competencies required to access and use electronic health services (Griebel et al., 2018).

Digital technologies, interventions and innovations have the potential to target and address a range of preventable public health issues and reduce risk factors for early mortality (Nasland and Aschbrenner, 2019). Box 11.2 details the possibilities for digital interventions at different levels.

---

**Box 11.2**

## The potential for digital interventions (Nasland and Aschbrenner, 2019)

*Individual Level* – for example, managing mental health symptoms, promoting healthy life-style behaviours, and targeting substance use concerns

*Health System Level* – for example, supporting the co-ordination of care, workforce training, and shared decision-making

*Social Determinants Level* – for example, facilitating opportunities for peer engagement in illness self-management and health promotion

---

As O'Neil (2019) argues, technology is rapidly changing the nature of health communication from more traditional methods to digital methods. This requires that health promotion, and those working to promote health, must be nimble, dynamic and proactive (Baldwin, 2020; Fleming et al., 2020).

---

**Research in Brief 11.2**

Morales et al. (2019) carried out a narrative review on the 'state-of-the-art and the future of technology used by researchers in the field of mobile health promotion' (p. 825) in the light of the ever-increasing prevalence and use of smartphones worldwide. Developments in mobile technology have great potential to improve health for people living in remote and rural areas around the world and the use of mobile technology has increased significantly. The authors reviewed research and literature relating to several different systems used to capture health data and to promote health and support health promotion via mobile interfaces. Mobile health promotion is a global phenomenon widely and relatively cheaply available with huge potential to influence health improvement and health outcomes via a range of interactive platforms including apps and diagnostic tools. This paper considers what mobile health promotion might look like in future, arguing that this is highly relevant to the field of health promotion. As Morales et al. (2019) state 'mobile technology ownership has increased substantially [...] providing an extraordinary opportunity for innovation in the delivery of tailored health promotion interventions [...] with the added advantage that it can be used by individuals in their natural environment' (p. 827).

*Source*: Morales, J., Unupakutika, D., Kaghyan, S., Akopian, D., Yin, Z, Evans, M. and Parra-Medina, D. (2019). Technology-based health promotion: Current state and perspectives in emerging gig economy. *Biocybernetics and Biomedical Engineering*, 39, 825–42.

The importance of research findings such as those described throughout this book, leads us to reflect upon the evidence-base underpinning health promotion practice, and education.

## Reflections on the Health Promotion and Health Education Evidence-base

One of the ways in which the discipline of health promotion has developed since its inception, is in relation to the evidence-base used to inform both practice, and education. Evidence and evaluation underpin the practice of the discipline. Woodall and Rowlands (2020) outline several ways in which evidence is used in the context of health-promotion practice:

- It is used to show what works to improve health through evaluation.
- Disseminating evidence into practice is useful for the development of guidelines for practitioners.
- It can inform decision-making to effect change.
- It can be a tool to inform policy.

However, evidence-based health promotion has been criticised on several levels, there have been debates about its effectiveness as well as usefulness. It faces political challenges in that it is increasingly expected to illustrate cost-effectiveness and value for money, and it is not always easy to provide evidence when measuring complexities. Evidence of course also remains useful in relation to nursing practice. Phillips (2019) argues that it is essential for nurses to embed health-promotion evidence into their practice, to empower patients and enable them to improve their health.

Evidence about models of health promotion indicates the continuing relevance of the discipline in tackling future challenges. Kickbusch (2021) argues that work to improve health in the future requires strong community involvement, which is exactly what health promotion has always provided. Furthermore, an area of the evidence-base that is rapidly expanding is of course in relation to Covid-19.

It is now hard to remember the world before the advent of Covid-19, which has impacted upon all people across the world, with societies most vulnerable and unequal experiencing the worst of these impacts in terms of higher death rates (Warwick-Booth, 2022). At the start of the pandemic, health promotion was at the forefront of government responses to the management of the outbreak in the form of strategies for the prevention of transmission. Given the absence of adequate vaccination and limited understandings of effective treatment to deal with Covid-19, health promotion was a much-needed tool. Furthermore, health promotion research has illustrated the usefulness of the discipline and associated practice in relation to disease outbreaks (Woodall and Freeman, 2020). Indeed, health promotion 'values can be the lens through which to understand both health and disease' (Woodall and Freeman, 2020: 629). Furthermore, Mainous et al. (2020: 373) state that 'the COVID-19 pandemic highlights the need for culturally competent health promotion and disease prevention programmes for noncommunicable diseases'. There are an increasing number of discussions in the literature that highlight lessons so far, from health promotion in the context of the Covid-19 pandemic.

## Case Study 11.1

### Lessons from health promotion in the wake of Covid-19

- Van den Broucke (2020) argues that given the ever-changing nature of Covid-19, and the limitations of health system capacity, health promotion is much needed. Downstream work focuses upon individual behaviour change; mid-stream efforts are about interventions within communities and organisations and upstream work relates to policy level approaches. Furthermore, the central value of health promotion in enabling people to take control over their health, remained essential during the pandemic.

- Simkhada et al. (2020) point out that as governments took unprecedented measures to try and control the spread of Covid-19, the role of health promotion was central within their responses. Communicating messages about how to stay safe, supporting behaviour change in day-to-day practice, and working to empower communities through education, all common health-promotion techniques, were evident. They also point out the importance of engaging local communities in health-promotion responses to Covid-19. Warwick-Booth and Coan (2021) evaluated a local city-wide response to Covid-19 in England, illustrating that this successful approach to health promotion involved funding local groups to design and deliver community interventions. A diverse variety of small-scale projects resulted, and an existing local network was used to link community members into information and support systems, raising morale at a much-needed time.

- Saboga-Nunes et al. (2020) argue that health promotion provides the ideal framework to bring together all the required elements that are needed to create a comprehensive approach to Covid-19 management, such as intersectorality, sustainability, empowerment, public health engagement, equity and a life course perspective.

- Ruggiero and Ardiles (2020) highlight how the discipline of health promotion has always been concerned with the unequal distribution of health, with the Covid-19 pandemic illustrating this ongoing need. They note that health promotion's concern with tackling inequalities as well as understanding context-specific needs is central to future disease responses.

- Baybutt and Dorris (2021) also outline five important areas that the pandemic illustrates in relation to health-promotion futures. First, effective health promotion needs integration as well as contextual appreciation of social, environmental and economic factors. Second, Covid-19 has highlighted the need to focus on health beyond the physical realm, because of growing evidence about the mental health impacts. Third, health promotion enables us to understand the importance of settings in responding to disease as well as tackling the social determinants of health. Fourth, Covid-19 has raised awareness of the complex relationships between human health, the ecology of our planet and a sustainable future. Finally, the ways in which governments attempted to contain the spread of Covid-19 have resulted in increased inequalities. Therefore, the future of health promotion needs to focus on transformative practice to ensure health for all.

## The Current Situation – Health Promotion Education for Healthcare Professionals, Possible Futures

Despite the clear definition of health promotion outlined within this book, as well as the discussions throughout about the importance of health education as part of the discipline, there are still some who argue that health promotion is in crisis, particularly in the global north (Woodall et al., 2018). These critical points have arisen from disciplinary debates about what the focus of health promotion should be, where it is going and what it has to offer (Woodall and Freeman, 2020), as well as a broader policy context in which the demand to train a specifically dedicated health-promotion workforce has been diminished, particularly in countries such as the UK (Warwick-Booth et al., 2018). However, counter to these critical debates we argue that there is hope for the future of health promotion as a discipline, and therefore a future too for health promotion education. Analyses of the uneven impacts from the Covid-19 pandemic are creating new opportunities for educators to understand and embody the values of the Ottawa Charter (WHO, 1986) because the need to tackle the social determinants of health and associated inequalities in health is clearer than ever (Warwick-Booth, 2022; Woodall and Freeman, 2020). The UK government's policy discourse has consequently changed in tone, focusing upon the need to level up via policy action, starting with the establishment of a task force of ministers who intend to begin tackling regional disparities (BBC News, 2020). Furthermore, the government is also restructuring the UK public health system with the intention of an increased focus on health promotion. Implementation will be through a newly established Office for Health Promotion, led by the Chief Medical Officer. There will also be a new UK Health Security Agency tasked with focusing upon infectious disease prevention (Department of Health and Social Care, 2021). Whilst the impacts of these changes are yet to be seen, there is potential for improvement given successful implementation, including addressing staff shortages (Kings Fund, 2021).

The role played by healthcare professionals during the pandemic is also likely to lead to changes, as there is increasing recognition that the world was not ready for Covid-19, with preparedness closely linked to the effectiveness of healthcare systems that were understaffed and underfunded. Investment in nursing and other healthcare professions is now on government agendas following the raised profile of the healthcare workforce around the world due to their commitment to care during the pandemic. The pandemic has further highlighted the need to increase workforce capacity (Catton and Iro, 2021). At the time of writing, there are significant health professional staff shortages across the globe. The WHO (2020) argues that nurse education, as well as leadership is essential in developing more equitable services, which lead to better patient outcomes. Given the pause in service provision during the pandemic, and the associated backlog of service need, demand for health care is not going to lessen, therefore increasing the number of global health care staff, who are educated and skilled to tackle the complexities of contemporary need is essential (Catton and Iro, 2021).

## Summary

This chapter has explored the future of health promotion and health education to outline the importance of both of these areas for achieving sustainable and equitable health outcomes on a global level. At the start of this book, Chapter 1: *Health and its determinants* highlighted the ways in which health is multidimensional and complex, as well as defining the importance of the social model in promoting health. This chapter has revisited these points, relating them to health education for professionals, the policy context in which health is promoted (or not) and the changing landscape of the discipline through technological developments as well as the impacts from Covid-19. The chapter concludes by making a strong case for the need for health promotion education for professionals working in care contexts.

──────── **Key Points** ────────────────────────────────────

- Effective education is needed for healthcare professionals who are, by definition of their roles, promoters of health.
- The policy context underpinning health promotion education and practice has varied considerably across the world but even in countries that have had a less positive policy environment such as the UK, encouraging changes are occurring.
- Technological developments are also enabling health to be promoted in new and innovative ways and expanding opportunities for education.
- Evidence from the Covid-19 pandemic is illustrating the importance of health promotion practice for the future.

# References

Annesley, S. (2019). The implications of health policy for nursing. *British Journal of Nursing 28*(8), 496–502.

Anugwom, E.E. (2020). *Health Promotion and Its Challenges to Public Health Delivery System in Africa.* doi: 10.5772/intechopen.91859

Baldwin, L. (2020). Sustaining the practice of health promotion. In M. Fleming and L. Baldwin (Eds), *Health Promotion in the 21st Century* (pp. 245–62). London: Allen & Unwin.

Bambra, C. (2019). *Health in Hard Times: Austerity and Health Inequalities.* Bristol: Policy Press.

Baybutt, M. and Dorris, M. (2021). COVID-19: a catalyst to transform our future? *International Journal of Health Promotion and Education 59*(1), 1–4.

BBC News (2020). Conservative MPs launch 'levelling up' taskforce 7 September 2020. Available at: www.bbc.co.uk/news/uk-politics-54049920. Accessed 25 January 2022.

Blakemore, K. and Warwick-Booth, L. (2013). *Social Policy: An Introduction.* Maidenhead: Open University Press/McGraw-Hill Education.

Catton, H. and Iro, E. (2021). How to reposition the nursing profession for a post-covid age *BMJ* 373, 1105. Available at: http://dx.doi.org/10.1136/bmj.n1105

Cross, R., Rowlands, S. and Foster, S. (2021a). The Foundations of Health Promotion. In R. Cross, L. Warwick-Booth, S. Rowlands, J. Woodall, I. O'Neil and S. Foster (Eds). *Health Promotion: Global Principles and Practice.* 2nd Ed. (pp. 1–40). Wallingford: CABI.

Cross, R., Warwick-Booth, L. and Foster, S. (2021b). Towards the Future of Health Promotion. In R. Cross, L. Warwick-Booth, S. Rowlands, J. Woodall, I. O'Neil and S. Foster. (Eds) *Health Promotion: Global Principles and Practice.* 2nd Ed. (pp. 186–231). Wallingford: CABI.

Department of Health and Social Care (2021). *Transforming the Public Health System: Reforming the public health system for the challenges of our times.* Available at: www.gov.uk/government/publications/transforming-the-public-health-system/transforming-the-public-health-system-reforming-the-public-health-system-for-the-challenges-of-our-times. Accessed 25 January 2022.

Di Ruggiero, E. and Ardiles, P. (2020). Health promotion perspectives on Covid-19. *Global Health Promotion* 1757-9759: *28*(1), pp. 3– 4; 1001005.

Dowding, K. (2020). *It is the Government Stupid: How Governments Blame Citizens for Their Own Policies.* Bristol: Policy Press.

Drennan, V.M. and Ross, F. (2019). Global nurse shortages – the facts, the impact and action for change. *British Medical Bulletin 130*(1), 25–37.

Ellenbecker, C.H. and Edward, J. (2016). Conducting nursing research to advance and inform health policy. *Policy, Politics & Nursing Practice 17*, 4, 208–17.

Evans, D., Coutsaftiki, D. and Fathers, C.P. (2017). *Health Promotion and Public Health for Nursing Students* 3rd Ed. London: Sage.

Fleming, M., Parker, E. and Baldwin, L. (2020). The changing nature of health promotion. In M. Fleming and L. Baldwin (Eds), *Health Promotion in the 21st Century.* (pp. 16–36). London: Allen & Unwin.

Fox, G., O'Connor, Y., Eze, E., Ndibuagu, E.O. and Heaving, C. (2020). End users' initial perceptions of mHealth in Nigeria: An investigation of primary healthcare workers' attitudes to the IMPACT App. *International Journal of E-Health and Medical Communications 11*(4), 50–65.

Griebel, L., Enwald, H., Golstad, H., Pohl, A., Moreland, J. and Sedlmayr, M. (2018). eHealth literacy research – Quo vadis? *Informatics for Health & Social Care 43*(4), 427–42.

Hajizadeh, A., Zamanzadeh, V., Kakemam, E., Bahreini, R. and Khodayari-Zarnaq, R. (2021). Factors influencing nurses' participation in the health policy-making process: a systematic review. *BMC Nursing 20*, 128. Available at: https://doi.org/10.1186/s12912-021-00648-6

Hubley, J., Copeman, J. and Woodall, J. (2021). *Practical Health Promotion* 3rd Ed. Cambridge: Polity.

Iriarte-Roteta, A., Lopez-Dicastillo, O., Mujika, A., Ruiz-Zaldibar, C., Hernantes, N., Bermejo-Martins, E. and Pumar-Méndez, M.J. (2020). Nurses' role in health promotion and prevention: A critical interpretative synthesis. *Journal of Clinical Nursing 29*(21–22), 3937–49.

Keshavarz Mohammadi, N. (2019). One step back toward the future of health promotion: complexity-informed health promotion. *Health Promotion International 34*, 635–9.

Kickbusch, I., Draper, R. and O'Neill, M. (1990). Healthy public policy: A strategy to implement the Health for All philosophy at various governmental levels. In A. Evers, W. Farrant and A. Trojon (Eds), *Healthy Public Policy at the Local Level* (pp. 1–6). Vienna: European Centre for Social Welfare Policy and Research.

Kickbusch, I. (2021). Visioning the future of health promotion. *Global Health Promotion 28*(4), 56–63.

Kings Fund (2021). *The Health and Care Bill: Six Key Questions.* 6th September. Available at: www.kingsfund.org.uk/publications/health-and-care-bill-key-questions. Accessed 24 January 2022.

Koh, A., Swanepoel, D.W., Ling, A., Ho, B.L., Tan, S.Y. and Lim, J. (2021). Digital health promotion: promise and peril. *Health Promotion International 36*, Supplement_1, i70–i80. Available at: https://doi.org/10.1093/heapro/daab134

Lipsky, M. (2010). *Street Level Bureaucracy, 30th Anniversary Edition: Dilemmas of the Individual in Public Service.* London: Russell Sage Foundation.

Liyanagunawardena, T.R. and Aboshady, O.A. (2017). Massive open online courses: a resource for health education in developing countries. *Global Health Promotion 25*(3), 74–6.

Mainous, A.G., Saxena, S., Beau de Rochars, V.M. and Macceus, D. (2020). Covid-19 highlights health promotion and chronic disease prevention amid health disparities. *British Journal of General Practice 70*(697), 372–3. doi: https://doi.org/10.3399/bjgp20X711785

Manning, V. (2017). Health promotion: A core role of the midwife. In J. Bowden and V. Manning (Eds), *Health Promotion in Midwifery: Principles and Practice* 3rd Ed. (pp. 19–32). London: CRC Press.

Morales, J., Inupakutika, D., Kaghyan, S., et al. (2019). Technology-based health promotion: current state and perspectives in emerging gig economy. *Biocybernetics and Biomedical Engineering 39*(3), 825–42.

Naslund, J.A. and Aschbrenner, K.A. (2019). Digital technology for health promotion: opportunities to address excess mortality in persons living with severe mental disorders. *Evidence-Based Mental Health 22*(1), 17–22.

NHS England (2014). *NHS Five Year Forward View*. Available at: www.england.nhs.uk/five-year-forward-view/. Accessed 24 January 2022.

National Midwifery Council (NMC) (2018). *Future Nurse: Standards of Proficiency for Registered Nurses*. Available at: <www.nmc.org.uk>. Accessed 25 May 2021.

O'Neil, I. (2019). *Digital Health Promotion*. Cambridge: Polity.

Palfrey, C. (2018). *The Future for Health Promotion*. Bristol: Policy Press.

Phillips, A. (2019). Effective approaches to health promotion in nursing practice. *Nursing Standard*. Available at: http://doi.org/10.7748/ns.2019.e11312

Public Health England (2018). *Improving People's Health: Applying Behavioural and Social Sciences*. Available at: www.gov.uk/government/publications/improving-peoples-health-applying-behavioural-and-social-sciences. Accessed 24 January 2022.

Saboga-Nunes, L., Levin-Zamir, D., Bittlingmayer, U., et al. (2020). *A Health Promotion Focus on COVID-19: Keep the Trojan horse out of our health systems. Promote health for ALL in times of crisis and beyond!* EUPHA-HP, IUHPE, UNESCO Chair Global Health & Education.

Simkhada, P., Mahato, P., Tamang, P., van Teijlingen, E. and Shahi, P. (2020). The role of health promotion during the Covid-19 pandemic. *Journal of Health Promotion 8*, 1–4.

UN (2022). *The 17 Goals. Sustainable Development*. Available at: https://sdgs.un.org/goals. Accessed 11 April 2022.

UNFPA, WHO & ICM (2021). *The State of the World's Midwifery 2021*. New York: United Nations Population Fund.

Van den Broucke, S. (2020). Why health promotion matters to the COVID-19 pandemic, and vice versa. *Health Promotion International 35*, 181–6 doi: 10.1093/heapro/daaa042

Van Winkle, B., Carpenter, N. and Moscucci, M. (2017). Why aren't our digital solutions working for everyone? *AMA Journal of Ethics 19*(1), 1116–24.

Walt, G. (1995). *Health Policy: An Introduction to Process and Power*. London: Zed Books.

Warwick-Booth, L. (2022). *Social Inequality*. 3rd Ed. London: Sage.

Warwick-Booth, L. and Coan, S. (2022). *Covid19 Grants Evaluation Communities of Interest Final Report*. December 2021, Leeds: Leeds Beckett University.

Warwick-Booth, L., Cross, R. and Lowcock, D. (2021). *Contemporary Health Studies: An Introduction*. 2nd Ed. Cambridge: Polity.

Warwick-Booth, L., Cross, R., Woodall, J., Bagnall, A.M. and South, J. (2018). Health promotion education in changing and challenging times: Reflections from England. *Health Education Journal 78*(6), 692–704.

Warwick-Booth, L. and Rowlands, S. (2020). Policies for Health in the 21st Century. In R. Cross, L. Warwick-Booth, S. Rowlands, J. Woodall, I. O'Neil and S. Foster.

(Eds) *Health Promotion: Global Principles and Practice* 2nd Ed. (pp. 75–105). Wallingford: CABI.

Watson, M.C., Tilford, S. and Lloyd, J. (2021). *Position Statement: Health Promotion (May 2021)*. Lichfield: Institute of Health Promotion and Education.

Whitehead, D. (2011). Health promotion in nursing: A Derridean discourse analysis. *Health Promotion International 26*, 117–27.

Whitehead, D. (2018). Exploring health promotion and health education in nursing. *Nursing Standard*. doi: 10/7748/ns.2018/e11220

WHO (1986). Ottawa Charter for Health Promotion. *Health Promotion*. Geneva, World Health Organization. *1*(4), pp. 405.

WHO (2015). *NURSES AND MIDWIVES: A Vital Resource for Health – European compendium of good practices in nursing and midwifery towards Health 2020 goals*. Geneva: World Health Organization.

WHO (2020). *The State of the World's Nursing 2020*. Geneva: World Health Organization.

WHO (2021). *New report sounds the alarm on global shortage of 900 000 midwives*. Joint News Release, New York: United Nations, 5 May. Available at: <www.who.int> Accessed 20 May 2021.

Wills, J. and Jackson, L. (2014). Health and health promotion. In J. Wills (Ed.). *Fundamentals of Health Promotion for Nurses*. 2nd Ed. (pp. 4–20). Chichester: Wiley Blackwell.

Woodall, J. and Freeman, C. (2020). Where have we been and where are we going? The state of contemporary health promotion. *Health Education Journal 76*(6), 621–32.

Woodall, J. and Rowlands, S. (2020). Professional Practice. In R. Cross, L. Warwick-Booth, S. Rowlands, J. Woodall, I. O'Neil and S. Foster (Eds). *Health Promotion: Global Principles and Practice*. 2nd Ed. (pp. 148–85). Wallingford: CABI.

Woodall, J., Warwick-Booth, L., South, J. and Cross, R. (2018). What makes health promotion distinct? *Scandinavian Journal of Public Health 46* (Suppl. 20), 118–22.

# Introduction to Section 3

# Health Promotion Through the Lifespan - Selected Stages and Issues

This third and final section of the book is designed to complement sections 1 and 2 by offering topic-based examples of potential and actual programmes of activity across the lifespan and in a variety of different settings. In this section several authors from different countries bring their expertise to bear on different subject matter relating this to the role of the nurse in health education and health promotion. This section begins with Chapter 12 which focuses on the maternal health part of the lifespan including pregnancy and its related morbidities. The chapter covers topics such as anaemia, HIV and female condom use, breast and cervical cancer, and violence against women within the context of low- and middle-income countries. Chapter 13 explores what makes a difference to children, young people and their families and how health promotion and health education during childhood life stage can help shape positive well-being across the lifespan. The chapter reimagines child and family health education and health promotion via a planetary health lens. Moving to the next life stage, adolescence, Chapter 14 looks at the important public health issue of unplanned teenage pregnancy using case study data and information from the Namibian context. The discussion is framed around the Socio-Ecological Model and the World Health Organization's framework for providing adolescents' and young people's services. Chapter 15 focuses on the young and middle-adult life stage. It highlights the demographic profile and risk behaviours that contribute to ill-health in this period, demonstrating how public policy and evidence-based strategies can be used in multi-sectoral health promotion interventions to address health issues in this life stage in settings such as communities, universities and workplaces. Chapter 16 considers older adult health in relation to the very important public health issue of falls prevention, presenting examples of effective health promotion and health education relevant to older people in retirement and residential care settings focusing specifically on the Australian context. The final chapter, Chapter 17, talks about health promotion in hospital and beyond focusing on the important issue of nutrition. Using a case study approach from the Norwegian context the chapter explores the transition from hospital to the community setting and the role that health promotion and health education must play in supporting people through this transition.

# 12

# Maternal Health

## Firoza Haffejee

### Introduction

This chapter offers context, practical guidance and examples of health promotion and education activities in the maternal health part of the lifespan, including pregnancy and its related morbidities. The chapter focuses on interventions to reduce maternal mortality and morbidity. Moreover, it explores the associated health-promotion interventions. Women during this phase of life are also vulnerable to HIV infection and non-communicable diseases such as breast and cervical cancer. In addition, particularly within the context of low socio-economic settings, pervasive violence against women is integral to their health-related outcomes. Addressing all these factors are important to the holistic well-being of women.

By the end of this chapter the reader will be able to:

1. Understand factors impacting on maternal mortality, particularly in low socio-economic environments.
2. Describe the factors contributing to high incidence of HIV among women of reproductive age.
3. Appreciate the need for, and describe, female initiated methods of HIV prevention.
4. Identify and understand cancers that primarily affect women of reproductive age.
5. Describe the link between violence against women and their well-being.

**Key terms**

Breast cancer, cervical cancer, female condom, HIV, PrEP, maternal morbidity, maternal mortality, violence against women

## Maternal Morbidity and Mortality

Maternal mortality and morbidity are pertinent indicators not only for maternal health, but for signifying the general health status of a country. Low- and middle-income countries (LMIC) continue to bear the burden of high maternal mortality rates. The Sustainable Development Goal 3, Good Health and Well-Being, first target is about maternal health. Target 3.1 aims to reduce the maternal mortality rate (MMR) to below 70 per 100,000 live births by 2030. However, many LMIC consistently remain far from this target. For instance, in South Africa the rate is currently 119 per 100,000 live births (WHO, UNICEF, UNFPA, The World Bank, & UNPD, 2019). Although this has reduced since 2010 when the MMR was 320 per 100,000 live births, the MMR still requires a further 50 per cent reduction in order to meet the SDG target within the next eight years.

Hypertensive disorders of pregnancy, haemorrhage, and non-pregnancy related infections, frequently due to HIV are causes of maternal mortality, which can be prevented using guidelines of the World Health Organization (South African National Department of Health, 2021). Early detection of hypertensive disorders, such as pre-eclampsia is vital in preventing the onset of potentially dangerous eclampsia. In addition, obstetric emergencies require competent specialists (Wium, Vannevel and Bothma, 2018). All women must therefore have access to maternal healthcare services during pregnancy, delivery and in the period after delivery.

Antenatal services are essential in promoting delivery at a healthcare facility, where skilled maternal care is provided (Smith, Portela, and Marston, 2017). In addition to providing routine examination and medication, healthcare workers are expected to provide family planning, maternal nutrition and infant feeding advice (South African National Department of Health, 2021). The service must be responsive to the individual patient's needs. In order to improve the childbirth experience, treating the patient with respect is important, especially during labour, delivery and the postnatal period. Where choices are available, for instance with the use of invasive procedures, the patient must be involved in arriving at a shared decision. This will empower women to take charge of their own health instead of being passive recipients of health services (Govender, Naidoo and Taylor, 2019).

In low-income countries, with limited funds and skilled personnel, it is often difficult to make healthcare services accessible to all women, particularly those from rural areas, who are more likely to die of complications related to childbirth (Lagese,

Abdulahi, and Dirar, 2016). In sub-Saharan Africa most women only attend antenatal clinics once during their pregnancy. These women receive inadequate counselling on birth preparedness and delivery at a healthcare facility (Brazier et al., 2014).

The long length of time to arrive at a facility where a skilled healthcare professional is available to assist with the delivery of a baby poses a massive problem to these women in the event of an obstetric emergency, such as eclampsia. Optimal referral pathways within these areas and between various levels of care are thus important (South African National Department of Health, 2021). Achieving positive outcomes in these settings may necessitate engagement by families and communities so that there is shared responsibility for maternal health outcomes.

Training of community healthcare workers is important to achieve this. Regular monitoring and communication by these community health workers with pregnant women is required. One such intervention, in Nigeria, provided pregnant women with mobile phones for communication with the community health worker, particularly in times of apparent emergency (Mimiko, 2017). However, that in itself cannot be sufficient if access to a healthcare centre is not available. These are required in underserved communities so that every pregnant woman has access to proper healthcare in close proximity to where she lives. In addition, staff and material resources need to be provided at these facilities (Ajayi and Akpan, 2020).

## Research in Brief 12.1

Facility-based child delivery requires upscaling in low- and middle-income countries. The "Abiye" (safe motherhood) initiative in Nigeria aimed to improve uptake of maternal healthcare. The intervention sought to address (1) the delay in seeking care; (2) the delay in reaching care; (3) delays due to financial difficulties and (4) delays in referrals.

To address the delay in seeking care, media warnings were used to inform women about the hazards of homebased deliveries. Trained community health workers were also used to convey this information. Building of new primary healthcare centres in underserved communities addressed the delay in reaching care. Furthermore, old centres were provided with new equipment and additional staff. Financial difficulties were addressed by exempting pregnant women from paying fees in government clinics and hospitals. The delays in referrals were addressed by providing community health workers with tricycles to transport women to hospitals during emergencies (Ajayi and Akpan, 2020). The latter intervention was used in the pilot study but subsequently discontinued as it was an inappropriate means of transferring pregnant women in areas with poor terrains. This initiative resulted in increasing facility-based child delivery from just over half to 85 per cent at the end of the initiative (Ajayi and Akpan, 2020).

Ajayi, A.I. and Akpan, W. Maternal healthcare services utilisation in the context of 'Abiye' (safe motherhood) programme in Ondo State, Nigeria. BMC Public Health 20, 362 (2020). https://doi.org/10.1186/s12889-020-08512-z

Maternity waiting homes in remote areas are important for women with limited access to healthcare services (Smith et al., 2017). These homes are near healthcare facilities and are used to house pregnant women with obstetric complications, close to time of delivery. This decreases possible delays in getting to the healthcare facility on time. Use of these maternity waiting homes in African countries such as Ethiopia, Zambia and Tanzania has resulted in decreased MMR (Dadi, Bekele, Kasaye and Nigussie, 2018). Organising transport schemes to transfer women to a healthcare facility may also be useful in this regard (Smith et al., 2017).

## Tutorial Trigger 12.1

As seen in Research brief 12.1, the tricycle was inappropriate to transport pregnant women during emergencies due to the poor road infrastructure. Thus, other methods are required to overcome the problem. Suggest alternative means of improving transport of pregnant women to healthcare facilities in the event of an emergency. Take into consideration areas where the road infrastructure is poor. What other methods or means might reduce MMR for women living in poorly resourced and/or rural areas?

Community engagement to increase health knowledge for patients and their families can impact on the quality of care that can be expected and hence received. Once knowledge of health is upscaled, decisions to access improved care can be made by the family and even community (Govender et al., 2019). This type of intervention was conducted in southeast Guinea in 2007 as well as more recently in Ethiopia. Motherhood committees were formed, comprising six to seven community members of both genders. They were trained on the importance of antenatal care, obstetric risks and the importance of skilled maternity care. The intervention was successful in that more women from these villages attended antenatal care and also delivered at a health facility (Ashebir, Medhanyie, Mulugeta, Persson and Berhanu, 2020; Brazier, Fiorentino, Barry and Diallo, 2014). Community involvement can lead to implementation of culturally appropriate services, which would be used by more people who in turn may have ideas to make the services more user friendly and accessible (Smith et al., 2017).

Partnerships can be fostered with traditional birth attendants, religious leaders and even men, to create greater awareness of maternal morbidity and mortality (Smith et al., 2017). Male involvement could lead to changes in the couple's relationship with improved communication, enhanced partner support, with implementation of health-promoting behaviours and care seeking, leading to improved maternal health outcomes (Tokhi et al., 2018). In Indonesia a similar health-promotion intervention involving men led to more deliveries with a skilled attendant and subsequently lowered maternal mortality rates (Ibid.). Uptake of routine post-partum care was also observed in some regions. Education for both men and women also has the potential to increase couple communication about sexually transmitted infections and family planning (Ibid.). Partnerships can be set up with traditional birth attendants and culturally appropriate but skilled maternal care can be provided (Smith et al., 2017).

In countries which experienced a dramatic decrease in maternal mortality rates, there was an increase in the number of women who were attended to by a skilled healthcare provider. There was also an increase in the number of women who gave birth at a hospital or other healthcare centre. These two factors resulted in a 65 per cent decrease in MMR in China between 1990 and 2008 (Paxton and Wardlaw, 2011). This is echoed in developed countries, such as the United States of America, where women who are economically disadvantaged have a three times higher MMR than those who are economically advantaged, as the latter are more likely to deliver their babies with the assistance of skilled healthcare professionals, indicating the importance of providing both skilled healthcare as well as well-equipped facilities for all populations (Ibid.).

## Anaemia

Iron deficiency anaemia is common in girls and women of reproductive age due to blood loss during menstruation and childbirth as well as insufficient iron in the diet. During periods of rapid growth as occur in young adolescent girls and throughout pregnancy, the demand for iron in the body increases. If the iron intake is lower than the body's demand for it, iron deficiency will ensue, leading to subsequent low levels of haemoglobin and red blood cells. Iron deficiency may also occur due to helminth infections and malaria, which causes destruction of red blood cells. Treatment of malaria, deworming, provision of clean water and improvement of handwashing practices are required at a community level, in areas where these parasitic infections are common. This will alleviate these infections and also reduce the prevalence of iron deficiency anaemia (World Health Organization, 2020).

Inadequate nutrition due to poverty and cultural norms deprives women of food rich in iron, affecting their overall health and well-being. In these women there is often an early age of childbearing and short birth spacing; factors that also lead to iron deficiency anaemia. The risk of haemorrhage and sepsis during childbirth is increased in those with anaemia. Collaborative efforts are required, to improve the diets of these women, so that they receive adequate nutrition. Iron supplementation may also be required (World Health Organization, 2020).

---

**Points to Ponder 12.1**

Daily iron supplementation is the most common intervention to treat as well as prevent iron deficiency in pregnancy. Hence early antenatal care visits are important. However, these are usually delayed in low socio-economic areas. Education, health, finance and nutrition programmes are required in these areas to alleviate pregnancy-related iron deficiency anaemia as well as other pregnancy related disorders.

1  Explain how each of the following types of intervention: education, health, finance and nutrition might improve anaemia outcomes.
2  How might socio-cultural factors deprive women of food rich in iron? How could this be prevented?

---

# Human Immunodeficiency Virus

In 2020, there were 37.7 million people living with Human Immunodeficiency Virus (HIV) worldwide, with a disproportionate representation of women particularly in sub-Saharan Africa (UNAIDS, 2021). Young age of sexual debut, lack of protection, multiple sexual partners who are often much older, make young women vulnerable to HIV infection (Haffejee, Koorbanally and Corona, 2018; Haffejee and Maksudi, 2020). In these countries, women aged 15–24 years have a fourfold increased HIV incidence compared to men (Martin, de Lora, Rochat and Andes, 2016). These women have reported difficulty in negotiating protection such as condom use, which is primarily controlled by the male partner (Haffejee and Maksudi, 2020). Female initiated methods of protection are thus required. These could include the female condom (FC) and the use of pre-exposure prophylaxis (PrEP).

The FC provides women with the ability to control their own sexual protection (Hoffman, Mantell, Exner and Stein, 2004). Awareness and knowledge of the FC and its use requires promotion (Mahlalela and Maharaj, 2015; Naidu, 2013). A recent study, in South Africa, indicated that many women did not know where to access the FC (Beksinska et al., 2017). Clinics could openly advertise FCs, to increase awareness of its availability.

Difficulty of FC use has been reported, with many claiming that the instructions on the package insert are difficult to understand, particularly when these were not in the home language of the client (Mahlalela and Maharaj, 2015; Naidu, 2013; Schuyler et al., 2016). Demonstration of condom insertion by healthcare workers will enhance uptake of FC use (Mantell, Scheepers and Abdool Karim, 2000). Pelvic models can be used for these demonstrations. A study in the United States of America reported that providing potential users with the opportunity to practise use on a pelvic model improves uptake as they perceive it favourably (Devanter et al., 2002).

However, difficulties in negotiating FC use with male partners, due to perceptions of reduced sexual pleasure and stigma, with some suggesting female infidelity, have been reported (Beksinska, Smit and Mantell, 2012; Mahlalela and Maharaj, 2015; Mantell et al., 2015; Schuyler et al., 2016). Only two-thirds (67.2 per cent) of service providers advise clients on condom negotiation skills (Beksinska et al., 2017). Interventions which involve promotion of the FC, together with teaching women on using it, is important in increasing uptake (Haffejee and Maharajh, 2019). A negotiation strategy used by some women was to suggest FC use as an alternative contraceptive method due to side effects of hormonal contraception (Mahlalela and Maharaj, 2015). In addition to training nurses, peer educator training may also be important, as social support improves uptake of condom use (Maksut and Eaton, 2015; Wiyeh, Mome, Mahasha, Kongnyuy and Wiysonge, 2020).

## Pre-Exposure Prophylaxis

The other female-initiated HIV protective mechanism is pre-exposure prophylaxis (PrEP), an oral medication that is taken daily. PrEP comprises of a combination of antiretroviral drugs, in a single tablet. The available combinations may differ in various countries. For instance, in South Africa the registered drug combination is Tenofovir and Emtricitabine, known as Truvada (Montjane, Dlamini and Dandara, 2018). Tenofovir disoproxil fumarate (TDF) and emtricitabine (FTC) are nucleoside reverse transcriptase inhibitors approved as pre-exposure prophylaxis (PrEP) against human immunodeficiency virus (Trang, Dong, Kojima and Klausner, 2016).

PrEP is suitable for use by HIV negative people who are at a high risk of contracting HIV and who are not regularly using another method of protection such as condoms. Since PrEP is taken orally, the fear of stigma, and disclosure to partners can be avoided. This is particularly useful for females whose partners are not willing to use either the male or female condom. A study in Malawi showed that females were willing to use PrEP (Maseko et al., 2020). However, some women did express that faithfulness to the partner negated the necessity to use PrEP. In a study in Durban, South Africa, almost a quarter of women in a PrEP trial discontinued use during the study and only half remained on PrEP after the trial ended, with the women citing difficulties in access to the prophylaxis (Beesham et al., 2020). Use in South Africa is reportedly too low to have any effect in decreasing the incidence of HIV in that country (Bekker et al., 2020). Barriers to using condoms can be overcome by the use of PrEP, as it can potentially be taken without partner knowledge (Haffejee, Fasanmi-Kana, Ally, Thandar and Basdav, 2022).

In the UK, a study on men who have sex with men (MSM) indicated an 86 per cent efficacy of sexual event-driven PrEP (Cambiano et al., 2018). This would be beneficial to those who do not wish to take the prophylaxis daily. In addition to the health benefits, the event-driven use is also cost effective. However, studies are required to show efficacy in women.

## Research in Brief 12.2

A study to assess the knowledge of PrEP among primary health clinic users and students in the province of KwaZulu-Natal, South Africa showed low levels of knowledge amongst both the clinic users as well as among the students. Approximately one tenth of both indicated awareness of PrEP. However, they only responded correctly to PrEP as a daily pill for prophylaxis but were unable to identify that PrEP could be used by sero-discordant couples to protect the uninfected partner. Students who were enrolled in the nursing programme did not fare better than other students. Neither did users of clinics, that were offering PrEP, have a greater knowledge than users of clinics not offering the prophylaxis. This indicates a gap in both the teaching programme as well as a service provider gap, where users are not informed of all services offered at clinics in the area (Haffejee et al., 2022). These gaps highlight the importance of providing current information to students as well as effective communication by healthcare workers to all patients at the clinics. The study reported that posters advertising PrEP were observed in the clinic waiting rooms, however, these are insufficient to provide information adequately, considering the low rate of literacy among the study population.

*Source*: Haffejee, F., Fasanmi-Kana, O., Ally, F., Thandar, Y. and Basdav, J. (2022), Four years later: Do South Africans know what pre-exposure prophylaxis for HIV is? *AIDS Care*, DOI: 10.1080/09540121.2022.2032573

## Points to Ponder 12.2

1  Including PrEP knowledge in a health science curriculum will increase the knowledge of PrEP amongst these students. What measures can be taken to increase this knowledge in students registered in other faculties?

2  Consider ways of improving PrEP knowledge among clinic users.

3  How has PrEP information been disseminated to people in developed countries?

## Cancer

Breast and cervical cancer cause high rates of morbidity and mortality, particularly in low- and middle-income countries. Inequalities in access to screening and early detection lead to large discrepancies in clinical outcomes and survival after treatment. Detection in these countries often occurs at advanced stages of cancer. With late detection, particularly of breast cancer, palliative care becomes the only treatment option, resulting in breast cancer being the second highest cause of cancer deaths (Alwan, 2016). It is important to teach women to examine their breasts. Training of community and healthcare workers to upscale this is required. This will in turn improve rates of seeking early diagnosis and treatment.

Cervical cancer is the third leading cause of death from cancer in women in low- and middle-income countries, where challenges in the provision of screening and treatment options are faced (Cubie and Campbell, 2020; World Health Organization, 2014). Cervical cancer usually affects women in low socio-economic groups who have inadequate health literacy, poor access to reproductive healthcare and screening, and who face many socio-economic challenges (World Cancer Research Fund, 2018). A recent study among women from a low socio-economic community in South Africa reported that knowledge and testing for cervical cancer was low (Ducray, Kell, Basdav and Haffejee, 2021).

An educational-based intervention on cervical cancer and women's reproductive health was provided, at a wellness day, to a marginalised community in the city of Durban, South Africa. Both the levels of knowledge and uptake of pap smears improved after the intervention. The women also showed a great enthusiasm to gain knowledge of the female reproductive system, its functioning and disorders. Some expressed a fear of the pap smear procedure, the potential result and subsequent treatment. Young health science students and graduates, most of whom were from similar ethnic backgrounds to the women, provided most of the educational intervention. This resulted in the women feeling comfortable, enabling uninhibited communication (Ducray et al., 2021). These types of interventions can be used in any communities with weak health systems. The human papillomavirus vaccine must also be promoted to make primary prevention widespread.

──────── Time to Reflect 12.1 ────────────────────────────

In Turkey, pap smear testing is low. A nursing intervention to improve uptake was conducted in three stages (Guvenc, Akyuz and Yenen, 2013). In stage 1, an education brochure was developed. It contained information on cervical cancer and created an awareness of screening with pap smear tests, which were recommended. An invitation to participate in screening with a free pap smear test was included along with relevant contact numbers. These brochures were then delivered to 2,500 women in their mailboxes. After the completion of this first stage, 510 women were screened.

In the second stage, 302 of those women who had not had a pap smear test after the first-stage intervention were interviewed telephonically, to ascertain why they had not tested. During this telephonic interview, they were also invited to screen. This second intervention resulted in a further 158 women being screened. Stage 3 included face-to-face interviews conducted in 54 women's homes to investigate the reasons for the non-uptake of free cervical cancer screening and another invitation to participate in the free screening. This resulted in a further 20 women being screened.

Reasons for non-screening included embarrassment, insufficient time, belief that they did not need the test, fear of a bad result, and fear that the pap smear test would be painful. Each stage resulted in more women being screened. This intervention indicates that whilst education through brochures is effective in increasing screening of women, providing further information telephonically and via face-to-face interviews intensifies the effect of the intervention. The second and third stages not only provided education, but also alleviated the concerns that women may have had about the screening procedure (Guvenc et al., 2013).

## Violence against Women

Violence against women and girls is another factor affecting the health of women. A third of women aged 15–49 years have experienced physical violence, sexual violence, or both by an intimate partner, with numerous adverse consequences to their health (Temmerman, Khosla, Laski, Mathews and Say, 2015). These women are more likely to have depression and alcohol use disorders and prone to experience sexual violence from their intimate partners, who often have multiple partners, thus increasing the risk for HIV and other sexually transmitted infections (Haffejee and Maksudi, 2020; Temmerman et al., 2015). Additionally, these women have adverse health outcomes during pregnancy and postpartum. A greater number of stressful symptoms are reported in the third trimester of pregnancy by victims of intimate partner violence (Gartland, Giallo, Woolhouse, Mensah, and Brown, 2019). Furthermore, there is a higher risk of pre-term deliveries and low birth weight infants (Do et al., 2021). Conversely, partner and social support during pregnancy has been shown to reduce antenatal distress and intimate partner violence (Ibid.). Health-promotion programmes that enhance social support for women could reduce the burden of physical and intimate partner violence with the concomitant reduction of adverse maternal health outcomes.

In order for the healthcare system to prevent and respond to violence against women and girls, healthcare workers must observe signs of violence, which could include unexplained bruises, cigarette burns, refusal to communicate and emotional withdrawal. Assistance needs to be provided to these women, however if the healthcare worker feels that this is out of her scope, then appropriate referrals must be made. Advice on emergency contraception, safe abortion, STI and HIV prophylaxis for post-rape care may also need to be provided (Temmerman et al., 2015).

Health promotion should not only target detection of violence but should aim for prevention of the perpetration of violence (Naidoo and Nadvi, 2013). Violence against women, in particular by an intimate partner, stems from the man's power and control over the woman and this needs to be challenged (Ibid.). Violence against women includes rape, sexual harassment in schools, female genital mutilation and forced marriage (Dustin, 2016). In Europe, feminist activism, through protests and raising awareness via social media facilitated the fight against rape and other forms of gender-based violence (Alldred and Biglia, 2015; Dustin, 2016). Similar activism in the United Kingdom (UK) resulted in legislation that protected women from violence. Gender equality was also formalised through the creation of equal opportunities for women, particularly with employment opportunities. Preventive measures include the promotion of research on gender-based violence and training of health workers, police, lawyers, teachers, trade unionists and employers to combat sexism (Alldred and Biglia, 2015).

Despite this having decreased overall GBV in the UK, forced marriages and female genital mutilations are prevalent within minority groups. These are often attributed to culture but need to be tackled (Dustin, 2016). In addition, GBV which can take the form of stalking, physical or sexual violence, harassment or other forms of abuse, has been reported to occur at institutions of higher education in developed countries such as the UK. This is a barrier to women's equality and could be reflective of GBV across a wider social sphere (Donaldson et al., 2018). Improvement of criminal justice, systems to apprehend and prosecute perpetrators of violence, is required.

Globally, gender inequality and subsequent GBV was exacerbated during the Covid-19 pandemic, which led to the breakdown of various social infrastructures (Mittal and Singh, 2020). It increased the exposure of women to sexual harassment and violence when they tried to procure essential supplies. Women were particularly vulnerable to domestic violence as they were unable to escape the perpetrator. Generally, more women are in informal employment and lost their jobs resulting in them becoming economically dependent on their male partners. This economic dependence increased their risk of GBV and also made it difficult to leave abusive partners. The quarantine led to difficulties in leaving the home environment and the constant close proximity with a violent partner increased domestic violence. In countries such as Australia, domestic violence increased by 5 per cent, while the USA saw an increase of up to 35 per cent in some states. Countries like India and China reported two- to threefold increases in domestic violence (Mittal and Singh, 2020). Abusers were able to enforce greater control over their victims by limiting access to telephones and the internet as well as to other people. Some countries, such as France, set up warning systems at grocery stores and pharmacies, so that victims could alert the necessary authorities. Healthcare workers must be able to recognise the signs of GBV. When women are asked if they feel safe at home, they may convey this in indirect ways, should GBV be prevalent. Healthcare workers should be able to provide therapeutic interventions, counselling, and social support. They can also set up on-line and telephonic services to assist these women. In addition to providing virtual emotional support, referrals to centres where further help is available can be made (Mittal and Singh, 2020).

───── Time to Reflect 12.2 ─────

Since nurses are integral to the healthcare team, how would they assist women against whom violence has been perpetrated to reaffirm the worth of these women?

## Tutorial Trigger 12.2

Twenty-one-year-old Jane has been dating Mark for the last two years. Her friend Teresa noticed that Jane has been feeling very sad lately and not communicating as she normally does. When she questions her, Jane confesses that Mark has been physically and sexually abusing her for the last four months. Teresa suggests that Jane seeks formal help.

1  How do you think Teresa can help Jane?
2  Design a referral pathway of formal support structures to assist Jane.
3  Identify informal support structures and describe how these would be able to assist Jane.
4  Identify any potential barriers that Jane may have in accessing formal support.

## Summary

This chapter has explored the factors affecting the reproductive health and well-being of women. As role models for health promotion, nurses can create a supportive environment for women as well as strengthen community engagement so that the health and well-being of women can be improved. It is also crucial to empower women with health information to enable them to have some control over their own healthcare needs.

───── Key Points ─────

- Many factors affect the health of women, and these can be exacerbated during this specific part of the lifespan.
- There is an increased risk of breast and cervical cancer, HIV, violence against women and anaemia at this stage in life.

- These factors are often intertwined. For example, violence against women may lead to an increased risk for HIV infection and sometimes cervical cancer, if the violence is sexual in nature. These then affect the overall health of the woman resulting in increased maternal morbidity and mortality.
- Nurses and other healthcare workers have a vital role to play in supporting women in maternal health and in reducing maternal morbidity and mortality.

# References

Ajayi, A.I. and Akpan, W. (2020). Maternal healthcare services utilisation in the context of 'Abiye' (safe motherhood) programme in Ondo State, Nigeria. *BMC Public Health 20*(1), 362. doi:10.1186/s12889-020-08512-z

Alldred, P. and Biglia, B. (2015). Gender-related violence and young people: An overview of Italian, Irish, Spanish, UK and EU legislation. *Children & Society 29*, 662–75.

Alwan, N.A.S. (2016). Breast cancer among Iraqi women: Preliminary findings from a regional comparative breast cancer research project. *Journal of Global Oncology*, *2*(5), 255–8. doi:10.1200/JGO.2015.003087

Ashebir, F., Medhanyie, A.A., Mulugeta, A., Persson, L.Å. and Berhanu, D. (2020). Women's development group leaders' promotion of maternal, neonatal and child healthcare in Ethiopia: A cross-sectional study. *Global Health Action 13*(1), 1748845. doi:10.1080/16549716.2020.1748845

Beesham, I., Welch, J.D., Heffron, R., Pleaner, M., Kidoguchi, L., Palanee-Phillips, T., ... Consortium, T.E.T. (2020). Integrating oral PrEP delivery among African women in a large HIV endpoint-driven clinical trial. *Journal of the International AIDS Society 23*(5), e25491. doi:10.1002/jia2.25491

Bekker, L.G., Brown, B., Joseph-Davey, D., Gill, K., Moorhouse, M., Delany-Moretlwe, S., ... Wallis, C.L. (2020). Southern African guidelines on the safe, easy and effective use of pre-exposure prophylaxis: 2020. *Southern African Journal of HIV Medicine 21*, 1–8. doi:10.4102/sajhivmed.v22i1.1295

Beksinska, M.E., Nkosi, P., Mabude, Z., Smit, J., Zulu, B., Phungula, L., ... Lazarus, N. (2017). Twenty years of the female condom programme in South Africa: past, present, and future. *South African Health Review 2017*(1), 147–56. Retrieved from https://hdl.handle.net/10520/EJC-c8100512a

Beksinska, M.E., Smit, J.A. and Mantell, J.E. (2012). Progress and challenges to male and female condom use in South Africa. *Sexual Health 9*(1), 51–8. doi:10.1071/SH11011

Brazier, E., Fiorentino, R., Barry, M.S. and Diallo, M. (2014). The value of building health promotion capacities within communities: evidence from a maternal health intervention in Guinea. *Health Policy and Planning 30*(7), 885–94. doi:10.1093/heapol/czu089

Cambiano, V., Miners, A., Dunn, D., McCormack, S., Ong, K.J., Gill, O.N., ... Phillips, A.N. (2018). Cost-effectiveness of pre-exposure prophylaxis for HIV prevention in men who have sex with men in the UK: a modelling study and health economic evaluation. *Lancet Infectious Disease 18*(1), 85–94. doi:10.1016/s1473-3099(17)30540-6

Cubie, H.A. and Campbell, C. (2020). Cervical cancer screening – The challenges of complete pathways of care in low-income countries: Focus on Malawi. *Women's Health 16*, 1745506520914804. doi:10.1177/1745506520914804

Dadi, T.L., Bekele, B.B., Kasaye, H.K. and Nigussie, T. (2018). Role of maternity waiting homes in the reduction of maternal death and stillbirth in developing countries and its contribution for maternal death reduction in Ethiopia: a systematic review and meta-analysis. *BMC Health Services Research, 18*(1), 748. doi:10.1186/s12913-018-3559-y

Devanter, N.V., Gonzales, V., Merzel, C., Parikh, N.S., Celantano, D. and Greenberg, J. (2002). Effect of an STD/HIV behavioral intervention on women's use of the female condom. *American Journal of Public Health 92*(1), 109–15. doi:10.2105/ajph.92.1.109

Do, H.P., Baker, P.R.A., Van Vo, T., Murray, A., Murray, L., Valdebenito, S., … Dunne, M.P. (2021). Intergenerational effects of violence on women's perinatal wellbeing and infant health outcomes: evidence from a birth cohort study in Central Vietnam. *BMC Pregnancy and Childbirth 21*(1), 648. doi:10.1186/s12884-021-04097-6

Donaldson, A., McCarry, M. and McCullough, A. (2018). Preventing gender-based violence in UK universities. The policy context. In A. Sundari and R. Lewis (Eds.), *Gender-Based Violence in University Communities: Policy, Prevention and Educational Intervention* 105–28. Bristol: The Policy Press.

Ducray, J.F., Kell, C.M., Basdav, J. and Haffejee, F. (2021). Cervical cancer knowledge and screening uptake by marginalized population of women in inner-city Durban, South Africa: Insights into the need for increased health literacy. *Women's Health 17*, 17455065211047141. doi:10.1177/17455065211047141

Dustin, M. (2016). Culture or masculinity? Understanding gender-based violence in the UK. *Journal of Poverty and Social Justice 24*(1), 51–62. doi:10.1332/1759827 16x14525979706964

Gartland, D., Giallo, R., Woolhouse, H., Mensah, F. and Brown, S.J. (2019). Intergenerational impacts of family violence – Mothers and children in a large prospective pregnancy cohort study. *EClinicalMedicine 15*, 51–61. doi:10.1016/j.eclinm.2019.08.008

Govender, D., Naidoo, S. and Taylor, M. (2019). Knowledge, attitudes and peer influences related to pregnancy, sexual and reproductive health among adolescents using maternal health services in Ugu, KwaZulu-Natal, *South Africa. BMC Public Health 19*(1), 928. doi:10.1186/s12889-019-7242-y

Guvenc, G., Akyuz, A. and Yenen, M.C. (2013). Effectiveness of nursing interventions to increase pap smear test screening. *Research in Nursing & Health 36*(2), 146–57. doi:10.1002/nur.21526

Haffejee, F., Fasanmi-Kana, O., Ally, F., Thandar, Y. and Basdav, J. (2022). Four years later: Do South Africans know what pre-exposure prophylaxis for HIV is? *AIDS Care 1*–8. doi:10.1080/09540121.2022.2032573

Haffejee, F., Koorbanally, D. and Corona, R. (2018). Condom use among South African university students in the province of KwaZulu-Natal. *Sexuality & Culture 22*(4), 1279–89. doi:10.1007/s12119-018-9523-5

Haffejee, F. and Maharajh, R. (2019). Addressing female condom use among women in South Africa: A review of the literature. *International Journal of Sexual Health 31*(3), 297–307. doi:10.1080/19317611.2019.1643813

Haffejee, F. and Maksudi, K. (2020). Understanding the risk factors for HIV acquisition among refugee women in South Africa. *AIDS Care 32*(1), 37–42. doi:10.1080/09540121.2019.1687833

Hoffman, S., Mantell, J., Exner, T. and Stein, Z. (2004). The future of the female condom. *Perspectives on Sexual and Reproductive Health 36*(3), 120–6. Retrieved from www.jstor.org/stable/3181284

Lagese, T., Abdulahi, M. and Dirar, A. (2016). Risk factors of maternal death in Jimma University specialized hospital: a matched case control study. *American Journal of Public Health Research 4*(4), 120–7. doi:10.2147/IJWH.S123455

Mahlalela, N.B. and Maharaj, P. (2015). Factors facilitating and inhibiting the use of female condoms among female university students in Durban, KwaZulu–Natal, South Africa. *The European Journal of Contraception & Reproductive Health Care 20*(5), 379–86. doi:10.3109/13625187.2015.1036415

Maksut, J.L. and Eaton, L.A. (2015). Female condoms – missed opportunities: Lessons learned from promotion-centered interventions. *Women's Health Issues 25*(4), 366–76. doi:10.1016/j.whi.2015.03.015

Mantell, J., Scheepers, E. and Abdool Karim, Q. (2000). Introducing the female condom through the public health sector: experiences from South Africa. *AIDS Care, 12*(5), 589–601. doi:10.1080/095401200750003770

Mantell, J., Smit, J.A., Exner, T.M., Mabude, Z., Hoffman, S., Beksinska, M., ... Stein, Z.A. (2015). Promoting female condom use among female university students in KwaZulu-Natal, South Africa: results of a randomized behavioral trial. *AIDS and Behavior 19*(7), 1129–40. doi: 10.1007/s10461-014-0860-6

Martin, J., de Lora, P., Rochat, R. and Andes, K.L. (2016). Understanding female condom use and negotiation among young women in Cape Town, South Africa. *International Perspectives on Sexual and Reproductive Health 42*(1), 13–20. doi:10.1363/42e0216

Maseko, B., Hill, L.M., Phanga, T., Bhushan, N., Vansia, D., Kamtsendero, L., ... Rosenberg, N.E. (2020). Perceptions of and interest in HIV pre-exposure prophylaxis use among adolescent girls and young women in Lilongwe, Malawi. *PLOS ONE 15*(1), e0226062. doi:10.1371/journal.pone.0226062

Mimiko, O. (2017). Experiences with universal health coverage of maternal healthcare in Ondo State, Nigeria, 2009–2017. *African Journal of Reproductive Health 21*(3), 9–26. doi:10.10520/EJC-b459ba0fc

Mittal, S. and Singh, T. (2020). Gender-based violence during COVID-19 pandemic: A mini-review. *Frontiers in Global Women's Health 1.* doi:10.3389/fgwh.2020.00004

Montjane, K., Dlamini, S. and Dandara, C. (2018). Truvada (emtricitabine/tenofovir) pre-exposure prophylaxis roll-out among South African university students: Lots of positives, but let us keep an eye on possible surprises. *SAMJ: South African Medical Journal 108*, 79–81. Retrieved from www.scielo.org.za/scielo.php?script=sci_arttext&pid=S0256-95742018000200005&nrm=iso

Naidoo, N. and Nadvi, L. (2013). Risk factor management and perpetrator rehabilitation in cases of gender-based violence in South Africa: Implications of salutogenesis. *Agenda 27*(1), 141–50. doi:10.1080/10130950.2013.801196

Naidu, M. (2013). Perceptions around second generation female condoms: Reporting on women's experiences. *Anthropological Notebooks 19*(1).

Paxton, A. and Wardlaw, T. (2011). Are we making progress in maternal mortality? *New England Journal of Medicine 364*(21), 1990–1993. doi:10.1056/NEJMp1012860

Schuyler, A.C., Masvawure, T.B., Smit, J.A., Beksinska, M., Mabude, Z., Ngoloyi, C. and Mantell, J.E. (2016). Building young women's knowledge and skills in female condom use: lessons learned from a South African intervention. *Health Education Research*, *31*(2), 260–72. doi:10.1093/her/cyw001

Smith, H.J., Portela, A.G. and Marston, C. (2017). Improving implementation of health promotion interventions for maternal and newborn health. *BMC Pregnancy and Childbirth 17*(1), 280. doi:10.1186/s12884-017-1450-1

South African National Department of Health. (2021). *South African Maternal, Perinatal and Neonatal policy.* Pretoria, South Africa: National Department of Health Retrieved from www.knowledgehub.org.za/elibrary/south-african-maternal-perinatal-and-neonatal-health-policy

Temmerman, M., Khosla, R., Laski, L., Mathews, Z. and Say, L. (2015). Women's health priorities and interventions. *BMJ : British Medical Journal 351*, h4147. doi:10.1136/bmj.h4147

Tokhi, M., Comrie-Thomson, L., Davis, J., Portela, A., Chersich, M. and Luchters, S. (2018). Involving men to improve maternal and newborn health: A systematic review of the effectiveness of interventions. *PLOS ONE 13*(1), e0191620. doi:10.1371/journal.pone.0191620

Trang, T.P., Dong, B.J., Kojima, N. and Klausner, J.D. (2016). Drug safety evaluation of oral tenofovir disoproxil fumarate-emtricitabine for pre-exposure prophylaxis for human immunodeficiency virus infection. *Expert Opinion on Drug Safety 15*(9), 1287–94. doi:10.1080/14740338.2016.1211108

UNAIDS. (2021). UNAIDS DATA 2021 Retrieved from www.unaids.org/en/resources/documents/2021/2021_unaids_data

WHO, UNICEF, UNFPA, The World Bank, and UNPD. (2019). *Trends in maternal mortality 2000 to 2017: estimates by WHO, UNICEF, UNFPA, World Bank Group and the United Nations Population Division.* Geneva, Switzerland: WHO Retrieved from www.unfpa.org/sites/default/files/pub-pdf/Maternal_mortality_report.pdf

Wium, L., Vannevel, V. and Bothma, S. (2018). Obstetric medical care and training in South Africa. *Obstetric Medicine 12*(1), 27–30. doi:10.1177/1753495X18783610

Wiyeh, A.B., Mome, R.K.B., Mahasha, P.W., Kongnyuy, E.J. and Wiysonge, C.S. (2020). Effectiveness of the female condom in preventing HIV and sexually transmitted infections: a systematic review and meta-analysis. *BMC Public Health 20*(1), 319. doi:10.1186/s12889-020-8384-7

World Cancer Research Fund. (2018). *Comparing more and less developed countries.* London, UK: WCRF Retrieved from www.crf.org/dietandcancer/comparing-more-and-less-developed-countries/

World Health Organization. (2014). *Comprehensive Cervical Cancer Control: A guide to essential practice*. Geneva, Switzerland: WHO. Retrieved from www.who.int/reproductivehealth/publications/cancers/cervical-cancer-guide/en/

World Health Organization. (2020). Global Anaemia Reduction Efforts among Women of Reproductive Age: Impact, achievement of targets and the way forward for optimizing efforts. Retrieved from www.who.int/publications-detail-redirect/9789240012202

# 13

# Reimagining Child and Family Health Education and Health Promotion Through a Planetary Health Lens

Lindsay Smith and Paula Nersesian

## Introduction

This chapter will explore what makes a difference to children, young people and their families and how health promotion and health education during childhood can help shape positive well-being outcomes across the lifespan. Through understanding what matters to children, health-promotion activities can encourage participation, collaboration and strengths that build resilience. Children and young people are at the front line of planetary health, and planetary health matters to them. In recent participatory research, children identified how planetary health is related to every domain of their well-being, making planetary health a new determinant of health and well-being.

By the end of this chapter the reader will be able to:

1. Discover the relationship between child health promotion and planetary health.
2. Discuss how health promotion and health education across six domains of child well-being enhance health and well-being outcomes across the lifespan.
3. Encourage children's participation in developing and implementing health promotion and health education.

---

### Key terms

Planetary health, domains of child well-being, participation, bioecological model, strengths, Anthropocene, disaster risk reduction, justice, equality, equity

---

## Understanding the Drivers of Health and Well-being Outcomes

Contemporary health education and health promotion for children require a deep understanding of the key drivers of health and well-being outcomes. Understanding the key drivers of health and well-being outcomes informs nurses and other healthcare providers on how to facilitate positive health outcomes through effective health promotion and health education. Key drivers of health and well-being are often understood through the four pillars of the bioecological model: person, process, context, and time (Bronfenbrenner, 2001; Bronfenbrenner and Ceci, 1994: 568; Xia, Li and Tudge, 2020).

- Person: a child-focused perspective respects the rights of the child and their decision-making ability; this promotes justice when barriers to health and well-being are removed, and determinants of health are addressed.
- Process: children need strong trusted enduring relationships with their family and other important people in their lives – including their nurse – who recognise their unique strengths and talents; promoting equality through recognising everyone has strengths.
- Context: family, in partnership with their community, provides the support every child needs to reach their potential health and well-being outcomes;

promoting equity and reorienting nursing and healthcare services to respond to the needs identified by children and their families, and supporting strength development.

- Time: child health and well-being outcomes develop over time and within the evolving point in time, for example the sudden emergence of the Covid-19 pandemic.

Robert Wood Johnson Foundation (RWJF) recently created a 'Framework for Understanding Human Well-Being' that includes multiple levels (Acharya and Plough, 2020) resembling the systems included in the domain of the context in Bronfenbrenner's model (2001). The RWJF framework levels are: Individual, Community, Civic, and Environment and Planet (Ibid.). The addition of well-being of the environment and the planet is an important acknowledgement of planetary health and a holistic expansion of the concept of well-being that child health nurses can translate to their health-promoting practice with children.

Considering the child and their family holistically requires the child health nurse to understand the domains of well-being and the external systems influencing well-being outcomes. A holistic interacting systems approach of the bioecological model enables nurses to provide health-promoting care addressing children's and families' priorities within the context of their environment. A bioecological approach guides care providers to understand the processes and contexts that support children and their families across the lifespan. It honours the past, present and future, supplying a means to understand the child's standpoint in their world.

Children, families and communities thrive when their strengths are operationalised to mitigate or adapt to challenges, overcome deficits, and build resilience. When nurses facilitate a health-promoting approach, listen to, respect, and respond to children in ways that facilitate participation in health decisions, then they are making important contributions to health and well-being among children, families, and communities. However, desired health and well-being outcomes for children depend on the context of a healthy environment for them to grow, develop, learn, and thrive over time. Because local environments are inextricably linked to the earth's ecosystems, health promotion exists within the context of a healthy planet. Recognising and acknowledging that people's actions affect the planet, and the health of the planet affects people's health is essential to achieving health and well-being outcomes. Honouring this ultimate contextual reality between people and the planet is essential for children's growth, development, and thriving across time.

## Children and Planetary Health

Planetary health is a foundational concept for this chapter about health promotion with children and their families since global climate change and its impacts on child health and well-being will be a predominant feature of the world children live in for the foreseeable future. All children on the earth today are living in the Anthropocene geological time period – 'a new geological epoch demarcated as the time when human activities began to have a substantial global effect on the Earth's systems' (Whitmee et al., 2015: 1975). What this means for children is that they will see ecosystem change and be affected by atmospheric and other changes throughout their childhood and adult life. They will be called upon to take critical action to reduce the speed of climate change and the degradation of the Earth's ecosystems. They will also learn about and probably experience disasters that can be associated with human activity on the planet.

As humans place greater pressure on the Earth's ecosystems, environmental change results in events ranging from those which are chronic, such as decreasing air quality, to immediate, such as flooding and fires. Some children will experience these events first-hand. And some will be gravely affected by chronic degradation of the atmosphere including increasingly poor air quality. For many children, poor air quality will silently wreak havoc on their respiratory system. Consider the example of Ella Kissi-Debrah who died of respiratory failure in February 2013 aged 9 years (Greenfield and Swallow, 2021). Her mother petitioned for a second coroner's examination and air pollution was found to be a contributing cause to her death. Ella and other children who live in crowded urban areas breathe unhealthy particulate matter all day long. Breathing low-quality air contributes to asthma, respiratory infections, chronic respiratory illness, and acute respiratory failure (Holst et al., 2020; Tiotiu et al., 2020). Among children, asthma is the leading disease globally (Asher, 2021). See the World Health Organisation Fact Sheet on Asthma for more information: https://www.who.int/news-room/fact-sheets/detail/asthma. Nurse home visitors are uniquely positioned to identify factors that place children at risk for chronic health problems and work with families to reduce exposure and manage symptoms when exposures are unavoidable.

## Research in Brief 13.1

Research exploring planetary health and child health is an emerging field. A vast body of research around climate change and human health often neglects to include a child health focus while studies that do, mainly include children as a minor sub-population with methodological concerns limiting transferability of results (Helldén et al., 2021). Nolan et al., (2021) reported on a youth participatory action research that engaged youths to research air quality. Results demonstrated marginalised people live with poorer air quality and greater planetary health stressors than non-marginalised people groups. Insights gained in this research further the understanding of the burden children can experience from planetary health challenges.

Deforestation can be characterised as a slow-moving disaster. The destruction of the Amazon rainforest, for example, is a slowly progressing disaster perpetrated by people who are converting forests to arable land. The result is devastating for indigenous communities as their traditional homeland is destroyed and they are forced to leave. The result is also devastating to people affected by the air pollution created by the fires used to destroy the forest. The Amazon rainforest is also important more broadly because it produces a substantial amount of oxygen through photosynthesis on land (Zimmer, 2019). Deforestation threatens child rights, especially those rights for indigenous children and their families (Bhérer-Magnan, 2022). For example, deforestation of sub-Saharan Africa is now associated with poorer diets in young children (Galway, Acharya and Jones, 2018).

Some disasters arrive swiftly and leave communities devastated, such as the 2021 sinkholes and flooding in Western Europe, or bush fires in Australia and California. Children and families are traumatised, and many are left with nothing except their will to recover and start over. Whether slowly or swiftly developing, disasters have lasting effects on children (Kousky, 2016; Lai and La Greca, 2020). Some children will only hear about disasters while others will struggle to live through them. Children who live in areas affected by natural or human-made disasters and those who experience disasters and atrocities first-hand may find the explanation that humans are responsible for the disasters difficult to accept. It is now understood that all disasters have a human element as a contributing factor (UNDRR, 2022). Richards et al., (2023) call on all nurses to adapt nurse education and practice in response to the Anthropocene. School, public health, and primary care nurses will all play roles in helping children make sense of what they live through and what they need to prepare for.

Children are at high risk of experiencing planetary health-related mental health challenges, with girls and First Nations peoples at particular increased risk (Gergis, et al., 2023).

───── Time to Reflect 13.1 ─────────────────────────────────

Think about a recent environmental disaster that occurred in your country or region of the world. Consider whether global climate change had an impact on the development of the disaster. What actions could you help children take to help mitigate further crises at the individual, family, national, or global levels? What specific policy action can you take now to help stem global climate change that contributes to disasters near you?

Children are learning how people on Earth are affecting the planet and the people, plants, and animals who call it home. Children will eventually develop into adults who will learn to mitigate disaster, adapt to a changing climate, and build resilience. Their goals and aspirations for health and well-being in the context of planetary health will be affected by what they experience (for example, local natural disasters), how they experience change, and whether they have a stable family structure and family members to support and guide them.

No doubt, children's lived experiences will surely influence their goals for health and well-being. Children who live in stable housing, have access to education, enjoy secure sources of food and a stable family are likely to have very different goals for health and well-being than those who lived through catastrophic events such as famine resulting from crop failure, drought, flooding from changes in the atmosphere, and parental loss due to a disaster event. Families affected by flooding suffer the loss of their homes, possessions and livelihoods. Disruptions such as these for families with young children can result in irreversible changes for children, depending on their access to resources and opportunities. For some, their early childhood education ends or is never allowed to start normally. For others, stable housing becomes perpetually unstable, family income is compromised, and community connections are fractured.

National, regional and local governments can influence mitigation, preparedness, response, and recovery from disasters. However, some disasters are hard to fathom, such as the cold snap in Texas during the winter of 2020 and the heatwaves of Europe and England of 2022 that left the electric grid unstable in some areas and unusable in others. Lack of foresight by policy makers into the implications of global climate change on infrastructure leaves communities – especially children – at risk. Nurses can partner with children and families in health-promotion and health-education activities to help reduce the risk of disaster and promote planetary health (Mort, Rodríguez-Giralt and Delicado, 2020). It is important for children to see that what matters to them also matters to the adults in their lives.

Health promotion can recognise the ability of children, respect their decision-making capacity in matters that impact on their lives, trust their strengths, and believe in their ability to adapt. For example, health education related to chronic respiratory conditions needs to account for the impact of pollution and help guide children and young people towards personal actions that may enhance both their respiratory health management and planetary health. A planetary health foundation for health promotion with children and their families broadens the role of nurses to holistically consider and independently act across all domains of well-being. Promoting outcomes in one domain important to children may be enhanced through concurrently promoting outcomes across other domains. In every episode of health promotion and nursing care, you can ask where is planetary health at play and how can planetary health support the health and well-being of the child? The immediate and the longer-term health promotion needs walk side-by-side.

## Child Health Promotion and the Domains of Child Well-being

Effective child health promotion requires a focus on two foundational elements. First, a holistic approach addressing the determinants of health and second, child and youth participation. Successful outcomes are dependent on the inclusivity of children and young people, in the broadest notion, at all stages during the planning and implementation of health-promotion activity. Children have a right to participate in decision-making concerning issues that affect them, and 'evidence shows that ... the incorporation of children's views is beneficial to project outcomes and to children directly' (Australian Research Alliance for Children & Youth, 2019).

### Research in Brief 13.2

Through research involving children and young people exploring the determinants of health and what matters to them by the Australian Research Alliance for Children & Youth (Goodhue, Dakin and Noble, 2021) the commonly understood determinants of health articulated by the World Health Organization (2017 https://www.who.int/news-room/questions-and-answers/item/determinants-of-health) are reimagined as outcomes that matter to children. ARACY and its flagship project, The Nest, identified Six Domains of Child and Youth Wellbeing (see Figure 13.1). This research project included two important actions of successful child health promotion. First, its aim was to understand what determinants of health are important to children. Second, it involved children's participation in many stages of the research. The success of the project is demonstrated by the wide acceptance and implementation of the research findings in practice and government policy. To explore this Research in brief further, view *It Takes a Tasmanian Village: The Nest in action* (https://youtu.be/tJbhl7INTqw) and see how the government in Tasmania, Australia adopted ARACY's Nest, then read Goodhue, Dakin and Noble (2021) *What's in the Nest* https://www.aracy.org.au/documents/item/700

## Upstream child health promotion conveys benefits across the lifespan

The current focus of health-promoting actions, programmes or services tends to be a response to different stages of identifiable biomedical needs (for example asthma and diabetes management), health related deficits (for example low activity level and poor dietary choices) and high-risk context of life experiences (for example

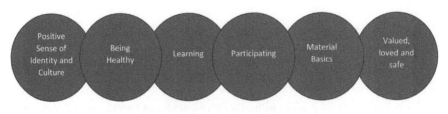

**Figure 13.1**   ARACY's Six domains of child and youth well-being

violence in the home). These can be considered downstream to the foundations of health and well-being that support a flourishing life journey and optimal outcomes. Services set up to address specific biomedical needs, reduce risks or build health-promoting behaviours and strengths are often empowered to respond in one or a few biomedical conditions and rarely have a holistic approach to address all six domains of child and youth well-being (see Figure 13.1). Services with a downstream approach to health and well-being are essential to support and further strengthen families and children to meet their acute health-promotion needs. Alongside downstream health promotion is the need to strengthen a holistic upstream approach to child and youth health promotion.

The impact of any health-promotion intervention is enhanced by a multi-domain approach to resilience building. The importance of a multi-domain approach has been demonstrated in that when children experience deprivation in one of the six domains of well-being, their outcomes are significantly enhanced through the strengths found in one or more of the other six domains of child and youth well-being (Sollis, 2019). Toxic stress related to more than one domain of well-being has an association to a prolonged biological state of inflammation leading to negative health and well-being outcomes and chronic disease (National Scientific Council on the Developing Child, 2020). School Nurses who work in health promotion targeted at mitigating toxic and chronic stress related to planetary health, can build school children's resilience and address their distress (Reiner and Haas-Howard, 2022). Child Health Nurses and other professionals undertaking health promotion and health education activities are helping to establish the future in which children will live (MacAskill, 2022), strongly promoting the Rights of the Child.

---

**Point to Ponder 13.1**

As you walk around your community, what opportunities, strengths and challenges do you see influencing child health and well-being outcomes? What health-promotion and health-education activities can you personally enact that will promote children's strengths in these areas and positively influence their future outcomes?

---

Understanding and supporting the bioecological determinants across the six domains of child and youth well-being is essential in promoting an upstream primary healthcare approach and reducing the pressure on current and future downstream acute care biomedical services. An example of a broad upstream approach to health and well-being is found in the Tasmanian Government's (2021) Child and Youth Wellbeing Strategy for 0–25-year-olds (see https://wellbeing.tas.gov.au/). The strategy is an exemplar of health promotion across the six domains of child and youth well-being (see Figure 13.1) and is a distinctive whole-of-government approach with an upstream focus on creating the context to support child and youth well-being. This strategy is creating the context for children and young people to flourish across the six domains of child and youth well-being and provides exciting areas for future nursing engagement.

### Research in Brief 13.3

Following the implementation of a School Health Nurse programme in Tasmania, Australia, a nurse-led research provided an opportunity for 12 School Health Nurses, 18 teachers and 6 school principals to evaluate the initial impact of the new programme in their school community. The evaluation followed a qualitative descriptive method using a naturalistic inquiry approach. The report 'Stories from the field: Evaluation of the School Health Nurse Programme in Tasmania' (Smith and Millward, 2019), demonstrated School Health Nurses regularly engage with children and youth to promote health across all six domains of child and youth well-being (see Figure 13.1). For example, related to the domain of being loved, safe and valued one teacher reported the School Health Nurse is another safe person for students to go to, that can help support with specific questions or issues. Improvement in child mental well-being following discussions on anxiety and feeling safe were reported. The results highlighted the multi-domain positive impact of school health nurses.

As the planetary health crisis unfolds, children and young people have a powerful and unique connection to the planet and ecology around them. Their future is entwined more in planetary health outcomes than any other age group. They will experience the success and challenges of planetary health well beyond their parents and older generations. Chronic stress as an outcome of children's concerns for planetary health is emerging.

Climate anxiety and distress were correlated with perceived inadequate government response and associated feelings of betrayal. Climate anxiety and dissatisfaction with government responses are widespread in children and young people in countries across the world and impact their daily functioning (Gergis et al., 2023). A perceived failure by governments to respond to the climate crisis is associated with increased distress (Hickman et al., 2021:). There is an urgent need for further research into the emotional impact of climate change on children and young people and for governments to validate their distress by taking urgent action on climate change.

Continuing with the Tasmania Child and Youth Wellbeing Strategy for 0–25-year-olds as an exemplar, in 2021 the Tasmania Government engaged with local children and young people seeking their voices on what matters to them in the determinants of health and well-being. Using the ARACY six domains as a framework (Figure 13.1) children and young people voiced their current understanding of what matters to them under each of the six domains. Unsurprisingly, yet previously unrecognised, children and young people identified how planetary health is foundational to every domain of well-being and underpins their determinants of health. Participatory research involving children is finding the association between planetary health and multi-domain chronic stress children may experience. The voices and concerns of children and young people are found in the adaptation of the ARACY six domains of well-being to include new planetary health descriptors under each of the six domains (see Figure 13.2).

Planetary health provides a way to see the interconnectedness of people and the Earth. The six domains of child and youth well-being is a framework for nurses to target health promotion and health education across the framework.

## Practice, Research and Policy Supporting Child Health Promotion

Nurses can contribute to children's health, well-being, and experience of the Earth through their roles as practitioners, researchers, and policy makers or policy influencers. The following are examples of how nurses can contribute to health promotion through a planetary health lens in each of the roles.

### Practice

Nurses working in school settings are crucial people in children's lives. Children spend a great deal of time embedded in the school setting. Health education on non-traditional topics such as mindfulness may help children develop skills that will allow them to be less anxious in the face of challenging circumstances, including hearing of planetary disasters around the globe (Reiner and Hass-Howard, 2022). School Health Nurses may be able to link health education sessions in school curricula related to the environment. Strategies may involve outside learning activities where nurses walk with children to explore the local environment for planetary health threats (such as plastic waste pollutants in the community) and collaboratively work in small groups to devise solutions the children, school and community could implement to mitigate what they see and experience.

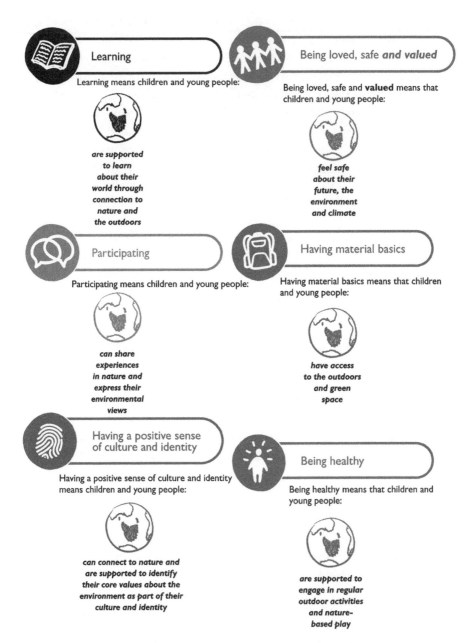

**Figure 13.2**  Planetary Health and the Domains of Child & Youth Well-being, adapted with permission from *It Takes a Tasmanian Village: Tasmania's Child and Youth Well-being Strategy 0 – 25 year olds*, Department of Premier and Cabinet, August 2021, pp. 14–15, ISBN 978-1-925906-34-9. https://hdp-au-prod-app-tas-shapewellbeing-files.s3.ap-southeast-2.amazonaws.com/2116/3159/8898/Child_and_Youth_Wellbeing_Strategy_Sept_2021_wcag_FINAL.pdf

---

**Research in Brief 13.4**

In a study with strong child participation conducted in the Republic of Moldova which included school-aged children as peers, health educators showed an improved understanding of antibiotics and their lack of efficacy in treating colds and flu (Cebotarenco and Bush, 2008). One element of the intervention was providing basic information on the appropriate use of medicines to children and their parents through peer education, meetings with parents, and the development and dissemination of a booklet, video vignettes, a newsletter, and a poster. The study team also facilitated children's participation and held a poster contest. This study demonstrated that children can be change agents for their health and well-being. By delivering health education to children, nurses and other healthcare providers can support individual and family-level behaviour change. Believing in children's abilities and trusting that they can be direct recipients of health-promoting information shows respect for children. Nurses play an important independent health-promotion and health-education role in talking with children about their medicines.

---

## Research

Nurses engaged in health promotion and health education require a strong evidence base arising from nurse-led research. Planetary health is an upstream determinant of health influencing both individual and population quality of life. Health promotion focused research can help understand the relationship between the Anthropocene and health and explore strategies to enhance eco-health literacy (Dos Santos et al., 2023).

The Covid-19 pandemic provides an example of children being disadvantaged by their age given their inability or barriers to be vaccinated against the SARS-CoV-2 coronavirus. We expect adults to actively protect children by getting vaccinated and practicing Covid-19 safe behaviours, yet some do not take this action and as a result place children at increased risk of the infection. Covid-19 vaccinations for younger children are being rolled out in some countries (for example in the USA Covid-19 vaccination is approved for use in children aged two years and older), however, this does not absolve adults from acting in the best interest of younger and vulnerable people. Nursing research on this conundrum could explore attitudes around vaccination and knowledge about how being unvaccinated places children at undue risk of infection.

Nurse researchers can help understand the relationship between individual behaviours, the interconnectedness of all people and the influence of the relationship on child health outcomes and health promotion strategies (LeClair and Potter, 2022). Including planetary health as a variable in nurse research with children and young people elevates nurses' leadership in research, health education, policy development and health promotion (Vandenberg, 2023). Creating sustainable health education and health promotion in nursing requires planetary health considerations in nurse research activity in the Anthropocene.

## Policy

Governments functioning for the well-being of their people provide direction through policy and legislation. Nurses as a professional group with a dedication to promoting health and well-being outcomes for children can make significant contributions to policy development. Yet nurses' potential to inform policy remains constrained by a lack of interprofessional recognition, limited government investment and challenges from within the healthcare system affecting job satisfaction and career advancement (Catton, 2022). Catton (2022) also believes 'nurses are a force for good and given the opportunity to contribute to the full scope of their commitments, knowledge and leadership insights, many of the failures in the health systems around the world [*during the COVID-19 pandemic*] would not have been so devastating'.

Children and young people globally have been deprived of opportunities causing a potential impact on their developmental outcomes during the Covid-19 pandemic. Nurses at the forefront of the Covid-19 pandemic advocated for a more child and family-friendly system response. For example, nurses were instrumental in facilitating family support and visiting during ICU admissions, during the pandemic when strict isolation was in place, helping children and families grieve, cope and be resilient during times of great family stress (Ning and Slatyer, 2021).

The International Family Nursing Association (IFNA) developed a position statement on planetary health that seeks to inform its members, educators, researchers, practitioners, other healthcare professionals, policy makers, and the public of the link between planetary health and family health. The position statement also offers practical support for family nursing education, research, and practice on the planetary health and family health through its nine essential activities and outcomes (IFNA, 2020). The associated blog series brings the essential activities and outcomes to life and serves as a launch pad for child health nurses to take direct action in their education, research, and practice (please see IFNA blog series on planetary health and family for more details – https://internationalfamilynursing.org/ps5).

---

### Tutorial Trigger 13.1

Name human activities that have contributed to global climate change. What impacts have changes in the Earth's atmosphere had on the health of young people in your area? How can we as a group collaborate to promote child health through promoting planetary health? For example, write a letter to your local parliamentary representative expressing how children's life outcomes will be affected by planetary health including an example from your practice or community to illustrate the personal impact of global climate change on a family from the local community that the parliamentarian represents.

## Summary

A universal, holistic supportive upstream well-being approach to health promotion and health education developed in collaboration with children and young people is required to help achieve lasting outcomes across the life course. The six domains of child and youth well-being challenge the current systems focusing on the problematisation of childhood and the life journey. In health education and health promotion a new approach that can provide focus on strengths, relationships, wholeness, and interconnectedness to planetary health is needed. The profession of nursing and the speciality areas related to child health are uniquely positioned to fulfil this need.

─────── Key Points ──────────────────────────────────

- Child health promotion and planetary health are interconnected across six domains of well-being. Health promotion and health education outcomes are enhanced by incorporating planetary health.
- Partnering with children and families in health promotion and health education strengthens outcomes of health-promoting activity.
- Child health promotion and health education can reduce toxic stress, positively influence the future chronic disease burden, and help create a context where children participate in decisions in areas that matter to them.
- Nurses engaging in policy development are engaging in health promotion giving voice to the often-ignored views of children.
- Child health promotion promotes the Rights of the Child and the future they will live in.

## References

Acharya, K. and Plough, A. (2020). Introduction: The imperative for well-being in an inequitable world. In A.L. Plough (Ed.), *Well-Being: Expanding the definition of progress.* (pp. xixviii). New York: Oxford University Press.

Asher, M.I., Rutter, C.E., Bissell, K., Chiang, C.Y., El Sony, A., Ellwood, E., ... Shah, J. (2021). Worldwide trends in the burden of asthma symptoms in school-aged children: Global Asthma Network Phase I cross-sectional study. *The Lancet 398*(10311), 1569–80.

Australian Research Alliance for Children & Youth (ARACY) (2019). Children's voice position statement. Canberra, Australia: ARACY. Available at: www.aracy.org.au/news/childrens-voice-position-statement

Bhérer-Magnan, F. (2022, June 19). 'The Amazon rainforest is disappearing quickly — and threatening Indigenous people who live there', *The Conversation*. Available at: https://theconversation.com/the-amazon-rainforest-is-disappearing-quickly-and-threatening-indigenous-people-who-live-there-185085

Bronfenbrenner, U. (2001). Bioecological theory of human development. In J.S. Neil and B.B. Paul (Eds), *International Encyclopaedia of the Social & Behavioural Sciences* (pp. 6963–70). Oxford, UK: Pergamon.

Bronfenbrenner, U. and Ceci, S. J. (1994). Nature-nurture reconceptualized in developmental perspective: A bioecological model. *Psychological Review 101*(4), 568.

Catton, H. (2022). International Nurses Day: Nurses can change the world, given the investment and support they deserve. *International Nursing Review 69*, 261–4.

Cebotarenco, N. and Bush, P.J. (2008). Reducing antibiotics for colds and flu: a student-taught program. *Health Education Research 23*(1), 146–57. Available at: https://doi.org/10.1093/her/cym008

Department of Premier and Cabinet (2021). *It Takes a Tasmanian Village: Tasmania's Child and Youth Wellbeing Strategy 0 – 25 year olds*. Tasmania, Australia: Department of Premier and Cabinet ISBN 978-1-925906-34-9. Available at: https://hdp-au-prod-app-tas-shapewellbeing-files.s3.ap-southeast-2.amazonaws.com/2116/3159/8898/Child_and_Youth_Wellbeing_Strategy_Sept_2021_wcag_FINAL.pdf

Dos Santos, O., Melly, P., Joost, S. and Verloo, H. (2023). Climate Change, Environmental Health, and Challenges for Nursing Discipline. *Int. J. Environ. Res. Public Health 20*(9): 5682. doi: 10.3390/ijerph20095682

Galway, L.P., Acharya, Y. and Jones, A.D. (2018). Deforestation and child diet diversity: A geospatial analysis of 15 Sub-Saharan African countries. *Health & Place 51*, 78–88.

Gergis, J., Blashki, G., Gardner, J. and Bradshaw S. (2023). Climate Trauma: The Growing Toll of Climate Change on the Mental Health of Australians. Melbourne, Australia: Climate Council of Australia.

Goodhue, R., Dakin, P. and Noble, K. (2021). *What's in the Nest? Exploring Australia's Wellbeing Framework for Children and Young People*. Canberra, Australia: ARACY. Available at: www.aracy.org.au/documents/item/700

Gergis, J., Blashki, G., Gardner, J. and Bradshaw S. (2023). Climate Trauma: The Growing Toll of Climate Change on the Mental Health of Australians. Melbourne, Australia: Climate Council of Australia.

Greenfield, D. and Swallow, V. (2021). All nurses should understand the principles of planetary health. *Nursing Times Opinion*. Retrieved from www.nursingtimes.net/opinion/all-nurses-should-understand-the-principles-of-planetary-health-08-02-2021/

Helldén, D., Andersson, C., Nilsson, M., Ebi, K.L., Friberg, P. and Alfvén, T. (2021). Climate change and child health: a scoping review and an expanded conceptual framework. *The Lancet Planetary Health 5*(3), e164–e175.

Hickman, C., Marks, E., Pihkala, P., Clayton, S., Lewandowski, R.E., Mayall, E.E., … and van Susteren, L. (2021). Climate anxiety in children and young people and their beliefs about government responses to climate change: a global survey. *The Lancet Planetary Health 5*(12), e863–e873.

Holst, G.J., Pedersen, C.B., Thygesen, M., Brandt, J., Geels, C., Bønløkke, J.H. and Sigsgaard, T. (2020). Air pollution and family related determinants of asthma onset and persistent wheezing in children: nationwide case-control study. *BMJ 370*, m2791. doi: 10.1136/bmj.m2791

International Family Nursing Association (IFNA). (2020). IFNA position statement on planetary health and family health. Available at: https://internationalfamilynursing.org/2020/04/18/ifna-position-statement-on-planetary-health-and-family-health/

Kousky, C. (2016). Impacts of natural disasters on children. *The Future of Children 26*, 73–92. Available at: www.jstor.org/stable/43755231

Lai, B. and La Greca, A. (2020). *Understanding the impacts of natural disasters on children. Child evidence brief No. 8.* Michigan, USA: Society for Research in Child Development. Accessed 12/09/2022, https://www.srcd.org/research/understanding-impacts-natural-disasters-children.

LeClair, J., and Potter, T. (2022). Planetary Health Nursing. *The American Journal of Nursing 122*(4): 47–52. doi: 10.1097/01.NAJ.0000827336.29891.9b

MacAskill, W. (2022). *What We Owe the Future.* New York: Basic Books.

Mort, M., Rodríguez-Giralt, I. and Delicado, A. (2020). *Children and Young People's Participation in Disaster Risk Reduction: Agency and resilience.* Bristol: Policy Press.

National Scientific Council on the Developing Child. (2020). *Connecting the brain to the rest of the body: Early childhood development and lifelong health are deeply intertwined. Working Paper No. 15.* Available at: www.developingchild.harvard.edu

Ning, J. and Slatyer, S. (2021). When 'open visitation in intensive care units' meets the Covid-19 pandemic. *Intensive & Critical Care Nursing 62*, 102969. doi: 10.1016/j.iccn.2020.102969

Nolan, J.E.S., Coker, E.S., Ward, B.R., Williamson, Y.A. and Harley, K.G. (2021). "Freedom to Breathe": Youth Participatory Action Research (YPAR) to Investigate Air Pollution Inequities in Richmond, CA. *International Journal of Environmental Research and Public Health 18*(2), 554. doi: 10.3390/ijerph18020554

Tiotiu, A.I., Novakova, P., Nedeva, D., Chong-Neto H.J., Novakova, S., Steiropoulos, P. and Kowal, K. (2020). Impact of air pollution on asthma outcomes. *International Journal of Environmental Research and Public Health 27*(17): 6212. doi: 10.3390/ijerph17176212

Reiner, K.L. and Haas-Howard, C. (2022). Essential strategies for School Nurses to move upstream in support of healthy students and a healthy planet. *NASN School Nurse 37*(4), 217–22. doi:10.1177/1942602X221078342

Renshaw, L. and Goodhue, R. (2022). The evidence for The Common Approach®. Canberra, Australia: ARACY. Available at: www.aracy.org.au/documents/item/715

Richards, C., Holmes, M., Nash, R., and Ward, A. (2023). Nursing in the Anthropo-cene–translating disaster nursing experience into climate crisis nurse education. *Teaching and Learning in Nursing*, doi: 10.1016/j.teln.2023.03.017

Smith, L. and Millward, A. (2019). Stories from the field: Evaluation of the School Health Nurse Programme in Tasmania. Unpublished report, Launceston, Australia: University of Tasmania.

Sollis, K. (2019). Measuring child deprivation and opportunity in Australia. *Applying the Nest framework to develop a measure of deprivation and opportunity for children using the Longitudinal Study of Australian Children*. Canberra, Australia: ARACY.

United Nations Office for Disaster Risk Reduction (UNDRR), Underlying disaster risk drivers. Available at: www.undrr.org/terminology/underlying-disaster-risk-drivers, Retrieved 23 September 2022.

Vandenberg, S. (2023). Planetary Health: Preparing Nursing Students for the Future. *Nurse Educator*, doi: 10.1097/NNE.0000000000001420

Whitmee, S., Haines, A., Beyrer, C., Boltz, F., Capon, A.G., de Souza Dias, B.F., ... Yach, D. (2015). Safeguarding human health in the Anthropocene epoch: Report of The Rockefeller Foundation–Lancet Commission on planetary health. *The Lancet* 386(10007), 1973–2028.

WHO (2017). Determinants of health. February 03. Availabe at: who.int/news-room/questions-and-answers/item/determinants-of-health

Xia, M., Li, X. and Tudge, J.R. (2020). Operationalizing Urie Bronfenbrenner's process-person-context-time model. *Human Development 64*(1), 10–20.

Zimmer, K. (2019). *Why the Amazon doesn't really produce 20% of the world's oxygen*. National Geographic. Available at: www.nationalgeographic.com/environment/article/why-amazon-doesnt-produce-20-percent-worlds-oxygen

# 14

# Adolescent Sexual Reproductive Health and Rights

Pandu Hailonga-van Dijk and Cloudina Venaani

## Introduction

The chapter draws from the social-ecological model to identify factors potentially associated with unintended adolescent pregnancies. It draws on the World Health Organization framework for providing adolescents and young people's services to guide nurses and people working with young people in implementing prevention and management programmes for unplanned pregnancies among adolescents. The chapter reiterates the fact that unplanned pregnancies among adolescents and young people are a major reproductive health concern with potentially detrimental personal and socio-economic consequences which may also affect their ability to contribute to the development of society. The chapter focuses on this issue in the context of low- and middle-income countries; however, the content has global relevance to the nurse's role in supporting adolescents and young people who experience unintended pregnancy.

By the end of this chapter the reader will be able to:

1. Describe the factors contributing to unplanned pregnancies among unmarried adolescents.

2. Understand the need for preventing unplanned pregnancies.
3. Apply the social-ecological framework and World Health Organization's framework to develop strategies for preventing and managing unplanned pregnancies among adolescents.

**Key terms**

Adolescence, sexual reproductive health, illegal abortion, adolescent unplanned pregnancies,[1] Rights

## Adolescent Pregnancies

The World Health Organization (WHO) estimates that, in 2019, 21 million girls aged 15–19 years in developing regions became pregnant and that approximately 12 million of them went on to give birth.[2] Globally, adolescent fertility was, and is still, the highest in Africa with West and Central Africa at 104 births per 1,000; East and Southern Africa at 92 per 1,000; Latin America and the Caribbean at 59 per 1,000; the Arab States at 45 per 1,000; Eastern Europe and Central Asia at 26 per 1,000; Asia and the Pacific at 21 per 1,000.[3]

A substantial number of adolescents experiment with sex at an early age, as early as 14 years or younger in southern Africa.[4] As of 2020, in Namibia, the global adolescent birth rate was estimated at 19 per cent (MoHSS, 2021). This is viewed as being the reason for a high level of school dropout globally, ranging from 15 per cent to 50 per cent, with the lowest rate among those under 15 years of age. Many societies report a high school enrolment rate but subsequent drop-off in enrolment into secondary level schooling. For example, in Namibia there is over 90 per cent enrolment at the primary school level but by the time young girls reached secondary school (ages 16–18 years) 50 per cent have dropped out of school due to pregnancies (EMIS, 2019).

Adolescents' sexual reproductive health and behaviours are influenced by several interactive factors that are beyond the individual's control. To explore this, this chapter draws from two frameworks – the Socio-Ecological Model (SEM) and the World Health Organization's framework for providing adolescents and young people's services. The Socio-Ecological Model (SEM) considers the complex interplay between individual, interpersonal, relationship, community, institutional and policy levels. The SEM enables service providers, such as nurses, to move beyond the biomedical model and to understand the determinants of unplanned adolescent pregnancy in a wider context, as reflected in Figure 14.1 which gives an overview of the Socio-Ecological model (SEM).

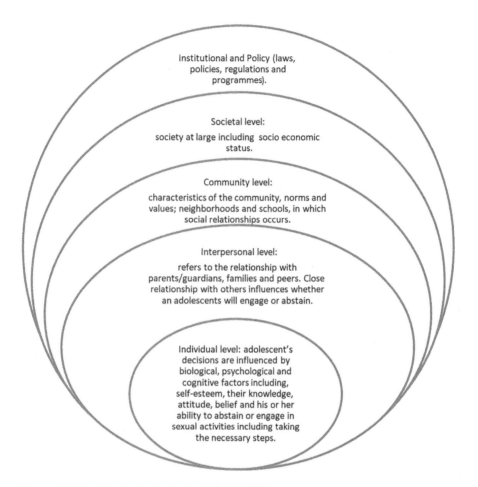

**Figure 14.1** The Socio-Ecological Model (SEM)

We now consider each level in turn in terms of the factors influencing unplanned adolescent pregnancies and the health-education and health-promotion strategies that might be adopted by nurses in order to address this issue.

## Individual Level

Adolescents aged 10–19 years have a higher risk of sexual and reproductive health issues, such as unplanned pregnancies, illegal abortion,[5] baby dumping, HIV and Gender Based Violence (GBV) partly due to their age, gender, im/maturity, self-esteem, knowledge about the self, body, reproductive health issues, including limited knowledge on the prevention, misconceptions and non-use of contraceptives, as well as a relative inability to negotiate for safe sex (Wood and Hendricks, 2017).

---

**Box 14.1**

---

## Sexual Reproductive Health (SRH) is defined as:

'a state of complete physical, mental and social well-being in all matters relating to reproduction, enabling people to have a satisfying safe sex life and the freedom to decide if, when and how often to reproduce, which implies the right of men and women to be informed and to have access to safe, effective, affordable and acceptable methods of family planning of their choice and the right of access to appropriate health care services that will enable women to go safely through pregnancy and childbirth and provide couples with the best chance of having a healthy infant' (UNFPA, 2014).

---

Unintended pregnancies among adolescents are associated with less desirable health, educational, social and economic outcomes. Pregnancy can disrupt education, reduce employment opportunity and may contribute to the cycle of poverty. Pregnant adolescents also have a high risk of eclampsia, post-partum complications and pregnancy-related issues, which also affect their infants. The ability to engage or not engage in unprotected sex is determined by the individual adolescents. Adolescents with higher levels of cognitive ability, academic achievement and aspiration were found to have the ability to avoid unplanned pregnancy (MoHSS, 2019: Wood, 2017).

Research shows that, in many African societies, females are expected to be sexually ignorant (MoHSS, 2019; Wood, 2017). Consequently, young women tend to have poor self-esteem, and rarely acknowledge that they are sexually active, which hampers their ability to access contraception and increases their risk of engaging in unprotected sex. This is further complicated by the perception among many young girls that they cannot get pregnant the first time they have sex (MoHSS, 2019; Wood, 2017).

Many health-promotion programmes have been implemented to address sexual and reproductive health challenges for young people. For example, in Namibia, there is the Comprehensive Sexuality Education (CSE), whose purpose is to educate adolescents about life skills including sexuality. CSE is offered as an integral part of the school curriculum and also for adolescents in the out-of-school environment. CSE has contributed to the knowledge about sexuality among young people which is made possible by well-trained and qualified teachers, and health providers (such as nurses) and is complemented by programmes using advocacy networks.

---

**Box 14.2**

---

Comprehensive Sexuality Education (CSE)UNESCO defines Comprehensive Sexuality Education (CSE) as a curriculum-based process of teaching and learning regarding the cognitive, emotional, physical and social aspects of sexuality. Its main goal is to equip children and young people with the knowledge, skills, attitudes and values that will empower them to realise their health, well-being and dignity; develop respectful social and sexual relationships; consider how their choices affect their own well-being and that of others; and understand and ensure the protection of their rights throughout their lives (UNESCO, 2019).

In Namibia, as a strategy to prevent unplanned pregnancies, some youth groups have developed social development programmes focusing on social and psychological skills (using fellow young people) as motivators, including emphasising the importance of having educational aspirations for their members. This has resulted in empowering young people and assisting them in making informed decisions, which has helped them understand that the age for sexual consent at 16 years did not imply that they could engage in risky sexual behaviours (Young Achievers Report, 2021). In their efforts to prevent unplanned pregnancies nurses should focus on strengthening the knowledge and self-esteem of adolescents, as well as strengthening their individual agency to plan and decide on their own sexuality and sexual practice.

## Tutorial Trigger 14.1

Consider the region and country where you live. What are the rates of unplanned teenage pregnancy? What measures are in place to support young people in making healthier choices? Can you find any examples of health-promotion programmes that are designed to provide high-quality sexual and reproductive health information and support at the individual level?

## Interpersonal Level

Relationships with others, whether formal or informal, including social support systems determine adolescents' ability and capacity to prevent pregnancy. Adolescent pregnancies are typically found to be highest among those living in compromised family structures with a lack of communication (about relationships, sex, abstinence, contraceptive usage), lack of family supervision and support, poor socio-economic status, low education levels, alcohol abuse, history of adolescent parenthood, lack of positive role models and poor parent-daughter/son relationships as well as pressure from friends/peers (MoHSS, 2019; MoE/UNESCO, 2021).

In southern Africa the ages of 14–18 years tend to coincide with a move to senior secondary schools which are often located away from home.[6] This situation gives young people a first taste of freedom away from the watchful eyes of their families, including wider community members. Young people often leave home with limited knowledge about life and look to peers for information which then shapes their knowledge, beliefs, attitudes and behaviours to navigate life outside with which they are unfamiliar. Research has noted that when friends or peers engage in any risky behaviour, be it unprotected sex, alcohol, drugs or crime, this influences the behavioural practices of those around them. Moreover, it has been noted by many that family have provided very little guidance to adolescents and that the majority of first adolescent sexual intimacy experience was because of peer pressure (Bongwong et al., 2019; Marravilla et al., 2017; MoHSS, 2019; UNESCO, 2021).

This highlights the importance of stakeholders' responsibility in ensuring that adolescents are well-informed and are able to resist or navigate peer pressure. The focus should be on promoting positive role models and addressing peer social norms, including engaging both young men and women as an effective way of preventing unplanned pregnancies. Nurses have an important role to play in this, in schools, healthcare settings and the wider community.

## Community and Societal Level

Community levels of influence include neighbourhoods, social/health services, transportation and social norms and they play a key role in the prevention of unplanned teenage pregnancies. Community norms[7] that are indifferent towards sexual debut, masculinity/femininity and multiple concurrent partners are the main driving force of HIV, STDs and high rates of unplanned adolescent pregnancies as well as gender-based violence (Maravilla et al., 2017; MoHSS, 2019).

In southern Africa, men are associated with power be it economic, emotional and or physical power, and manhood is also defined by sexual experiences. This includes the number of children men have as well as the number of sexual partners. Conversely, women are relatively passive and powerless, and comparatively unable to protect themselves against unwanted sexual intercourse or to negotiate for safer sex (MoHSS, 2019; MOE and UNESCO, 2021). Moreover, communities tend to hold an embedded sense of disapproval of adolescent sexual activities as well as the perceived notion that contraceptives are reserved for married women and those with children.[8] This is further complicated by a culture of silence and the promotion of different and unequal value systems which contributes to young women's vulnerability to becoming pregnant. These socially constructed cultural beliefs of what it means to be a man may reinforce double standards that boys and men may be sexually active with multiple partners while expecting girls to abstain and remain 'innocent'.

---

### Point to Ponder 14.1

In southern Africa, the transition from primary school to secondary school coincides with the adolescence phase of the lifespan. A substantial number of learners, in Namibia, leave their parental home to attend school somewhere else, mainly because of the limited number of secondary schools and the geographical distances between schools and villages. These learners are often forced to *rent rooms by themselves*, because of limited school hostels and host families. They are likely to live in poor neighbourhoods, renting in or near alcohol outlets, with a high rate of alcohol abuse, gender inequality, unemployment, poverty and lack of education opportunities resulting in a high rate of adolescent pregnancy. This type of situation also leads to girls being preyed upon by older men. This is further worsened by the economic status of the adolescents, who often come from poor backgrounds. Consequently, adolescent girls engage in transactional sex for money, basic needs, school fees, and other luxury items to meet their needs, and often to feel part of the crowd.

*Source*: (MoHSS, 2019; UNESCO, 2021).

---

## Research in Brief 14.1

Research into interpersonal relationships noted that the positive engagement of parents/adult and adult-child communication has a positive impact on the adolescent. In line with the African concept of 'it takes a village to raise a child' in situations where the family structure has disintegrated, strategies need to be developed to support young women. For example, the Philani Mentor Mother model (PMMM) in South Africa empowers, informs, educates and supports behaviour change and encourages health in multiple ways (Le Roux et al., 2013). The PMMM is inspired by the Positive Deviant Model, which focuses on finding solutions within the communities and is based on the philosophy that even in very poor communities, parents can develop coping mechanisms to raise healthy children.

Strengthening community structures is key to the protection of vulnerable girls and young women, who are confronted with strong patriarchal norms in more traditional societies. Developing and promoting positive enhancing extracurricular activities, and identifying and engaging adult community members to act as mentors for young people who are on their own are important. In addition, the provision of financial support, including job opportunities, is proven to result in economically empowered girls and young women which, in turn, helps to reduce the rates of unplanned adolescent pregnancy. Using boys and men as allies in preventing unplanned pregnancies and building gender-equitable relationships is fundamental to addressing the issue. Nurses can work with young women and young men in different community settings to achieve this.

---

## Tutorial Trigger 14.2

Choose a city or region in the country you live in. Try to find out what you can about the incidence and prevalence of adolescent pregnancies in that city or region. Are you able to identify areas with the highest and lowest numbers? What are the differences between the areas? Consider the wider social factors that might impact on the rates of teenage pregnancies in those areas such that have been discussed within this chapter.

## Institutional and Policy Level

Sexual Reproductive Health and Rights (SRHR) is a fundamental human rights issue. The Namibian government, like many, has put in place numerous conventions, policies, international commitments and legal instruments aimed at safeguarding the healthy transition from being a child to adulthood.[9] The UN Convention on the Rights of the Child (CRC) states that children and young people have the right[9] to access health facilities, and the right to information to decide on their health, about sexuality, and about reproductive health including family planning (Articles 17 & 24).[11] The minimum legal age for sexual consent and marriage is between 16–18 years according to the federal law of many African countries. For example, in Botswana, Senegal and Namibia a child can consent to sex from the age of 16 years. In countries like Kenya, Tanzania and Rwanda the age of consent is 18 years[12] (GRN Gazette, 2000).

Notwithstanding laws, adolescents as young as 14 years old have given birth, sometimes younger. In 2019 the World Health Organization reported that, globally, 777,000 births were by adolescent girls under the age of 15 years impregnated by older men[2] in developing countries who were often more than three years older. Impregnating a girl under age 16 years is the violation of law in Namibia pertaining to age of consent; however, paradoxically, no man has been detained for statutory rape (MoHSS, 2021). To further complicate things, research has found barriers to young people's access to contraceptive services, health workers who are not comfortable in dealing with sexuality issues, and that also refuse to give family planning to young people (MoHSS, 2019).

### Tutorial Trigger 14.3

At age 16 the rationale for engaging in sexual activities is usually not for procreation but for fun or out of curiosity.

Make a list of the laws that relate to SRH in your country and comment on their effectiveness in relation to the following:

- age of consent for sex and marriage
- age to access contraceptives
- age for HIV testing with no parental permission.

Research has found that translating policy into action is a challenge. Faced with the adolescent pregnancies, and with the sometimes judgemental attitudes of health workers who refused to give contraception to adolescents, government and partners have integrated sexual and reproductive health into the pre- and in-service curriculum of health providers such as nurses. Interventions that take a multidisciplinary approach such as engaging family, community members, and traditional religious (including political leaders) has also been found to be effective. For example this was the case with the Comprehensive Sexuality Education programme mentioned earlier in this chapter which initially faced resistance and was later supported by key stakeholders, and eventually removed the stigmatisation of adolescent sexuality and their use of sexual and reproductive services (MoHSS, 2019). Engaging and supporting non-governmental and third sector organisations is also a proven effective way to provide youth-friendly services to young people.

## World Health Organization Framework for Providing Adolescent-friendly Health Services

The World Health Organization's framework provides six key components for the provision of youth and adolescent-friendly health services. They are (1) accessibility, which includes location and opening hours; (2) availability of services, including commodities; (3) acceptability of services offered in non-judgemental attitude,

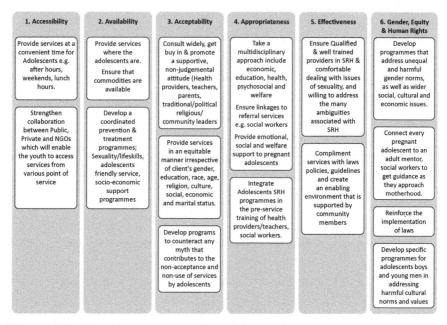

**Figure 14.2**   Key elements in providing adolescent SRH services

supportive and supported by key stakeholders (community, traditional, political and religious leaders); (4) effectiveness, the providers' (such as nurses) ability to provide services in a comfortable way, addressing sensitive issues and knowing where necessary to make relevant referrals; (5) appropriateness, right services supported by laws, policies and guidelines; and (6) Equity, Gender, and Human Rights. Figure 14.2 provides an overview of the 6 components of the framework.

## Summary

This chapter has explored factors that determine adolescents' sexual reproductive health and behaviour in relation to unplanned adolescent pregnancy and has noted that they are influenced by several interactive factors that are often beyond the individual's control. The discussion shows that prevention and management of unplanned pregnancies should take into consideration the interplay of factors between individual, interpersonal, relationship, community, institutional and policy level, recognising the structural constraints adolescents face in negotiating for safer sex and accessing contraceptives, as well as the potential lack of support they might get from parents and healthcare providers, all of which can act as barriers to youth-friendly health services. Services for young people should address issues of acceptability, availability, effectiveness and most importantly integrate equity, gender and human rights. Preventive intervention programmess should be implemented not as sporadic measures, but as systematic and long-term actions. The nurse has an important role to play in settings where adolescents live their lives. All of this supports the aim stated within the Sustainable Development Goal agenda which seeks to ensure universal access to sexual and reproductive healthcare services, including family planning services, information, and education by 2030.

———— Key Points ————

- Prevention of unplanned pregnancies among adolescents is only effective if providers take a multidisciplinary approach and address the different levels of influence:
  - Focus on strengthening the knowledge and self-esteem of adolescents, strengthening their agency to plan and decide on their own sexuality. Develop empowerment programmes that include conflict resolution, social-emotional learning, safe dating and healthy relationship skill programmes, including the promotion of positive role models and healthy peer social norms.
  - Develop programmes that give young people educational aspirations, a vision and a purpose in life.
- Key to the protection of vulnerable girls and young women, who are confronted with strong patriarchal norms including toxic masculinity, is enhancing community

structures (sports activities, youth programmes, economic opportunities; reducing alcohol outlets in communities and creating safe places).

• Reinforcing laws and policies through political commitment, adequate resource allocation, capacity building, and the creation of systems of accountability will also have a positive impact.

---

# Notes

1  For this chapter the focus is on adolescents who are not married and whose pregnancy was not planned.

2  https://www.who.int/news-room/fact-sheets/detail/adolescent-pregnancy

3  Statista Adolescent fertility rate worldwide as of 2020, by region (*per 1,000 girls*) Downloaded 20 Sept. 2022 https://www.statista.com/statistics/1228319/adolescent-fertility-rate-worldwide/

4  UNFPA eastern and southern Africa reported that the age of first intercourse was 14 years in Angola: https://esaro.unfpa.org/en/news/day-life-sexual-and-reproductive-health-activist-angola-how-young-people-are-leading-change

5  Anecdotal evidence reported that young people 15-24 years are responsible for the majority of unsafe abortions and baby dumping. For example, the number of Dilation and curation (D &C) performed on this group.

6  Lack of secondary schools country wide, as well as distances, have contributed to many young people moving closer to the schools, in boarding schools, and sometimes renting nearby shebeens/alcohol selling bars/outlets.

7  Community social norms are rules and standards that guide or constrain social behaviours and often relate to a perceived social pressure to engage or not engage in a specific behaviour (Ajzen, 1991).

8  A study in northern Namibia found that health providers in Ohangwena region refused to give contraceptives to young people with no child due to a widespread myth of infertility (MoHSS, 2019).

9  The UN Convention on the Rights of Children; ICPD; Maputo Plan of action; Sustainable Development Goals; Convention on the Elimination of All Forms of Discrimination Against Women (CEDAW); The Bill of Rights; The European Convention on Human Rights; The Beijing Declaration & Program of Action. The United Nations' 2030 Agenda for Sustainable Development Goals (SDGs), which are collections of interlinked goals designed to achieve a better sustainable future for all. Related to SRH are SDGs 3 & 3.7, which focus on ensuring healthy lives and promote well-being for all ages; universal access to services including family planning, information and education and the integration of reproductive health into national strategies and programmes.

10  Young people also have the right to be heard, express opinions, and be involved in decision-making (Article 12). They have the right to education which will

help them learn, develop and reach their full potential and prepare them to be understanding and tolerant towards others (Article 29).

11 https://www.equalityhumanrights.com/en/our-human-rights-work/monitoring-and-promoting-un-treaties/convention-rights-child

12 https://www.africanchildforum.org/clr/Harmonisation%20of%20Laws%20in%20Africa/other-documents-harmonisation_7_en.pdf

## References

Ajzen, I. (1991). The theory of planned behaviour. *Organizational Behavior and Human Decision Processes 50*(2), 179–211.

Bongwong, Bruno and Monju, Patrick Mbicho (2019). Peer Pressure as a Determinant for Young People's Sexual Behaviour in the University of Buea. Available at: https://doi.org/10.5281/zenodo.3255025. Accessed August 2022.

Education Management Information System (EMIS) (2019). Ministry of Education, Arts and Culture Government of the Republic of Namibia, Windhoek, https://www.moe.gov.na

Government of the Republic of Namibia (GRN) (2000). Government Gazette No. 7 of 2000: Combating of immoral Practices Amendment Act, 2000 No. 2325. Available at: www.lac.org.na/laws/2000/2325.pdf downloaded May 2019.

Le Roux, I.M., Tomlinson, J.M., Harwood, M.J., et al. (2013). Outcomes of home visits for pregnant mothers and their infants: A cluster Randomized Controlled Trial. *AIDS* (London, England) *27*(9), 1461–71.

Maravilla, J.C., Betts, K.S., Couto, E., Cruz, C. and Alati, R. (2017). Factors influencing repeated teenage pregnancy: A review and meta-analysis. *American Journal of Obstetrics and Gynecology*. doi: 10.1016/j.ajog.2017.04.021. https://pubmed.ncbi.nlm.nih.gov/28433733/ Retrieved May 2022.

Ministry of Education, Arts and Culture & UNICEF (2015). School Drop-Out and Out-Of-School Children in Namibia: A National Review. Available at: www.unicef.org/namibia/na.OutofSchoolReport_Final_WEB.pdf Retrieved January 2022.

Ministry of Health and Social Services (MoHSS) (2019). Geographic And Programmatic Scoping/Mapping For Adolescents Girls And Young Women In Rural Namibia (Kavango East, Kavango West, Ohangwena And Zambezi). Windhoek, Namibia: MoHSS.

Ministry of Health and Social Services (MoHSS) (2021). Programme Data, DHIS 2 database 2018–2020. Windhoek, Namibia: MoHSS.

Ministry of Higher Education, Technology and Innovation, Namibia, and United Nations Educational, Scientific and Cultural Organization (UNESCO) ( 2021). Situation analysis on the status of SRH of students in Higher Education and Tertiary institutions in Namibia. Windhoek, Namibia.

The Namibia Ministry of Health and Social Services (MoHSS) and ICF International (2014). *Namibia Demographic and Health Survey 2013*. Windhoek, Namibia, and Rockville, Maryland, USA: MoHSS and ICF International.

Statista (2020). Adolescent fertility rate worldwide as of 2020, by region *(per 1,000 girls)*. Available at: www.statista.com/statistics/1228319/adolescent-fertility-rate-worldwide/ Accessed 18 June 2022.

Stoner, M.C.D., Rucinski, K.B., Edwards, J.K., et al. (2019). The relationship between school dropout and pregnancy among adolescent girls and young women in South Africa: A HPTN 068 Analysis. *Health Education & Behaviour 46*(4), 559–68. doi: 10.1177/1090198119831755. Epub 2019, Feb. 28. PMID: 30819011; PMCID: PMC6625926.

Wood, L. and Hendricks, F. (2017). A participatory action research approach to developing youth-friendly strategies for the prevention of teenage pregnancy. *Educational Action Research 25*, 103–18

United Nations, Department of Economic and Social Affairs (UNESCO), Population Division (2019). *World Population Prospects 2019*: Data Booklet. ST/ESA/SER.A/424.

UNFPA (2014). and International Conference on Population and Development (ICPD), Program of Action, UN Doc.A/CONF.171/13 1994, chap. 7.

UNFPA eastern and southern Africa https://esaro.unfpa.org/en/news/day-life-sexual-and-reproductive-health-activist-angola-how-young-people-are-leading-change. Accessed September 2022.

WHO Adolescent pregnancy (2022). Available at: www.who.int/news-room/fact-sheets/detail/adolescent-pregnancy. Accessed August 2022.

Wood, K. and Jewkes, R. (2006). Blood blockages and scolding nurses: Barriers to adolescent contraceptive use in South Africa. *Reproductive Health Matters 14*, 27, 109–18. doi: 10.1016/S0968-8080(06)27231-8

# 15

# Young to Middle Adult Health

## Antoinette Barton-Gooden and Jasneth Mullings

## Introduction

This chapter focuses on health promotion for the young and middle-aged adult. It highlights the demographic profile and risk behaviours contributing to ill-health and related psychological theories of the characteristics of the young to middle adulthood period. The chapter discusses the age parameters and the lack of consensus on the age definition for young adults and middle adulthood. Globally, vast resources are being utilised in health-promotion programmes; however, implementation challenges result in less than desired outcomes in some instances. This chapter will demonstrate how public policies and evidence-based strategies are utilised in multi-sectoral health-promotion interventions to address this group in settings such as communities, universities and workplaces. The discussion will also include the strengths and weaknesses of these programmes and the application to health and allied professions. This will assist students, healthcare workers, industry leaders and policy makers in the decision-making process to promote efficiency and effectiveness in targeted health promotion programmes.

By the end of this chapter the reader will be able to:

1. Describe three (3) psychosocial developmental theories, age parameters and risk behaviours specific to young and middle adulthood.
2. Describe the global demographic profile and health risks for young to middle adults.

3. Identify the key health-promotion strategies used in targeting young and middle-aged adults in diverse settings.
4. Demonstrate how targeted health-promotion policies, strategies and programmes have impacted the health and well-being of these groups.

### Key terms

Youth, young adults, middle-age, middle-aged adults, inter-disciplinary teams, evidence-based strategies

## Young-middle Adulthood Parameters and Related Psychosocial Developmental Theories

Health-promotion practitioners have long recognised the importance of development theories in guiding health care programmes. Erik Erikson is a mainstay in biomedical sciences, however more recently, psychologists Jeffrey Arnett and Daniel Levinson have also been recognised. Arnett (2000) highlighted the concept of the emerging adult which occurs between ages 18–25 years. Like adolescence, health risk behaviour at this stage may contribute to unintentional injuries sometimes with serious or fatal consequences (WHO, 2011). Erikson described the period of adulthood as being mainly focused on building relationships and goal attainment (Erikson, 1950, 1963). Risk behaviours may include multiple intimate relationships, occupational exposure and lifestyle behaviours that contribute to chronic non-communicable diseases (CNCDs). Additionally, Daniel Levinson's theory of adult development examined gender differences as each strives to attain culturally ascribed roles and goals (Levinson, 1986). Commonalities between these theorists includes the need for independence, loving relationships, a sense of achievement and well-being (Feldman, 2011). This illustrates the salient perspectives of the developmental theorists.

---

### Tutorial Trigger 15.1

Society shapes our views about normative behaviours and virtues during adulthood. The need for independence, relationship and achievement supports well-being during this period. Supportive networks are integral for adaptation because change is a constant as individuals mature and face life challenges.

The virtues in each stage of development are often integrated in health-promotion programmes. As younger adults are driven by different values, which is partly due to brain development (Sowell et al., 2001), it is also important to recognise the contribution of gender differentials. Research seems to support the fact that men have poorer health-seeking behaviour than women (Galdas, Cheater and Marshall, 2005; Good, Dell and Mintz, 1989). Despite women having greater health-seeking tendencies (Thompson et al., 2016; Tong, Raynor and Aslani, 2014), oftentimes they report poorer health related quality of life (HRQoL) and are more prone to depressive symptoms. It is theorised that brain size, cortical and limbic changes between the genders might account for differences in behaviour and health status (Giedd et al., 1997; Lenroot et al., 2007; Raznahan et al., 2014; Simmonds et al., 2013).

───── Time to Reflect 15.1 ─────────────────────────────────────

Drawing on your experience reflect on potential gendered difference in health-seeking behaviours and coping strategies. Identify contrasts in behaviour according to socio-demographic characteristics such as country of origin, rural-urban populations, race and/or ethnicity.

There is no clear consensus about the age group that constitutes young adults. The United Nations [UN] (1981) defined youth as the period from ages 15–24 years (UN, 1995), yet other literature defines young adulthood as the period between 18 and 25 years (Society for Adolescent Health and Medicine, 2017) and middle adulthood from 40–65 years (Feldman, 2011). Adulthood can be filled with great expectation as the young adult transitions into college, university, skills training institution or the workforce. However, it can be a tumultuous period characterised by lifestyle behaviours that can have lasting health impact into middle adulthood and beyond.

## Tutorial Trigger 15.2

Differences in the definitions of 'youth' and 'young adult' are evident in the literature. What definition do you find acceptable? Can you justify your choice/response? How might the variation in the definition of 'youth' and 'young adult' impact on the delivery of care or health-promotion interventions?

## Global Demographic Profile for Young to Middle Adults and Health Risk Behaviours

The overlap with adolescent and young adult years (ages 12–26 years) is a critical period for health promotion because behaviours established during these years are then integral to health, well-being, and productivity in later life. The World Health Organization (2011) has highlighted the main risk factors for young adults are unintentional injuries and violence, mental and neurological conditions, sexual and reproductive health problems including human immunodeficiency virus (HIV), nutrition, alcohol, and illicit drug use (UNDESA, 2012; WHO, 2011). The world population reached 8 billion persons in November 2022 (UNDESA, 2022: 3). Population estimates for 2020 and each decade up to 2050 indicate that the 15–59 year age group will constitute some 62 per cent, 60 per cent, 59 per cent in each subsequent decade and will, by 2050, represent 58 per cent of the world's population (UN, 2019). This volume of people has the potential to enhance national development. However, this could be thwarted if the population is unhealthy as many unhealthy youthful lifestyle behaviours may become entrenched and thus will subsequently burden healthcare systems as those people age.

## Key Health Promotion Interventions Impacting the Health and Well-being of Young and Middle-aged Adults in Diverse Settings

Most chronic non-communicable diseases (CNCDs) in adulthood are associated with modifiable lifestyle behaviours such as poor diet, tobacco usage and inadequate physical activity (WHO, 2005), with many of these risks being enhanced by multiple social determinants of health (SDoH). Health inequity and the SDoH contribute to health disparities that may result in lower life expectancy in selected groups. Although some SDoH may be modified by public policies, it is argued that pre-conception factors and socio-economic position also influence the development of CNCDs according to evidence from cohort studies (Barker, 2004; Power, Kuh and Morton, 2013). It is for that reason that primordial public health interventions such as folic acid supplementation to address developmental illnesses and congenital heart disease, are so impactful (Czeizel et al., 2013). Adults have a personal responsibility for maintaining individual health, however it is also a government mandate to maintain a healthy population. Therefore, multiple programmes and strategies are a necessity across the lifespan as health equity is paramount for national development and meeting the Sustainable Development Goals

2030. Using the social-ecological model for young and middle adult intervention programmes is strategic, because humans are social beings who function in diverse settings such as homes, schools, communities and workplaces (Stokols, 2000; Wold and Mittelmark, 2018).

───── Time to Reflect 15.2 ─────────────────────────────────────────

Currently, approximately 62 per cent of the global population are aged 15–59 years. This makes the young and middle-aged adults the largest cohort of the world's population, and it is projected that this momentum will continue. Globally, CNCDs are the leading cause of illness and death in adulthood. Health promotion programmes often focus on lifestyle prevention strategies and the SDoH. Identify two SDoH or lifestyle behaviours that are possible drivers for any CNCD. *How might that CNCD be addressed using the social-ecological approach?*

Health systems are designed and delivered by nursing and allied health professions, utilising inter-professional teams to address needs across the lifespan. Strategies to target young and middle-aged adults include several integrative approaches some of which will be highlighted in these targeted programmes:

- peers and youth engagement and advocacy
- technology integration such as digital health
- evidence-based methods such as motivational interviewing
- policy framework; multi-disciplinary teams; community-based and culturally appropriate settings.

Peer relationships and social support are integral for psychological development in young adults. Therefore, using peer engagement in health promotion activities can yield positive change, by promoting inclusivity and embracing diversity. Healthcare workers can liaise with student-led organisations (i.e., college/university level) to share information from reputable sources to keep the communities aware of health information and threats. Pinto-Foltz, Logsdon and Myers (2011) demonstrated the feasibility, acceptance, and improved knowledge in addressing mental health stigma in adolescents using the *In Our Voice* community-based intervention among young people. Although this study did not see a reduction in stigma over the intervention period, as was seen in college-aged students (Pittman, Noh and Coleman, 2010), the intervention was deemed feasible. It was possible that the length of the intervention, sample size and age of participants might have been major factors affecting that outcome. In the United States of America, California integrated a social marketing approach aimed at reducing mental health stigma mandated by the Mental Health Service Act (Clarke et al., 2013), with positive outcomes.

Given the ubiquitous use of technology, young adults live technology-driven lives and are often early adopters of technology, spending a tremendous amount of time on their devices either for learning or social interaction. They are not averse to its use for providing health information (Kee Low and Manias, 2019) and it is for this reason that health-promotion interventions have utilised this medium. Digital health is a key consideration in improving access to health care and this has proven to be advantageous for the integration of health-promotion programming. Using multiple digital technologies and platforms (e.g., social media, mobile health, wearable and digital devices, and games for health), healthcare delivery and community health education services can be extended to the population at large, including, young and middle-aged adults. Unfortunately, some marginalised populations have limited access and are not benefiting from such promotion activities.

---

## Point to Ponder 15.1

Health-promotion programmes which recognise generational differences and integrate specific strategies are more likely to be effective. In particular, programmes for young adults that are inclusive, embrace diversity, and which utilise a multiplicity of strategies including technology, have yielded positive outcomes in some conditions. However, planning health-promotion programmes that will reach under-served or marginalised groups can be challenging if they are transient or undocumented. *What suggestions do you have to reach such groups?*

---

Dunn-Navarra et al.'s (2017) integrative review demonstrated the feasibility of using SMS text messaging and computer-based support in antiretroviral therapy (ART) adherence in adolescents and young adults (AYAs) with human-immunodeficiency virus (HIV). The integration of tele-health/tele-medicine and virtual educational workshops has taken on greater significance for service delivery, especially since the advent of the Covid-19 pandemic. The American College Health Association [ACHA] conducted a survey on the effects of the Covid-19 pandemic on campus health services (ACHA, 2020) and reported that 71 per cent of institutions were using Telemedicine with limited face-to-face visits.

Newer evidence-based approaches for behaviour change have been integrated in clinical practice. In a systematic review and meta-analysis on integrating motivational interviewing (MI) in lifestyle disease management, it was shown to be highly effective across many conditions including CNCDs, substance abuse and medication adherence (Rubak, Sandbæk and Christensen, 2005). Motivational interviewing is grounded in the transtheoretical model (TTM) of behaviour change.

Recognition that behaviour change is often non-linear, relapses and termination are possible before reaching the final stage of TTM. Therefore, modifications to the model have been proposed to support the provider-patient interactions (Goldstein, DePue, Kazura et al., 1998). The healthcare provider who uses MI demonstrates empathy, while evoking the individual's intrinsic values to promote and sustain behaviour change (Miller and Rollnick, 2002). Heckman, Egleston and Hofmann's (2010) systematic and meta-analysis of MI efficacy in smoking cessation across the lifespan demonstrated the efficacy when used by nurses and other healthcare members. They reported that MI had a significant effect on adolescents, young adults and pregnant smokers. This strategy is one which can be integrated into nursing, medical and allied professional curricula (Jacobs, Calvo, Dierenger et al., 2021; Schoo et al., 2015), and seamlessly utilised in healthcare delivery in the chronic disease care model (Tuccero et al., 2016). Unfortunately, nursing and allied health professional curricula integration is limited in developed countries such as the United States of America and Canada (Sarna et al., 2009; Schultz et al., 2015). It is possible that a similar trend exists elsewhere.

---

## Point to Ponder 15.2

The use of motivational interviewing (MI) supports provider-patient interactions, if it is evidence-based and is highly effective for behaviour change in CNCDs, substance abuse, smoking cessation, and mediation adherence. Unfortunately, integration in nursing and allied health professionals' curricula globally is lagging. The diffusion of evidence-based information can be slow and may lead to a lag in practice integration. A point to ponder is *'Do healthcare workers have the skill set to evaluate these interventions?'* Having policy support and curricula integration are strategies that can enhance the implementation of efficacious interventions in healthcare settings.

---

Policy enforcement is more likely to sustain widespread change when the ecological approach is utilised. One example is the World Health Organization (WHO) Framework Convention on Tobacco Control (FCTC) which has led to a significant reduction in tobacco smoking globally. The evolution of electronic nicotine device systems (ENDS) has emerged, and its appeal is spreading across the lifespan. McDonald (2000) identified that persons with severe mental illness (SMI) are more likely to smoke. In a systematic review, it was shown that persons with SMI benefited from randomised control trials (RCTs) using Bupropion and Varenicline (Peckham et al., 2017). In England, a nurse-led smoking-free hospital initiative has been impactful for patients, staff and visitors at the South London and Maudsley NHS Foundation Mental Health Trust (SLaM). Using a multidisciplinary model, persons with SMI were identified via electronic health records (EHR), given brief smoking cessation referral services and nicotine replacement therapy. Additionally, a smoke-free environment was integrated at the agency (NHS, 2018). Policy support in the form of a smoke-free environment provided cues for staff, patients and visitors to quit smoking. Anecdotal reports are that the returns on investment (ROI) have been positive as there has been a reduction in the need for psychotropic drugs, inhalers, antibiotics, and tranquillisation medications. Monitoring and evaluation are ongoing as data are being collected (NHS, 2018).

### Research in Brief 15.1

Nurse-led interventions are impactful in chronic disease management. McDonald (2000) identified that persons with severe mental illness (SMI) are more likely to smoke. Oftentimes, persons with SMI are marginalised and may not benefit from smoking cessation interventions if they are homeless or lack social support. One success story was a nurse-led smoking-free hospital initiative in England for patients, staff and visitors at the South London and Maudsley NHS Foundation Mental Health Trust (SLaM). Nurse-led interventions are increasing in chronic illnesses in various regions and healthcare settings (Massimi, De Vito, Brufola et al., 2017).

*Source*: Massimi, A. et al. (2017). Are community-based nurse-led self-management support interventions effective in chronic patients? Results of a systematic review and meta-analysis. *PLoS One*, *12* (3).

## Health Promotion Interventions in Middle Adulthood – Some Examples

Hypertension is a leading cause of morbidity and mortality in middle adulthood as many people go undiagnosed. In the United Kingdom (UK), the National Health Service (NHS) community pharmacy blood pressure check service, integrates pharmacists to do blood pressure checks, health education, and referral to general physicians. This programme targeted middle-aged adults who utilised the community pharmacy, and was guided by the National Institute for Health and Care Excellence (NICE) evidence-based guidelines. According to the NHS website, this multidisciplinary approach supports the NHS mandates by strengthening the synergy amongst the Department of Health and Social Care (DHSC), NHS England and NHS Improvement, and the Pharmaceutical Services Negotiating Committee (PSNC) which is based on the new Community Pharmacy Contractual Framework 2019–2024 (NHS, 2021). This programme is supported by systematic review and meta-analysis and is deemed to be feasible (Cheema, Sutcliffe and Singer, 2014; Santschi et al., 2014). Health promotion programmes are enhanced by using a multiplicity of strategies. This programme uses health communications, health education, health-related community service strategies and health policy that enforces action towards hypertension management using the multidisciplinary team approach. This requires strong government financial commitment, health systems strengthening and removal of implementation barriers.

## Research in Brief 15.2

Pharmacists play an important role in hypertension management in adults. Working in inter-disciplinary teams, sometimes they are not often highlighted as they work behind the scene in chronic disease management. The National Health Service (NHS) community pharmacy blood pressure check service integrates pharmacists to do blood pressure checks, health education, and referral to the general physicians. This programme targeted middle-aged adults who utilised the community pharmacy and was guided by the National Institute for Health and Care Excellence (NICE) evidence-based guidelines. Support for such interventions are supported by systematic reviews (Cheema, Sutcliffe and Singer, 2014; Santschi, Chiolero, Colosimo et al., 2014). They evaluated studies which utilised multiple strategies that led to significant changes in the systolic and diastolic blood pressures as the outcome variable. Interdisciplinary collaboration and evidence-based hypertension guidelines integration enhanced hypertension management in at-risk groups in diverse settings.

*Source*: Cheema, E., Sutcliffe, P. and Singer, D.R. (2014). The impact of interventions by pharmacists in community pharmacies on control of hypertension: a systematic review and meta-analysis of randomized controlled trials. *Br. J. Clin. Pharmacol.* 78(6), 1238–47.

Santschi, V. et al. (2014). Improving blood pressure control through pharmacist interventions: a meta-analysis of randomized controlled trials. *J. Am. Heart Assoc.* Apr 10, 3(2), e000718.

While there is no universal blueprint for worker wellness programmes, various models have been utilised. The generally accepted potential benefits of workplace wellness programmes include increased productivity, reduced presenteeism, lowered absenteeism and heightened morale and engagement and reduction of healthcare costs. A 2018 global survey of workforce well-being reported stress (95 per cent) as the leading factor driving employee well-being. Other top issues included work-life issues (94 per cent), depression, anxiety, and weight-management (93 per cent) healthcare service access (92 per cent) (Buck Consultants, 2012). Jirathananuwat and Pongpirul's (2018) systematic meta-review of physical activity (PA) highlighted the requirements for successful workplace programmes. They identified five domains that enhance implementation using the PRECEDE-PROCEED model. The strategies identified across diverse workplaces were categorised in domains:

predisposing, enabling, reinforcing, policy regulatory and environmental development strategies. Predisposing strategies were targeted knowledge, attitude and skills towards PA. Enabling strategies were aimed at increasing access to PA in individuals and communities, and increasing motivation (Jirathananuwat and Pongpirul, 2018). Reinforcing strategies were aimed at social support, changing social norms, and using incentives to promote PA. A policy regulatory framework supported PA as they were integrated as protocols and environmental development included modifications in the workspace that promoted PA among employees (Jirathananuwat and Pongpirul, 2018). They summarised that all programmes used multiple strategies, but those that integrated multidisciplinary strategies were the most impactful in increasing PA in these workplaces.

Another example of a workplace intervention programme was the *iThrive* workplace wellness programme at the University of Illinois at Urbana-Champaign. The intervention included educational sessions (in-person) on chronic disease and weight management, physical fitness classes, hotline for tobacco cessation and online, self-paced wellness programme (Jones, Molitor and Reif, 2019). Jones, Molitor and Reif's (2019) randomised control trial study of the intervention concluded that while some changes in health beliefs, disease management, and self-reported outcomes were reported, the programme produced no changes in key outcomes such as clinical health measures, healthcare expenditure, healthcare utilisation and employment outcomes such as absenteeism and productivity. Similarly, another large-scale randomised trial of a workplace wellness programme of 26,000 employees of the BJ's Wholesale Club in the USA further suggested that the return on investment (ROI) for wellness programmes might not be as significant as expected or demonstrated in previous studies (Song and Baicker, 2019). Mixed reviews of workplace interventions are not always poor. Sandercock and Andrade (2018) reported some benefits with reductions in body mass index, waist circumference and body fat composition. They concluded that incorporating a motivational theory and having individualised plans are beneficial over the long term as building self-efficacy is necessary for long-term behaviour change.

## Summary

Health-promotion programming which targets lifestyle behaviours in colleges, universities and workplaces in young and middle adulthood are deemed to be beneficial. However, the inconsistent findings and outcomes reported in systematic reviews and meta-analyses raise questions about their effectiveness and long-term impact. Those that report positive results are often supported by policies and multidisciplinary teams, use a multiplicity of strategies such as technology or mass communication, engagement and advocacy, and have sustained funding. In other cases, challenges included inadequate motivation among participants, low returns on investment (ROI), and inadequate monitoring and evaluation processes. It was recommended that these programmes benefit by including the policy framework, motivation theory, planned formative and summative evaluation processes during implementation to enhance effectiveness and ROI. Additionally, to improve the relevance and applicability of interventions, they should be tailored to the specific setting in which they are being implemented. Also, continuous assessment and evaluation of outcomes are necessary for the refinement of health promotion programmes (McKenzie, Neiger and Thackeray, 2009).

Nurses have opportunities to integrate evidence-based practice, policies and public health theories during care delivery. Their role as care coordinator creates a bridge for the sharing of health-promotion information across the lifespan. Hence, this discussion is relevant to the development of nursing in the areas of (a) training and curriculum development; (b) clinical practice and service delivery; and (c) nursing research and evidence-based practice. The active engagement of nurses in health promotion, while utilising the technological advances in digital health, holds significant potential for improving patient and community health outcomes.

—— **Key Points** ————————————————————————

- Nurses as care coordinators have an opportunity to integrate evidence-based practice, policies and public health theories into nursing care delivery.
- Actively engaging nurses through technological advances in digital health care holds significant potential for increasing access to young and middle-aged adults in diverse settings.
- The policy framework and multidisciplinary teams are critical support systems for health interventions such as physical activity and smoking cessation programmes in the workplace. These have been reported to positively contribute to positive behaviour change in adults.

# References

American College Health Association Covid-19 Task Force Survey Sub-Committee. The Covid-19 Pandemic's Effect on Campus Health Services – A Snapshot of Operating Status and Response. April 6–9, 2020. Available at: www.acha.org/documents/Resources/COVID_19/COVID-19_Effect_On_Campus_Health_Services_April6-9_Survey_Report.pdf

Arnett, J.J. (2000). Emerging adulthood: A theory of development from late teens to early twenties. *American Psychologist 55*(5), 469–80.

Barić, L. (1993). The settings approach – implications for policy and strategy. *Journal of the Institute of Health Education 31*, 17–24.

Barker, D.J. (2004). The developmental origins of chronic adult disease. *Acta Paediatrica Supplement 93*, 26–33.

Buck Consultants (2012). Fifth Edition Global Survey of Health Promotion and Workplace Wellness Strategies. Available at: www.bucksurveys.com/bucksurveys/product/tabid/139/p-115-working-well-a-global-survey-of-healthpromotion-and-workplace-wellnessstrategies-2012.aspx. Accessed March 2013.

Cheema, E., Sutcliffe, P. and Singer, D.R. (2014). The impact of interventions by pharmacists in community pharmacies on control of hypertension: A systematic review and meta-analysis of randomized controlled trials. *British Journal of Clinical Pharmacology,* Dec. *78*(6), 1238–47. doi: 10.1111/bcp.12452. PMID: 24966032; PMCID: PMC4256613.

Clarke, W., Welch, S.N., Berry, S.H. et al. (2013). California's historic effort to reduce the stigma of mental illness: The Mental Health Services Act. *American Journal of Public Health 103*, 786–94. doi:10.2105/ AJPH.2013.301225.

Czeizel, A.E., Dudás, I., Vereczkey, A. and Bánhidy, F. (2013). Folate deficiency and folic acid supplementation: The prevention of neural-tube defects and congenital heart defects. *Nutrients.* Nov. *215*(11), 4760–75. doi: 10.3390/nu5114760. PMID: 24284617; PMCID: PMC3847759.

Dooris, M., Poland, B., Kolbe, L.J., De Leeuw, E., McCaw, D. and Wharfe Higgins, J. (2007). Healthy settings building evidence for the effectiveness of whole system health promotion – Challenges and future directions. In D.V. McQueen and C.M. Jones (Eds), *Global Perspectives on Health Promotion Effectiveness* (pp. 327–52). New York: Springer. Available at: http://eknygos.lsmuni.lt/springer/672/327-352.pdf

Dunn-Navarra, A-M., Viorst Gwadz, M., Whittemore, R., et al. (2017). Health technology-enabled interventions for adherence support and retention in care among US HIV-infected adolescents and young adults: An integrative review. *AIDS Behavior* Nov. *1*(11), 3154–71. doi:10.1007/s10461-017-1867-6.

Erikson, E. (1950/1963). *Childhood and Society.* 2nd Ed. New York: W. W. Norton.

Feldman, R.S. (2011). *Development across the Life Span.* 6th Ed. New Jersey: Pearson Education.

Galdas, P.M., Cheater, F. and Marshall, P. (2005). Men and health help-seeking behaviour: Literature review. *Journal of Advanced Nursing.* March *49*(6), 616–23. doi: 10.1111/j.1365-2648.2004.03331.x.

Giedd, J.N., Castellanos, F.X., Rajapakse, J.C., Vaituzis, A.C. and Rapoport, J.L. (1997). Sexual dimorphism of the developing human brain. *Progress in Neuro-Psychopharmacology and Biological Psychiatry 21*(8), 1185–201.

Goldstein, M.G., DePue, J., Kazura, A. and Niaura, R. (1998). Models for provider–patient interaction: Applications to health behavior change. In S.A. Shumaker, E.B. Schron, J.K. Ockene and W.L. McBee (Eds), *The Handbook of Health Behavior Change* (pp. 85–113). Springer Publishing Company.

Good, G.E., Dell, D.M. and Mintz, L.B. (1989). Male role and gender role conflict: Relations to help seeking in men. *Journal of Counseling and Development 36*(3) 295–300.

Heckman, C.J., Egleston, B.L. and Hofmann, M.T. (2010). Efficacy of motivational interviewing for smoking cessation: A systematic review and meta-analysis. *Tobacco Control* Oct. *19*(5), 410–16. doi: 10.1136/tc.2009.033175. Epub 2010 Jul 30. PMID: 20675688; PMCID: PMC2947553.

Irwin, C.E. Jr. (2020). Using technology to improve the health and well-being of adolescents and young adults. *Journal of Adolescent Health* . *67*(2), 147–8. doi: 10.1016/j.jadohealth.2020.05.019. PMID: 32739018; PMCID: PMC7388009.

Jacobs, N.N., Calvo, L., Dieringer, A., Hall, A. and Danko. R. (2021). Motivational interviewing training: A case-based curriculum for preclinical medical students. *MedEdPORTAL* Feb. *12*(17),11104. doi: 10.15766/mep_2374-8265.11104. PMID: 33598544; PMCID: PMC7880250.

Jirathananuwat, A. and Pongpirul, K. (2017). Promoting physical activity in the workplace: A systematic meta-review. *Journal of Occupational Health* Sep. 28, *59*(5), 385–93. doi: 10.1539/joh.16-0245-RA. Epub 2017 Jul 21. PMID: 28740029; PMCID: PMC5635147.

Jones, D., Molitor, D. and Reif, J. (2019). What do workplace wellness programs do? Evidence from the Illinois Workplace Wellness Study. *Quarterly Journal of Economics* (forthcoming).

Kee Low, J. and Manias, E. (2019). Use of technology-based tools to support adolescents and young adults with chronic bisease: Systematic review and meta-analysis. *JMIR Mhealth Uhealth* Jul. *18*(7), e12042.

Lenroot, R.K., Gogtay, N., Greenstein, D.K., et al. (2007). Sexual dimorphism of brain developmental trajectories during childhood and adolescence. *NeuroImage 36*(4), 1065–73.

Levinson, D.J. (1986). A conception of adult development. *American Psychologist 41*(1), 3–13.

Massimi, A., De Vito, C., Brufola, I., et al. (2017). Are community-based nurse-led self-management support interventions effective in chronic patients? Results of a systematic review and meta-analysis. *PLoS One* Mar. *10*(12), 3, e0173617. doi: 10.1371/journal.pone.0173617. PMID: 28282465; PMCID: PMC5345844.

McDonald, C. (2000). Cigarette smoking in patients with schizophrenia. *British Journal of Psychiatry* 176, 596–7.

McKenzie, J.F., Neiger, B.L. and Thackeray, R. (2009). *Planning, Implementing and Evaluating Health Promotion Programs: A primer.* 5th Ed. Benjamin Cummings.San Francisco, CA: Pearson.

Miller, W.R. and Rollnick, S. (2002). *Motivational Interviewing: Preparing people for change.* New York: Guilford Press.

National Health Service (2018). A case study: Introducing a comprehensive Tobacco Dependence Treatment policy in South London and Maudsley NHS Foundation Trust. Retrieved on 20 April 2022 from www.england.nhs.uk/atlas_case_study/introducing-a-comprehensive-tobacco-dependence-treatment-policy-in-south-london-maudsley-nhs-foundation-trust/

National Health Service (2021). Community pharmacy contractual framework. Retrieved on 20 April 2022 from www.england.nhs.uk/primary-care/pharmacy/community-pharmacy-contractual-framework/

Peckham, E., Brabyn, S., Cook, L., Tew, G. and Gilbody, S. (2017). Smoking cessation in severe mental ill health: what works? An updated systematic review and meta-analysis. *BMC Psychiatry* Jul. *14*, 17(1), 252. doi: 10.1186/s12888-017-1419-7. PMID: 28705244; PMCID: PMC5513129.

Pinto-Foltz, M.D., Logsdon, M.C. and Myers, J.A. Feasibility, acceptability, and initial efficacy of a knowledge-contact program to reduce mental illness stigma and improve mental health literacy in adolescents. *Social Science & Medicine 72*(12), 2011-9. doi: 10.1016/j.socscimed.2011.04.006.

Pittman, J.O.E., Noh, S. and Coleman, D. (2010). Evaluating the effectiveness of a consumer delivered anti-stigma program: Replication with graduate-level helping professionals. *Psychiatric Rehabilitation Journal 33*(3), 236–8. doi: 10.2975/33.3.2010.236.238.

Power, C., Kuh, D. and Morton, S. (2013). From developmental origins of adult disease to life course research on adult disease and aging: Insights from birth cohort studies. *Annual Review of Public Health 34*, 7–28.

Raznahan, A., Shaw, P.W., Lerch, J.P., et al. (2014). Longitudinal four-dimensional mapping of subcortical anatomy in human development. *Proceedings of the National Academy of Sciences of the United States of America 111*(4), 1592–7.

Rubak, S., Sandbæk, A. and Christensen, B. (2005). Motivational interviewing: A systematic review and meta-analysis. *British Journal of General Practice 55*(513), 305–12.

Sandercock, V. and Andrade, J. (2018). Evaluation of worksite wellness nutrition and physical activity programs and their subsequent impact on participants' body composition. *Journal of Obesity* 3 Dec. 2018:1035871. doi: 10.1155/2018/1035871. PMID: 30631593; PMCID: PMC6304910.

Santschi, V., Chiolero, A., Colosimo, A.L., et al. (2014). Improving blood pressure control through pharmacist interventions: a meta-analysis of randomized controlled trials. *Journal of American Heart Association* Apr. *10* 3(2), e000718. doi: 10.1161/JAHA.113.000718. PMID: 24721801; PMCID: PMC4187511.

Sarna, L., Bialous, S.A., Rice, V.H. and Wewers, M.E. (2009). Promoting tobacco dependence treatment in nursing education. *Drug and Alcohol Review* Sep. *28*(5), 507–16. doi: 10.1111/j.1465-3362.2009.00107.x. PMID: 19737209.

Schoo, A.M., Lawn, S., Rudnik, E. and Litt, J.C. (2015). Teaching health science students foundation motivational interviewing skills: Use of motivational interviewing treatment integrity and self-reflection to approach transformative learning. *BMC Medical Education*. Dec. *21*(15), 228. doi: 10.1186/s12909-015-0512-1. PMID: 26689193; PMCID: PMC4687369.

Schultz, A.S.., Dunford, D., Atout, R. and Grymonpre, R. (2015). Situating tobacco dependency education in health professional prelicensure curricula: An interprofessional learning opportunity. *Canadian Journal of Respiratory Therapy* Fall, *51*(4), 86–8. PMID: 26566378; PMCID: PMC4631134.

Simmonds, D., Hallquist, M.N., Asato, M. and Luna, B. (2013). Developmental stages and sex differences of white matter and behavioral development through adolescence: A longitudinal diffusion tensor imaging (DTI) study. *NeuroImage 92*, 356–68.

Song, Z. and Baicker, K. (2019). Effect of a workplace wellness program on employee health and economic outcomes: A randomized clinical trial. *JAMA 321*(15), 1491–501. doi: 10.1001/jama.2019.3307. Erratum in: *JAMA*. Apr 17; PMID: 30990549; PMCID: PMC6484807.

Stokols, D. (2000). The social ecological paradigm of wellness promotion. In M.S. Jamner and D. Stokols (Eds), *Promoting Human Wellness* (pp. 21–37). Berkeley: University of California Press.

The Society of Adolescent Health and Medicine (2017). Young adult health and well-being: A position statement of the Society for Adolescent Health and Medicine. *Journal of Adolescent Health 60*, 758–9.

Sowell, E.R., Thompson, P.M., Mattson, S.N., Tessner, K.D., Jernigan, T.L., Riley, E.P., Toga, A.W. (2001). Voxel-based morphometric analyses of the brain in children and adolescents prenatally exposed to alcohol. *Neuroreport 12*(3), 515–23. doi: 10.1097/00001756-200103050-00018.

Thompson, A.E., Aniscimowicz, Y., Miedema, B., Hogg, W.P. and Aubrey-Bassler, K. (2016). The influence of gender and other patient characteristics on health care-seeking behaviour: a QUALICOPC study. *BMC Family Practice 17*(38). doi 10.1186/s12875-016-0440-0.

Tong, V., Raynor, D.K. and Aslani, P. (2014). Gender differences in health and medicine information seeking behaviour – A review. *Journal of the Malta College of Pharmacy Practice*. Summer *20*, 14–16.

Tuccero, D., Railey, K., Briggs, M. and Hull, S.K. (2016). Behavioral health in prevention and chronic illness management: Motivational interviewing. *Primary Care* Jun, *43*(2), 191–202. doi: 10.1016/j.pop.2016.01.006. PMID: 27262001.

United Nations (1995). World programme of action for youth. General Assembly Resolution, A/RES/50/81, 1995. Retrieved on 13 May 2021 from www.un.org/esa/socdev/unyin/documents/wpay_text_final.pdf

United Nations Department of Economic and Social Affairs, Population Division (2012). *World Population Monitoring Adolescents and Youths. A concise report.* https://www.un.org/development/desa/pd/content/world-population-monitoring-adolescents-and-youth-concise-report

United Nations Department of Economic and Social Affairs (2019). World Population Prospects 2019. Population Dynamics. Available at: https://population.un.org/wpp/DataQuery/

Wold, B. and Mittelmark, M.B. (2018). Health-promotion research over three decades: The social-ecological model and challenges in implementation of interventions. *Scandinavian Journal of Public Health 46* (Suppl. 20), 20–26.

World Health Organization (2011). Youth and health risks. Sixty-four World Health Assembly. A64/25. Retrieved on 13 May 2021 from https://apps.who.int/gb/ebwha/pdf_files/WHA64/A64_25-en.pdf

World Health Organization (2005). Preventing chronic diseases: A vital investment. Retrieved on 19 May 2021 from www.who.int/chp/chronic_disease_report/contents/en/

# 16

# Older Adult Health: Retirement Communities and Residential Aged Care Homes

Jed Montayre and
Tiffany Northall

## Introduction

This chapter presents examples of effective health promotion and health education relevant to older people in retirement and residential aged care settings, with a focus on health promotion and health education as part of falls prevention. Fall incidents are one of the most common preventable healthcare adverse events. They also lead to severe health outcomes, particularly in populations with chronic conditions and those who are considered frail. Over the years, several falls prevention campaigns and strategies have been implemented. These interventions range from global or national strategies to locally implemented initiatives. This chapter presents the most common approaches to falls prevention through education and health promotion targeted at a population level, as well as healthcare professionals providing care to those who are at a high risk of falling.

Progressing a strong falls prevention agenda for older people in residential aged care settings or long-term care is crucial to their quality of life and their added years aimed at healthy longevity. With increasing life expectancy and rising incidence of chronic conditions, healthcare practice and policies have emphasised preventive measures in the communities to prevent negative health outcomes, particularly from the consequences of avoidable events, such as falls. Health-promotion strategies for falls prevention encompass a range of approaches such as physical strengthening exercises, healthy eating and active lifestyles. Health education about falls targets patients and their families as well as healthcare providers to be knowledgeable about the common factors contributing to falls incidence. One relevant factor to older people living in retirement and residential aged care facilities is the association of polypharmacy and falls. These issues, as well as the strategies, will be covered in this chapter.

By the end of this chapter the reader will be able to:

1. Develop a practical understanding of the impact of falls to the health and well-being of older people in aged care settings.
2. Apply principles of health promotion towards relevant falls prevention strategies for older people.
3. Apply principles of health education among patients, families and healthcare professionals towards falls prevention for older people.
4. Analyse the impact of health promotion and health education to the outcomes of falls prevention strategies in older people living in aged care settings.

## Key terms

Falls, older people, aged care, long-term care, falls prevention strategies, risk factors

## Falls in Older People

Globally, falls are becoming an increasing problem, especially for older people. This is because as we age, we are more likely to experience illness and disability associated with age. This can include vision impairment, reduced strength and mobility, cognition problems and at least one or more chronic illness. In many countries, there is no standard definition of a fall; however, in this section, we use the World Health Organization's (WHO) definition of a fall which is as follows:

*A fall is an event which results in a person coming to rest inadvertently on the ground or floor or other lower level* (WHO, 2021).

According to the World Health Organization falls are the second leading cause of injury and death globally with an estimated 684.000 fatal falls each year (WHO, 2021). Age is a risk factor for falls as older people are more likely to experience falls, which increases the risk of serious injury or death. In Australia, people aged over 65 make up 15.9 per cent of the population (ABS, 2019). The cost of attempting to prevent falls in an Australian context is $590 million Australian dollars per year (Mitchell et al., 2018). While many older people live active lives well into their old age, others may have more than one chronic disease. The burden of disease shows the years lost due to poor health or premature death. For people aged over 65 the fatal burden of disease made up 61 per cent of the total burden of disease (AIHW, 2019). Due to the incidence of disability and disease associated with age, older people may experience a reduction in their strength which can contribute to the increased incidence of falls.

Nurses have a key role in falls prevention. Falls are more likely to occur in hospitals, possibly because people are recovering from an illness in an unfamiliar environment. Strategies that could be used in hospitals to reduce falls include alarms that trigger when the patient attempts to get out of bed; encouraging patients to use the call bell to get assistance; improved nurse-patient ratios, less crowded hospital rooms and brighter lighting (Chu, 2017). While these strategies are useful within a confined environment (i.e., hospital wards), nurses oftentimes are confronted with issues on how to effectively plan implementing falls prevention strategies when patients are discharged home (Walker et al., 2007). Moreover, the number of falls in homes and in the community is increasing, which highlights the importance of nurses' roles in education and health promotion beyond the hospital bedside.

In an Australian context, strategies to minimise falls include falls prevention guidelines; being active and healthy; staying on your feet; a stepping on program; and Falls SA (South Australia).

---

## Tutorial Trigger 16.1

Nurses take an active role in preventive strategies in their workplace, such as preventing falls occurring. Practice is informed by best-practice guidelines, which also aim to educate healthcare professionals.

What do you think should be emphasised in falls prevention practice guidelines? Are there any specific areas that need to be highlighted in older people?

The following section of this chapter, 'Health Education on Falls Prevention', may assist your thoughts on the important aspects of falls prevention guidelines.

## Health Education on Falls Prevention

### Falls prevention guidelines

In Australia 80 per cent of older people will have a fall or fall-related injury which requires an admission to hospital (Kannus, Khan and Lord, 2006). The impact of a fall for older people can be life changing. The most common injury for older people following a fall is hip and thigh injuries. A hip fracture for an older person can lead to an increased risk of death and decreased level of function and independence as well as a higher chance of entering a residential aged care facility (Brennan-Olsen, 2019; Rapp, et al., 2019). While there are multiple contributing factors to falls, the Australian Commission of Safety and Quality Health Care (ACSQHC) (2009) produced a report that examined the impact of falls and strategies to minimise them. These strategies included balance and mobility; identifying risk factors, and discharge planning. The following are important key areas for nurses to consider when providing education to patients and staff.

### Balance and mobility

Balance and mobility are important, as balance problems and cognitive impairment are often precursors to falls for older people (Pieruccini-Faria et al., 2019). There are a range of assessments for balance and mobility, most of which can be used in a variety of settings. Balance is a key part of falls prevention, yet as people age, they are more likely to have weakened muscles which can make standing, getting up from a chair or climbing stairs difficult (ACSQHC, 2009). This is particularly relevant for older people who are discharged from hospital as they are more likely to have a fall at home as their mobility and balance may have deteriorated during the hospital admission.

### Identifying risk factors

There are several risk factors that contribute to falls such as: cognition problems; continence; feet and footwear; medications and vision impairment (ACSQHC, 2009). Older people are more likely to have a cognitive impairment than younger people. Whether the cognitive impairment is related to dementia or delirium, an older person with either condition has an increased risk of falling. This is because older people with a cognitive impairment are more likely to have difficulty maintaining balance, possibly because they are not always able to interpret the environment they are in and recognise hazards (Casey et al., 2020). Validated falls risk screens for people with dementia are minimal yet older people with cognition problems may benefit from exercise to restrengthen and improve balance (Casey et al., 2020). Polypharmacy is also one factor that led to people experiencing falls. Although evidence has indicated that polypharmacy is an independent factor contributing to falls incidence in older people, there has been some significant association between falls and the type of medications, which results in increased risk (Hammond and Wilson, 2013). Attention to specific Fall Risk Increasing Drugs (FRIDs) is important, particularly when older people are taking medication such as anti-depressants (Ie, Chou, Boyce and Albert, 2021).

## Point to Ponder 16.1

The risk factors contributing to falls are considered 'multi-factorial'. For older people, there are some complexities or factors that might not be present in younger populations. For example, the occurrence of chronic conditions in advanced age will lead older people to be taking multiple medications for these conditions, and will also affect their physical functioning, stability and gait. It is important that a comprehensive geriatric assessment among older people is undertaken, which looks into the factors that contribute to a high falls risk. For instance, paying attention to 'polypharmacy' and how we can better educate clinicians, patients and their families to address this issue and outline strategies to prevent polypharmacy causing falls.

## Discharge planning

When a person is discharged from hospital there is usually some form of discharge planning. Older people who have been admitted due to a fall, or who have had a fall in hospital, are more likely to require discharge planning. This is because older people are more likely to have risk factors related to falls such as poor eyesight, muscle weakness and multiple medications. Ideally discharge planning should be multidisciplinary and begin on admission to hospital which may include exercises for older people post-fall to build up their strength and balance (ACSQHC, 2009). Discharge plans should also consider options for older people to continue to restrengthen once at home as well as considering short-term home support and rehabilitation.

## Point to Ponder 16.2

Falls prevention extends from hospital care settings. It is important that nurses and fellow clinicians are able to educate and involve patients and their families towards falls prevention upon discharge to the community. The same way that falls are caused by different factors, prevention strategies could be multidimensional, and personal circumstances, such as living situation (living alone) is crucial when considering falls prevention strategies. While clinicians are skilled in undertaking risk assessments in healthcare settings, it would be important that monitoring for these risks continue in the community to avoid hospital re-admissions and the negative health outcomes that can result from falls.

## Falls prevention strategies

*Falls risk screening:* Risk screening for falls usually includes selecting a validated falls screening tool and should be considered for all patients in hospital. This is particularly important for those people who have already had one or more falls. The risk screen may well be completed in hospital, but it is not always clear whether interventions from the falls screen are implemented. Ideally there should be a falls care plan developed for the person's specific needs.

### Research in Brief 16.1

The aim of a study by Chidume (2021) was to implement a nurse-led intervention using a falls prevention toolkit (FPT), which included falls screening and prevention education. The use of toolkits for falls prevention has been proven to be helpful. For Chidume's study, a pre-test – post-test approach was undertaken with the implementation of the nurse-led intervention – FPT. The intervention involving falls risk assessment and falls prevention education was implemented with 30 people who were 65 years old and over, who attended mobile Interprofessional Education (IPE) clinics in community settings. The main findings from the study suggested that the longer period a person was involved with the intervention, the greater likelihood that their falls risk assessment score lowered, which meant lower falls risk. A 'Check for Safety' home safety brochure aided the identification of potential falls at home. The overall conclusion and recommendations of the study asserted that falls prevention and awareness should be assessed to decrease falls in all population groups. The mobile IPE community clinics brought a positive impact to their health, social and nutritional assessments. Nurses have an important role in the implementation of the intervention and promoting and educating older people to prevent them from falling.

*Source*: Chidume (2021). Promoting older adult fall prevention education and awareness in a community setting: A nurse-led intervention. *Applied Nursing Research* https://doi.org/10.1016/j.apnr.2020.151392

## Health Promotion Addressing Falls

### Active and healthy

The New South Wales government in Australia initiated an 'Active and Healthy' website that encourages older people to exercise in an effort to reduce falls (see www. activeandhealthy.nsw.gov.au). The website supports older people to stay active by accessing exercise and falls prevention programmes close to home. The resources provide information on 'Staying steady and preventing falls'. This involves booklets on staying active and on your feet as well as a range of exercise programmes which include Tai Chi, warm water exercise, chair yoga, healthy and active life online (Clinical Excellence Commission, 2013). The programmes are offered in person or online and are aimed at supporting older people to remain active and healthy as they age.

---

### Tutorial Trigger 16.2

There are different community-based campaigns for falls prevention; however, you will notice that these campaigns have similar elements in terms of aspects these approaches are trying to address. Can you find a specific focus or item that these campaigns for falls prevention have in common?

In the next part of this chapter, you will be able to explore different falls prevention community initiatives and their focus on promoting 'sense of independence'.

---

### Stay on your feet

A programme developed in Australia by Queensland Health aims to reduce falls by supporting people to be active, independent and on their feet. This programme offers ideas and ways that older people can remain active, healthy and independent. The comprehensive falls checklist is part of this programme and supports older people to identify any potential falls risks so they can remain at home longer (Falls Injury Prevention, 2021). This also includes a clear outline of what a person should do if they fall at home and provides images to depict how to get up following a fall. Strategies such as this enable older people to be in charge of their own health and mobility.

### Stepping On

In Australia the Stepping On programme offers a seven-week programme to support older people following a fall. The programme includes strategies to empower older people to remain independent, active and stepping on by using evidence-based strategies. The Stepping On programme covers risk assessment, exercise, hazards, safety and footwear, vision and falls, medication management, and planning ahead. Research indicates that the Stepping On programme had an impact on falls prevention for people aged over 65 and has reduced falls by 31 per cent in the community (Tiedemann et al., 2021). The programme is free and is part of a New South Wales initiative 'Active and Healthy'.

───── Time to Reflect 16.1 ──────────────────────────────────

A fall is a completely preventable incident, still it happens and is one of the most common types of healthcare-related harm experienced by patients, particularly among older people. From this chapter, knowing the different strategies for falls prevention, how do you think health-education and health-promotion measures might support such strategies to be effective and sustainable?

## Falls South Australia

In 2017 there were 21,120 people who were admitted to hospital following a fall. Those who were 65 years and over made up 65 per cent of these falls and 395 older people died in hospital following a fall (SA health, 2017). Some of these falls may have been prevented due to strategies such as: rapid review post-falls to reduce further falls, regular rounds in hospitals and staff completing falls prevention courses (SA health, 2017). In South Australia a programme was developed to support older people to do exercises at home to maintain their independence. Reducing the risk of falls involves a range of strategies which include assessing risk factors, environment, minimising injury from falls and making a plan to help if a person has a fall (themselves or others) (Department of Health and Ageing, 2011).

Falling is connected to risk, especially as people age. There are programmes that can reduce the risk of falls through balance training, exercise, monitoring the environment and promoting safer footwear. Yet, there continues to be falls in older people. Accessing falls prevention support and training may reduce the risk of falls, even though it remains a worldwide problem.

─── Research in Brief 16.2 ───────────────────────────────

A systematic review by Sherrington et al. (2020) examined the effects of exercise interventions for preventing falls in older people in the community. The review included randomised controlled trials that evaluated the effect of exercise (single intervention) on falls in older populations (60+ years). The review found that exercise reduces the rate of falls by 23 per cent in 59 studies with high-certainty evidence. Multiple types of exercise reduce the rate of falls by 34 per cent in 11 studies. The review concluded that with the positive effect of exercise on falls, exercise programmes should be implemented and recommended to older people.

*Source*: Sherrington, C., Fairhall, N., Wallbank, G., Tiedemann, A., Michaleff, Z.A., Howard, K., ... and Lamb, S. (2020). Exercise for preventing falls in older people living in the community: an abridged Cochrane systematic review. *British Journal of Sports Medicine, 54*(15), 885–91. Available at: http://dx.doi.org/10.1136/bjsports-2019-101512

## Summary

This chapter has considered the role of the nurse in health education and health promotion for falls prevention. It has presented several different interventions and strategies that have been implemented in the Australian context as examples of how falls prevention can be initiated in effective and sustainable ways. The implications for the health of older people particularly, are significant, given that falls are potentially avoidable through a variety of measures. This is more salient given the impact that falls often have on the person concerned. The health trajectory for someone who has experienced a fall is much worse than for someone who has not. Understanding the evidence about what works is vital in falls prevention.

——— Key Points ————————————————————————

- Nurses have a key role in falls prevention. The number of falls occurring in the community has highlighted the importance of nurses' roles in providing education and health promotion beyond the hospital bedside.
- The common falls prevention strategies include balance and mobility, identifying risk factors, and discharge planning. These are important key areas for nurses to consider when providing education to patients and staff.
- Older people can remain active and be engaged in exercises; these are factors that have the huge potential of reducing the incidence of falls in aged care and community settings.

## References

Australian Bureau of Statistics (ABS) (2019). *Twenty Years of Population Change*. Available at: www.abs.gov.au/ausstats/abs@.nsf/0/1cd2b1952afc5e7aca257298000f2e76

Australian Commission of Quality and Safety in Health Care (2009). *Preventing Falls and Harm From Falls in Older People*. Available at: www.safetyandquality.gov.au/sites/default/files/migrated/GuidelinesHOSP.pdf

Australian Institute of Health and Welfare (2019). *Health of Older People*. Available at: www.aihw.gov.au/reports/australias-health/health-of-older-people

Brennan-Olsen, B. (2018). Why hip fractures in the elderly are often a death sentence. *The Conversation*. Available at: https://theconversation.com/why-hip-fractures-in-the-elderly-are-often-a-death-sentence-95784

Casey, C.M., Caulley, J. and Phenlan, E.A. (2020). The intersection of falls and dementia in primary care. *Medical Clinical North America* 104, 791–806. Available at: https://doi.org/10.1016/j.mcna.2020.06.003

Chidume, T. (2021). Promoting older adult fall prevention education and awareness in a community setting: A nurse-led intervention. *Applied Nursing Research* 57, 151392. Available at: https://doi.org/10.1016/j.apnr.2020.151392

Chu, R.Z. (2017). Preventing in-patient falls. *Nursing* 47(3), 24–30. doi:10.1097/01.NURSE.0000512872.83762.69

Clinical Excellence Commission (2013). *Staying active and on your feet*. Centre for Population Health Resource Distribution Unit.

Department of Health and Ageing (2011). *Falls can be Prevented! A guide to preventing falls for older people*. Commonwealth of Australia. Available at: www.health.gov.au/sites/default/files/documents/2021/04/don-t-fall-for-it-falls-can-be-prevented.pdf

Falls Injury Prevention Collaborative, Education and Resource Working Group (2021). Queensland How to Stay On Your Feet® Checklist v5. Patient Safety and Quality Improvement Service, *Clinical Excellence Queensland, Queensland Health*. © State of Queensland.

Government of South Australia (2017). *Falls Prevention*. South Australian Health.

Hammond, T. and Wilson, A. (2013). Polypharmacy and falls in the elderly: a literature review. *Nursing and Midwifery Studies* 2(2), 171. doi: 10.5812/nms.10709

Ie, K., Chou, E., Boyce, R.D. and Albert, S.M. (2021). Fall risk-increasing drugs, polypharmacy, and falls among low-income community-dwelling older adults. *Innovation in Aging* 5(1), igab001. Available at: https://doi.org/10.1093/geroni/igab001

Kannus, P., Khan, K. and Lord, S. (2006). Preventing falls among elderly people in the hospital environment. *Medical Journal of Australia* 184(8), 372–3.

Mitchell, D., Raymond, M., Jellet, J., et al. (2018). Where are falls prevention resources allocated by hospitals and what do they cost? A cross sectional survey using semi-structured interviews of key informants at six Australian health services. *International Journal of Clinical Studies* (86), 52–9.

Pieruccini-Faria, F., Lord, S.R., Tonson, B., Kemmler, W. and Schoene, D. (2019) Mental flexibility influences the association between poor balance and falls in older people – A secondary analysis. *Frontiers in Ageing Neuroscience* 11(33), 1–10.

Rapp, K., Büchele, G., Dreinhöfer, K., Bücking, B., Becker, C. and Benzinger, P. (2019). Epidemiology of hip fractures. *Zeitschrift Fur Gerontolgie Und Geriatrie 52*(1), 10–16. doi:10.1007/s00391-018-1382-z

South Australia Health (2017). Fall and Fall Injury Prevention and Management Policy Directive. Available at: https://www.sahealth.sa.gov.au/wps/wcm/connect/public+content/sa+health+internet/clinical+resources/clinical+programs+and+practice+guidelines/older+people/falls+prevention/falls+prevention+policy+directive+and+toolkit

Sherrington, C., Fairhall, N., Wallbank, G., et al. (2020). Exercise for preventing falls in older people living in the community: An abridged Cochrane systematic review. *British Journal of Sports Medicine 54*(15), 885–91. Available at: http://dx.doi.org/10.1136/bjsports-2019-101512

Tiedemann, A., Purcell, K., Clemson, L., Lord, S.R. and Sherrington, C. (2021). Falls prevention behaviour after participation in the Stepping On Program: A pre-post study. doi.org/10.17061/phrp30122004

Walker, C., Hogstel, M.O. and Curry, L.C. (2007). Hospital discharge of older adults: how nurses can ease the transition. *The American Journal of Nursing 107*(6), 60–70.

World Health Organisation (2021). *Falls*. World Health Organisation. Retrieved from www.who.int/news-room/fact-sheets/detail/falls

# 17

# Health Promotion in Hospital and Beyond

## Kari Ingstad and Trude Wille

## Introduction

This final chapter uses a case study approach to explore the transition from the hospital to the community setting and the role that health promotion and health education have to play in supporting people through this transition. The chapter focuses on nutrition, a vital aspect of patient care during hospitalisation. Drawing on health-education and health-promotion principles the chapter centres on healthy nutrition as a case study exploring the opportunities for health promotion and health education during the hospital stay and beyond. The case study is discussed specifically in the Norwegian context.

By the end of this chapter, the reader will be able to:

1. Appreciate the complex reasons underlying malnutrition.
2. Understand cooperation and communication among healthcare providers to ensure that patients receive proper and coordinated nutritional treatment and care.
3. Understand that caring for patients with multifaceted nutritional issues is considerably more complex than merely addressing the failure to eat.
4. Describe how optimum nutrition can be promoted.

## Key terms

Health-promoting hospitals, nutrition, malnutrition, transitional care, hospital-to home transition

## Health-promoting hospitals

Hospitals must adapt and expand their efforts to focus on health-promotion activities given that integrated health promotion improves clinical outcomes after hospital treatment (Oppedal, Pedersen and Skjøtskift et al., 2010; Whitehead, 2005). Health-promoting hospitals place greater emphasis on health promotion and disease prevention than on diagnostic and curative services alone (Groene and Garcia-Barbero, 2005). However, many hospitals across Europe struggle to comply with standards and regulations, and health promotion is often seen as a luxury (Groene, 2008). In 1986, World Health Organization (WHO) initiated the International Health Promoting Hospital Network (HPH Network) as a setting approach for the reorientation of health services and a structured process for health promotion action (Whitehead, 2005). Today, the network consists of almost 600 healthcare institutions worldwide and aims to support members to systematically incorporate health-promotion concepts, values, frameworks, and evidence into the governance, management, structure, culture and operations of hospitals and health services (HPH, 2021).

The HPH network is one of the largest health-promoting hospital movements, especially across Europe. However, this network has not been without criticism. The main criticism is that work in this area tends to centre on the small projects, often not evaluated, rather than systematic and comprehensive programmes or whole organisational policy change (McHugh, Robinson and Chesters, 2010; Watson, 2020). For example, although some services such as nutritional counselling and patient education are provided in some hospitals, there is no defined structure for much of this provision.

Hospitals provide an important setting for health-promotion interventions (Groene, Alonso and Klazinga, 2010). Health promotion in hospitals is an opportunity to work with people whilst they are in-patients to educate and empower them in relation to individual behaviour change, an opportunity that no longer exists once the person has recovered and returned to work or their usual routine. Hospitals must approach health promotion reform in a realistic, consistent and concerted manner, driven by evidence and advocacy (Whitehead, 2004). Healthy nutrition is one area where hospitals can focus on health promotion projects/activities to prevent malnutrition. This chapter focuses on healthy nutrition as an illustrative case study exploring the opportunities for health promotion and health education during the hospital stay and beyond.

## Malnutrition: An Issue for Health Promotion

Malnutrition is a common condition in the elderly population that often results in adverse health events, including decreased physical function, prolonged hospital stay, morbidity, and mortality (Allard et al., 2016; Bell et al., 2016; Marshall et al., 2014). Notably, the prevalence of malnutrition has been reported to be as high as 20–45 per cent after hospitalisation (Allard et al., 2015; Kondrup and Sorensen, 2009). Malnutrition in hospitals is often overlooked, underdiagnosed, and left untreated (VanBlarcom and McCoy, 2018). This highlights the need to improve the quality of nutritional treatment, both in the hospital and post discharge, as typical hospital stays are relatively short. Currently, dietary changes are the primary treatment for malnourished patients who can eat on their own. Nurses often educate patients about the nutritional content of food and encourage them to make health-promoting choices. By contrast, nurses may need to intravenously feed patients who do not or cannot eat. Preventive measures, such as early and prolonged nutritional interventions, may be effective in avoiding nutrition-related conditions and tend to be rooted in a medical approach to promoting health (Wills, 2023) (please see Chapter 4 for more detail about different approaches to health promotion). Specifically, hospital-initiated care plans with post-discharge follow-ups conducted by qualified healthcare providers may constitute effective approaches to improve nutritional status, reduce complications, and decrease readmission rates among older adult patients (Ha et al., 2010; Pedersen et al., 2017).

The ESPEN (European Society for Clinical Nutrition and Metabolism) guidelines on clinical nutrition and hydration, claim that a range of effective interventions is available to support adequate nutrition in older persons to maintain or improve their nutritional status, clinical course, and quality of life. Their evidence-based recommendations for nutritional care include the following:

- All older adults, regardless of diagnosis and including overweight and obese persons, should be routinely screened for malnutrition to identify those with an existing risk.
- Nursing interventions, education, nutritional counselling, and food modification can all support oral nutrition. Oral nutritional supplements should be offered when dietary counselling and food fortification prove insufficient in increasing dietary intake and reaching nutritional goals.
- Older persons with a reasonable prognosis should be offered enteral nutrition if oral nutrition is insufficient or impossible.
- Dietary restrictions that may limit dietary intake are potentially harmful and should be avoided. Weight-reducing diets should only be considered for obese older persons with weight-related health problems and combined with physical exercise.

- All older adults should be considered at risk of low-intake dehydration because of insufficient fluid consumption, and they should be encouraged to drink adequate amounts of liquid.
- Generally, nutritional and hydration care should be individualised, comprehensive, and part of a multimodal and multidisciplinary team approach.

(Volkert et al., 2019)

---

**Box 17.1**

---

### The World Health Organization's definition of malnutrition (WHO, 2021):

Malnutrition refers to deficiencies or excesses in nutrient intake, imbalances of essential nutrients, or impaired nutrient utilisation.

---

## A Full Life-All Your Life: Health-Promoting Policy in Norway

*A full life-all your life* has been used as a quality reform for older persons in Norway (Norwegian Ministry of Health and Care Services, 2020). In addition to various health-related concepts, it focuses on food and meals to create healthy meal experiences and reduce the risk of undernourishment. In the light of this reform, this chapter discusses how healthcare personnel can promote nutrition for patients during their hospital-to-home transition.

The need for health-promoting interventions is substantial in Norwegian hospitals across all specialities (Oppedal et al., 2010), and municipalities (Hagen, Øvergård, Helgesen, Fosse and Torp, 2018). In the future, patients will be transferred earlier from specialised hospitals to health services in municipalities, where the main focus will be on health promotion in a broad sense. Although none of the Norwegian hospitals are members of the International Health Promoting Hospital Network, health promotion is, and has been, at the forefront of governance, and new whitepapers have been passed in Norway to ensure increased attention to health promotion in health services. As a result of this, several reforms in the sphere of older adult care and healthcare have been launched.

One of these is the quality reform *A full life-all your life*, which aims to help people stay in control of their lives for longer and ensure a good and secure lifestyle for all older adults. Previous reforms have primarily dealt with systems; however,

*A full life-all your life* deals with the people and things that matter the most in life (Norwegian Ministry of Health and Care Services, 2020). This government reform is directed at a new and sustainable policy meant to ensure the wellbeing and security of all older adults. The programme comprises 25 specific solutions in areas where services for older adults are inadequate. This involves better services and activities and a society in which older adults can use their strengths and abilities. The programme identifies the following five target areas:

- an age-friendly Norway
- activity and socialisation
- food and meals
- health care
- continuity of services.

This chapter focuses on the third target: food and meals. The reform aims to improve meal enjoyment for people living at home, in nursing homes, or in hospitals.

## The Role of Food and Meals in Preventing Undernutrition

In the last decade, nutrition and mealtimes have been on the agenda for older persons in Norway. However, significant gaps remain between the recommendations of health and care authorities and the services offered to older persons. The main challenges are summarised as follows:

- lack of systematic follow-up
- lack of social community and emphasis on mealtime surroundings
- few meals per day and long nightly fasts
- little variation and freedom of choice
- large distance between production and service.

Five solutions have been recommended to address these challenges: good mealtimes, mealtimes, freedom of choice and variation, systematic nutritional measures, and local kitchens and competency. The goal is to reduce undernutrition and create good food and mealtime experiences.

Health promotion is best served as an integral part of regional health service strategies, when integrated into regional policies in an explicit and structured manner (Whitehead, 2004). The *A full life-all your life* reform has been implemented in municipalities, county councils, health trusts, and among the public. The government has established a support network to inform and inspire municipalities to put the contents of this reform on their agendas, with additional tasks including the development of relevant tools, methods, and materials for local implementation (Norwegian Ministry of Health and Care Services, 2020).

# Nutrition during the Hospital-to-Home Transition: The International Context

Since 2000, the average length of hospital stay has declined in most countries (Organisation for Economic Co-operation and Development, 2019). Based on the 36 member countries of the OECD, the average length of hospital stay for all causes was approximately eight days in 2015 (Organisation for Economic Co-operation and Development, 2017, 2019). Shorter hospital stays have led to an increased need for nutritional treatment post discharge, thus promoting overall nutritional status (e.g., sufficient energy intake and proper body mass index) to prevent complications and readmission (Beck et al., 2013; Beck et al., 2015; Pedersen et al., 2017). However, lack of continuity in care and poor communication during transitions from hospital, are critical risk factors for malnutrition (Allen et al., 2017; Håkonsen et al., 2018; Munk et al., 2016).

---

### Research in Brief 17.1

Hospitals across the world struggle to prevent malnutrition, especially among older hospitalised adults (Abd Aziz et al., 2017; Meijers et al., 2009; Rasheed and Wood, 2013). Studies have reported a prevalence of malnutrition as high as 20–45 per cent at the time of discharge (Allard et al., 2015; Kondrup and Sorensen, 2009). Incomplete nutritional treatment may adversely impact health outcomes for patients, as malnutrition increases the risk of complications, loss of function, prolonged hospital stays, morbidity, and mortality (Allard et al., 2016; Badgwell et al., 2013; Bell et al., 2016). This emphasises the need to improve the quality of nutritional education and treatment both in the hospital and during the hospital-to-home transition (Ingstad et al., 2020).

---

## Tutorial Trigger 17.1

Mr Olsen is rushed to the hospital with urosepsis. As there is only one nurse on duty at the municipal health service centre where Mr Olsen lives, she does not have the time to write a transfer to send with the ambulance personnel. There is no form of collaboration between the documentation systems at the hospital and the municipal health service centre, implying that the nurses who provide hospital care to Mr Olsen do not know that he has a nutrition plan.

If you are the nurse at this municipal health service centre, do you have any responsibility for Mr Olsen now that he is a patient at the hospital? What can you do to let the nurses at the hospital know about Mr Olsen's nutrition plan? What could have been done to avoid this situation in the future?

## The Nurse's Role in Preventing Malnutrition

Integrated health promotion improves clinical outcomes after hospital treatment. Therefore, patients should be given recommendations, guidance, and support regarding health promotion in hospitals. Health promotion ensures that risk conditions are identified and that the patient is aware of the significance of these conditions, recommendations for change, and that they receive active support for carrying out these changes (Groene and García-Barbero, 2005).

Nurses work near patients and are often described as patient advocates, as they promote patient safety and quality care. Given repeated direct contact, nurses play a key role in preventing and treating malnutrition and coordinating nutritional care (Cate et al., 2019). Nurses are responsible for addressing patients' nutritional needs by conducting screenings, performing assessments, and administering interventions. They can provide oral nutritional supplements and food fortification or enrichment and often provide dietary counselling and education (Xu et al., 2017).

Initiation of relevant nutritional treatment and continued observation of body weight and food intake should be performed throughout the patient's stay in the hospital (Groene and García-Barbero, 2005). Treatment options vary depending on the cause of malnutrition. Nutritional and hydration care should be individualised and comprehensive (Volkert et al., 2019). Individualised care acknowledges the uniqueness of each patient and may be implemented to improve the quality of nutritional care for cases involving complex problems. Therefore, patients who are at risk of undernutrition require individualised nutrition care plans upon hospital discharge. These plans are developed based on detailed individual assessments of nutritional needs, conditions and desires (Dorner and Friedrich, 2018; Volkert et al., 2019). An individualised care plan includes the patient's nutritional status, individual nutritional treatment measures, dietary intake, and requirements. A nutrition care plan contains documented nutritional interventions that are designed to achieve defined treatment goals; they are continually revised to assess their effectiveness and can be adjusted as needed throughout the treatment (New South Wales Nutrition Care, 2017; Volkert et al., 2019).

─────── Time to Reflect 17.1 ───────────────────────────────

Mrs Hansen has been hospitalised for a long time because of a brain haemorrhage. She has large sequelae and is somnolent. As Mrs Hansen has a feeding tube and a pain pump, there are concerns about overmedication. Her relatives and doctor hope for rehabilitation when she steps down on painkillers. During the transition between the hospital and the municipal health service, Mrs Hansen pulls out the nutrition probe and clearly states that she does not want it. She is discharged to the care of the municipal health service on the same day without a feeding tube. Later, she is sleepy and does not eat or drink by herself. What do you think about Mrs Hansen's ability to absorb nutrition? What measures would you recommend? What do you think about her chances of rehabilitation?

---

Malnutrition prevention is a social and economic issue. This condition may be ameliorated by increasing economic levels and supporting individuals who live alone, whether single, widowed or divorced. Older adults who reside in areas far from grocery stores have limited food choices, whereas low-income families may go hungry because of limited funds. There are many possible reasons for malnutrition. In such cases, nurses may make a difference through health-promoting means. For example, they can inform people and communities about eating healthy foods and direct them towards available nutritional programmes and services (Besora-Moreno et al., 2020). Effective malnutrition management requires collaboration among multiple clinical disciplines (Tappenden et al., 2013) and between hospitals and communities (Keller, 2021). Information communication on discharge to homecare services or nursing homes is important. The advantages of nutritional interventions initiated during a hospital stay may be lost if care continuity is not adequately addressed when patients are discharged. More direct contact between hospital-based and community nurses can promote a better mutual understanding of the journeys experienced by older patients during transitions, with an emphasis on improving care coordination (Gautun et al., 2020).

High performing hospitals attain excellence across multiple measures of performance and multiple departments. A qualitative systematic review identified seven themes representing factors associated with high performing hospitals: positive organisational culture, senior management support, effective performance monitoring, building and maintaining a proficient workforce, effective leaders across the organisation, expertise-driven practice, and interdisciplinary teamwork (Taylor, Clay-Williams, Hogden, Braithwaite and Groene, 2015). The factors that lead to high performance are complex and rely on a different set of contextual factors. Insights into high-performing hospitals and factors important for success can be valuable if these factors can be identified and applied. Learning from high-performing hospitals, factors associated with high performers, and practical strategies for improvement can lead to better nutritional treatment for patients during their stay in the hospital and the hospital-to-home transition (Taylor, Clay-Williams, Hogden, Braithwaite and Groene, 2015).

---

## Point to Ponder 17.1

Due to illness or impaired health, some patients completely depend on the nurses' help and time to obtain adequate nutrition. Are such cases caused by a lack of knowledge, or are moral issues at play? Can you imagine other reasons why older patients do not want to eat?

---

## Point to Ponder 17.2

We invite you on a journey into your fantasy. Close your eyes and take three deep breaths. Set your mind free and imagine yourself at a party – a real feast with friends, family, and loved ones. The band is playing your favourite music, and you can hear friendly chatter. You can feel the warm breeze through the open doors. You see a beautiful, covered table and smell fantastic food from the kitchen. How do you think your patient's appetite would be affected by the environment and those around them? How do you stimulate your patient's senses? How can you have a party for your patients at the municipal health service centre?

---

### Research in Brief 17.2

One randomised controlled trial (RCT) indicated that individualised nutritional treatment improves energy intake and the activities of daily living (ADLs) for older acute stroke patients with malnutrition risk, compared with a standard care group (Otsuki, 2019).

In the present study, nutritional screening and treatment were started on the seventh hospital day. The results implied that nutritional management in early stage of stroke, might lead to more improvements in the ADL.

Nutritional problems do not occur overnight, nor are they resolved in such a brief amount of time. Caring for patients with multifaceted nutritional issues is considerably more complex than merely addressing a failure to eat. Promoting nutritional health may involve psychological, physical and social issues, including dental problems, addiction, dementia, dysphagia, depression and loneliness, all of which can affect the appetite and ability to eat (Hestevik et al., 2019). Cooperation and communication among healthcare providers are important to ensure that patients receive proper and coordinated nutritional treatment and care (Håkonsen et al., 2018). Just as general individualised care targets a patient's unique needs, individualised nutrition care plans can reduce the risk of malnutrition for those at risk upon hospital discharge. Hospital policies should highlight the processes, requirements, roles and responsibilities concerning nutrition and hydration care to ensure that all patients receive nutrition and hydration in a form that is acceptable to them and meets their needs. Furthermore, health-promoting hospitals should also ensure proper transitions to maintain or improve nutritional status and the clinical course and quality of life post-hospital discharge.

## Summary

This chapter has considered the role of the health-promoting hospital in relation to nutrition. Specifically, it has focused on nutrition and malnutrition in older people in the hospital setting. Drawing on current policy from the Norwegian context the chapter has discussed a number of important requirements for promoting the nutritional health of older people whilst in hospital and beyond.

――――― Key Points ―――――――――――――――――――――――――――――――――――

- Nutrition is a key area in which nurses working in hospital settings have an important role to play in the promotion of health.
- Nurses have many skills to bring to nutritional support including those that underpin health education and health-promotion efforts, both in the acute hospital setting and beyond.
- Hospitalisation provides an opportunity for nursing staff to work with people to improve and promote their nutrition.
- With the international decrease in average hospital stays, time is of the essence in ensuring that patients attain optimal nutritional status.

## References

Abd Aziz, N.A.S., Teng, N.I.M.F., Abdul Hamid, M.R. and Ismail, N.H. (2017). Assessing the nutritional status of hospitalized elderly. *Clinical Interventions in Aging 12*, 1615–25. Available at: https://doi.org/10.2147/CIA.S140859

Allard, J.P., Keller, H., Teterina, A., Jeejeebhoy, K.N., Laporte, M., Duerksen, D.R., et al. (2015). Factors associated with nutritional decline in hospitalised medical and surgical patients admitted for 7 d or more: A prospective cohort study. *British Journal of Nutrition 114*(10), 1612–22. Available at: https://doi.org/10.1017/S0007114515003244

Allard, J.P., Keller, H., Jeejeebhoy, K.N., Laporte, M., Duerksen, D.R., Gramlich, L., et al. (2016). Malnutrition at hospital admission—contributors and effect on length of stay: A prospective cohort study from the Canadian Malnutrition Task Force. *Journal of Parenteral and Enteral Nutrition 40*(4), 487–97. Available at: https://doi.org/10.1177/0148607114567902

Allen, J., Hutchinson, A.M., Brown, R. and Livingston, P.M. (2017). User experience and care integration in transitional care for older people from hospital to home: A meta-synthesis. *Qualitative Health Research 27*(1), 24–36. Available at: https://doi.org/10.1177/1049732316658267

Badgwell, B., Stanley, J., Chang, G.J., Katz, M.H.G., Lin, H.Y., Ning, J., et al. (2013). Comprehensive geriatric assessment of risk factors associated with adverse outcomes and resource utilization in cancer patients undergoing abdominal surgery. *Journal of Surgical Oncology 108*(3), 182–6. Available at: https://doi.org/10.1002/jso.23369

Beck, A.M., Holst, M. and Rasmussen, H.H. (2013). Oral nutritional support of older (65 years+) medical and surgical patients after discharge from hospital: Systematic review and meta-analysis of randomized controlled trials. *Clinical Rehabilitation 27*(1), 1–927. https://doi.org/10.1177/0269215512445396

Beck, A., Andersen, U.T., Leedo, E., Jensen, L.L., Quvang, M., Rask, K.Ø., et al. (2015). Does adding a dietician to the liaison team after discharge of geriatric patients improve nutritional outcome: A randomised controlled trial. *Clinical Rehabilitation 29*(11), 1117–28. Available at: https://doi.org/10.1177/0269215514564700

Bell, J.J., Pulle, R.C., Crouch, A.M., Kuys, S.S., Ferrier, R.L. and Whitehouse, S.L. (2016). Impact of malnutrition on 12-month mortality following acute hip fracture. *ANZ Journal of Surgery 86*(3), 157–61. Available at: https://doi.org/10.1111/ans.13429

Besora-Moreno, M., Llauradó, E., Tarro, L. and Solà, R. (2020). Social and economic factors and malnutrition or the risk of malnutrition in the elderly: A systematic review and meta-analysis of observational studies. *Nutrients 23*(3), 737.

Cate, D., Ettema, R.G.A., Waal, G.H., Bell, J., Verbrugge, R., Scoonhoven, L. et al. (2019). Interventions to prevent and treat malnutrition in older adults to be carried out by nurses: A systematic review. *Journal of Clinical Nursing 29*(11–12), 1883–902. Available at: https://10.1111/jocn.15153

Dorner, B. and Friedrich, E.K. (2018). Position of the Academy of nutrition and dietetics: Individualized nutrition approaches for older adults: Long-term care, post-acute care, and other settings. *Journal of the Academy of Nutrition and Dietetics 118*(4), 724–35. Available at: https://doi.org/10.1016/j.jand.2018.01.022

Gautun, H., Bratt, C. and Billings, J. (2020). Nurses' experiences of transitions of older patients from hospitals to community care. A nation-wide survey in Norway. *Health Science Reports 3*(3), e174. Available at: https://doi.org/10.1002/hsr2.174

Groene, O. and García-Barbero, M. (2005). *Health Promotion in Hospitals: Evidence and quality management.* Copenhagen – the European Regional Office for WHO.

Groene, O. (2008). Health promotion in hospital quality and governance systems: addressing the missing link. (Online), 18 May 2022. Hospital Healthcare Europe. Available at: https://hospitalhealthcare.com/news/health-promotion-in-hospital-quality-and-governance-systems-addressing-the-missing-link/

Groene, O., Alonso, J. and Klazinga, N. (2010). Development and validation of the WHO self-assessment tool for health promotion in hospitals: Results of a study in 38 hospitals in eight countries. *Health Promotion International 25*(2), 221–9. Available at: https://doi.org/10.1093/heapro/daq013

Ha, L., Hauge, T., Spenning, A.B. and Iversen, P.O. (2010). Individual, nutritional support prevents undernutrition, increases muscle strength, and improves QoL among elderly at nutritional risk hospitalized for acute stroke: A randomized, controlled trial. *Clinical Nutrition 29*(5), 567–73. Available at: https://doi.org/10.1016/j.clnu.2010.01.011

Hagen, S., Øvergård, K.I., Helgesen, M., Fosse, E. and Torp, S. (2018). Health promotion at local level in Norway: The use of public health coordinators and health overviews to promote fair distribution among social groups. *International Journal of Health Policy and Management 7*(9), 807–17.

Hestevik, C.H., Molin, M., Debesay, J., Bergland, A. and Bye, A. (2019). Healthcare professionals' experiences of providing individualized nutritional care for older people in hospital and home care: A qualitative study. *BMC Geriatrics 19*(1), 1–9. Available at: https://doi.org/10.1186/s12877-019-1339-0

HPH (2021). *International Network of Health Promoting Hospitals and Health Services.* International Network of Health Promoting Hospitals and Health Services. [Brochure]. Hamburg, Germany: International HPH Network. Available at: https://www.hphnet.org/wp-content/uploads/2022/01/HPH_Brochure_2021-November.pdf

Håkonsen, S.J., Pedersen, P.U., Bjerrum, M., Bygholm, A. and Peters, M.D.H. (2018). Nursing minimum data sets for documenting nutritional care for adults in primary healthcare: A scoping review. *JBI Evidence Synthesis 16*(1), 117–39. Available at: https://doi.org/10.11124/JBISRIR-2017-003386

Ingstad, K., Uhrenfeldt, L., Kymre, I.G., Skrubbeltrang, C. and Pedersen, P. (2020). Effectiveness of individualised nutritional care plans to reduce malnutrition during hospitalisation and up to 3 months post discharge: a systematic scoping review. *BMJ Open 9*(9), 10:e040439. Available at: https://doi.org/10.1136/bmjopen-2020-040439

Keller, H., Donnelly, R., Laur, C., Goharian, L. and Nasser, R. (2021). Consensus-based nutrition care pathways for hospital-to-community transitions and older adults in primary and community care. *Journal of Parenteral and Enteral Nutrition,* Early View. Available at: https://doi.org/10.1002/jpen.2068

Kondrup, J. and Sorensen, J.M. (2009). The magnitude of the problem of malnutrition in Europe. In M. Elia and B.R. Bistrian (Eds), *The Economic, Medical/scientific, and Regulatory Aspects of Clinical Nutrition Practice: What impacts what?* (Vol. 12, pp. 1–14). Berlin: Karger Publishers. Available at: https://doi.org/10.1159/000235664

McHugh, C., Robinson, A. and Chesters, J. (2010). Health promoting health services: a review of the evidence. *Health Promotion International 25*(2), 230–7. doi: 10.1093/heapro/daq010

Marshall, S., Bauer, J. and Isenring, E. (2014). The consequences of malnutrition following discharge from rehabilitation to the community: A systematic review of current evidence in older adults. *Journal of Human Nutrition and Dietetics 27*(2), 133–41. Available at: https://doi.org/10.1111/jhn.12167

Meijers, J.M.M., Schols, J.M.G.A., van Bokhorst-de van der Schueren, M.A.E., Dassen, T., Janssen, M.A.P. and Halfens, R.J.G. (2009). Malnutrition prevalence in the Netherlands: Results of the annual Dutch national prevalence measurement of care problems. *British Journal of Nutrition 101*(3), 417–23. Available at: https://doi.org/10.1016/j.nut.2008.11.004

Munk, T., Tolstrup, U., Beck, A.M., Holst, H.H., Rasmussen, K. and Hovhannisyan, T.T. (2016). Individualised dietary counselling for nutritionally at-risk older patients following discharge from acute hospital to home: A systematic review and meta-analysis. *Journal of Human Nutrition and Dietetics 29*(2), 196–208. Available at: https://doi.org/10.1111/jhn.12307

New South Wales Nutrition Care. Policy Directive. (2017). New South Wales Government Health. Retrieved from https://intranet.nnswlhd.health.nsw.gov.au/docs/PD2017_041-nutrition-care-v-002.pdf

Norwegian Ministry of Health and Care Services. (2020). *A full life – all your life: A Quality Reform for Older Persons*. Retrieved from https://www.regjeringen.no/contentassets/196f99e63aa14f849c4e4b9b9906a3f8/en-gb/pdfs/stm201720180015000engpdfs.pdf

Oppedal, K., Nesva, S., Pedersen, B., Skjøtskift, S., Aarstad, A.K.H., Ullaland, S., et al. (2010). Health and the need for health promotion in hospital patients. *European Journal of Public Health 21*(6), 744–9.

Organisation for Economic Co-operation and Development. (2017). *Health at a Glance 2017: OECD indicators*. Paris: OECD Publishing.

Organisation for Economic Co-operation and Development. (2019). Length of hospital stay (indicator). Retrieved from https://data.oecd.org/healthcare/length-of-hospital-stay.htm

Otsuki, I., Himuro, N., Tatsumi, H., Mori, M., Niiya, Y., Kumeta, Y. et al. (2019). Individualized nutritional treatment for acute stroke patients with malnutrition risk improves functional independence measurement: A randomized controlled trial. *Geriatrics & Gerontology International 20*(3), 176–82. Available at: https://doi.org/10.1111/ggi.13854

Pedersen, J.L., Pedersen, P.U. and Damsgaard, E.M. (2017). Nutritional follow-up after discharge prevents readmission to hospital—A randomized clinical trial. *Journal of Nutrition, Health & Aging 21*(1), 75–82. Available at: https://doi.org/10.1007/s12603-016-0745-7

Rasheed, S. and Woods, R.T. (2013). Predictive validity of 'Malnutrition Universal Screening Tool' ('MUST') and Short Form Mini Nutritional Assessment (MNA-SF) in terms of survival and length of hospital stay. *e-SPEN Journal 8*(2), e44–e50. Available at https://doi.org/10.1016/j.clnme.2013.01.001

Tappenden, K., Quatrara, B., Parkhurst, M., Malone, A., Tanjang, G. and Ziegler, T. R. (2013). Critical role of nutrition in improving quality of care: An interdisciplinary call to action to address adult hospital malnutrition. *Journal of the Academy of Nutrition and Dietetics 113*(9), 1219–37. Available at: https://doi.org/10.1016/j.jand.2013.05.015

Taylor, N., Clay-Williams, R., Hogden, E., Braithwaite, J. and Groene, O. (2015). High performing hospitals: a qualitative systematic review of associated factors and practical strategies for improvement. *BMC Health Services Research 15*(1), 1–22. Available at: https://doi.org/10.1186/s12913-015-0879-z

VanBlarcom, A. and McCoy, M.A. (2018). New nutrition guidelines: Promoting enteral nutrition via a nutrition bundle. *Critical Care Nurse 38*(3), 46–52. Available at: https://doi:10.4037/ccn2018617

Volkert, D., Beck, A.M., Cederholm, T., Cruz-Jentoft, A., Goisser, S., Hooper, L. et al. (2019). ESPEN guideline on clinical nutrition and hydration in geriatrics. *Clinical Nutrition 38*(1), 10–47. Available at: https://doi.org/10.1016/j.clnu.2018.05.024

Watson, M.C. (2020). Improving workplace health in the NHS. *BMJ* 368. doi: https://doi.org/10.1136/bmj.m850 (Published 9 March 2020).

Whitehead, D. (2004). The European Health Promoting Hospitals (HPH) project: How far on? *Health Promotion International 19*(2), 259–67.

Whitehead, D. (2005). Health promoting hospitals: The role and function of nursing. *Journal of Clinical Nursing 14*(1), 20–7.

WHO (2021). Nutrition. Available at: https://www.who.int/health-topics/malnutrition#tab=tab_1

Wills, J. (2023). *Foundations for Health Promotion.* 5th Ed. London: Elsevier.

Xu, X., Parker, D., Ferguson, C. and Hickman, L. (2017). Where is the nurse in nutritional care? *Contemporary Nurse 53*(3), 267–70. https://doi.org/10.1080/10376178.2017.1370782

# Index

Note- Page number with 'f' indicates figure, 't' indicates table.